Poor People's Medicine

Poor People's Medicine

Medicaid and American Charity Care since 1965

JONATHAN ENGEL

DUKE UNIVERSITY PRESS   DURHAM & LONDON

2006

© 2006 Duke University Press

All rights reserved

Printed in the United States of America on acid-free paper ∞

Designed by Rebecca M. Giménez

Typeset in Minion by Keystone Typesetting, Inc.

Library of Congress Cataloging-in-Publication Data appear

on the last printed page of this book.

IN MEMORY OF MY FATHER

Contents

Preface

This is a story of ambivalence, for no other word better describes efforts at charity medical care in the United States over the past half-century. Unwilling to wholly abandon the poor to private charities and municipal relief efforts, but at the same time unwilling to provide full access to the private health system through a fully funded state insurance program, the nation has provided health insurance to the poor, coupled with an array of loosely coordinated community health centers, public hospitals, and neighborhood health clinics. The result has been imperfect, and frequently unsatisfactory, yet the effort has also produced startling successes. America's poor today live nearly as long as the nonpoor, survive infancy at rates approaching those of the population at large, and use private physicians and hospitals at least as much as the privately insured do. Even as they complain, accurately, of being shunted to a second-tier medical system, the poor are granted access to some of the best hospitals and physicians in the country.

Moreover, by most any measure the system has improved continuously for forty years. Starting with the legislation which created the modern Medicaid program in 1965, the nation has increased federal subsidies to the states which administer the Medicaid programs, implemented new early screening and care programs, expanded eligibility, and subsidized services unimaginable at the time of the program's construction. Dental, prenatal, and nutritional benefits were added at various points, along with innovative managed-care programs to ensure access to primary-care physicians. With the widespread move toward managed care in the private insurance sector, Medicaid recipients found themselves, paradoxically, fought over by private hospitals and outpatient treatment facilities. Indeed, in half a dozen states Medicaid recipients brought to their physicians more generous reimbursements than Medicare or privately insured patients did.

Yet even as federal and state governments continually fine-tuned eligibility levels and benefit packages under Medicaid, they rarely funded the program adequately to compete with private insurers. Thus, rather than wholly supersede the existing system of public hospitals and clinics, Medicaid actually strengthened that system by bringing federal funds to institutions which had hitherto existed solely on state and municipal largesse. In this the program failed badly, as for most of its history its recipients disproportionately sought care from doctors with exclusive or near exclusive Medicaid practices, and checked themselves into public hospitals which cared almost exclusively for Medicaid patients or self-payers. Medicaid, unintentionally, opened a new tier of American medicine: one populated by foreign medical graduates with urban practices, who treated patients in small "Hill-Burton" rural hospitals or aging municipal or Catholic hospitals in downtown precincts. At the same time, it brought funds to experimental community and neighborhood health centers, and community mental health centers, none of which were intended to treat the full economic spectrum of patients. Medicaid, in short, further locked America's poor into a separate and inferior tier of medical care, even as it aimed to obviate entirely just such a tier.

In maintaining this lukewarm commitment to charity care, the United States is exceptional. No other industrialized nation has been as reluctant to federalize or nationalize its system of medical care or medical payment. The United States alone allows a large number of its citizens to live without health insurance, even as it maintains coverage for the poorest and most vulnerable. Yet it has been unwilling to allow medical care and medical products to simply fall to the vagaries of the markets as well. Without committing itself to universal coverage, the United States has committed itself to rigorous review and standardization of medical practice, hospital organization, drug development and marketing, professional licensing, and insurance sales. A health care professional in America can scarcely speak to a patient without appropriate licensure and accreditation, yet the government has been unwilling to guarantee its citizens, even many of the poorest citizens, funds to exploit those professionals' services. It is a strange picture.

Yet in a larger sense, this nation's ambivalence toward charity medical care mirrors its historically ambivalent commitment to poor relief generally. While other nations developed comprehensive and generous social welfare systems in the early decades of the twentieth century, the United States proved strangely reluctant to adopt similar ones. Old-age pensions, disability insurance, unemployment insurance ("the dole"), widows' pensions, and child welfare services, all of which undergirded the great social welfare projects of Western European democracies through the twentieth century, have all proven contentious here. Americans have looked askance at most every one of these programs and products, and have adopted them in small, incremental measures when they adopted them at all. Sometimes the country has taken substantial steps back, terminating existing programs in a flurry of tax-cutting devolution and states' rights rhetoric. And the sentiment continues to this day. As this preface is being written, the federal government is attempting to impose an increasing share of the costs of Medicaid on state governments, even as those states face looming budget shortfalls and expanding populations of indigent residents.[1] America has proven itself consistent, if not compassionate.

Charity Medicine?

The medical profession has incorporated eleemosynary efforts into its enterprise for as long as we have records. The Hippocratic Oath demands that physicians heal when able to, regardless of a patient's ability to pay, and archival records suggest that both physicians and whole communities have made substantial efforts to provide care to the impoverished sick since at least the Middle Ages. Public health agencies and offices are some of the oldest extant bureaucracies in Europe, and almshouses which house the sick as well as the poor rank among the longest-lasting of civic institutions. Of the two great publicly provided human services, public health care preceded public education by at least half a millennium.

Early Americans made efforts to care for the poor through philanthropy and community largesse. David Rothman writes that colonial efforts at alleviating poverty grew naturally from Protestant dictates of charity and self-improvement. A minister in Boston, Samuel Cooper, wrote: "[Relief of the needy] ennobles our nature, by conforming us to the best, the most glorious patterns. . . . Charity conforms us to the Son of God himself."[2] This Christian and community-minded spirit began to express itself in the form of institution building in the Jacksonian era, during which America began to construct—along with prisons— almshouses, orphanages, and asylums. Although Rothman warns us that this spree of institution building was impelled as much by a yearning for social order as it was by charity, these efforts at communal largesse were mirrored in the development of the general hospital, which civic-minded citizens began constructing as early as the eighteenth century.[3] A century later, immigrant ethnic groups and religious denominations established hospitals intended in large part to serve the poor among them. These efforts in turn were followed by a spate of municipally funded public hospital building at the beginning of the twentieth century.

The history of these early efforts at hospital building and care of the poor is well documented.[4] For present purposes the reader should appreciate that providing charity medical and hospital care to the destitute has been an omnipresent and essential civic endeavor since the earliest days of this country, and that until relatively recently most of the work has been done by private groups, with some state and municipal money donated to build municipal hospitals and state lunatic asylums.

Thus far, the American story parallels the European one with some minor divergences. But as of the beginning of the twentieth century America went in its own direction. While most Western European states began to develop comprehensive national health plans, hospital systems, and health payment systems, the United States almost singly left the production, distribution, and payment of medical care in private hands, with government efforts limited to public hospitals, hospital care for war veterans, and sporadic school-based immunization programs.[5] This decision created fundamentally different charity care systems. While the European nations, along with New Zealand, Australia, and Japan, folded their poor into the health payment platforms they had devised for the general populations, the United States incrementally expanded and enriched its charity care programs to create a health system parallel to the main one. That system, made of public hospitals, physicians with lesser or foreign training, community and neighborhood health clinics, and discount pharmacies and treatment centers, remains with us today.

Stumbling toward Social Welfare

America's tepid efforts at charity health care have been consistent with its tepid efforts at social welfare provision in general. Emerging scholarship points to a constant American ambivalence toward funding social welfare programs along European lines. Whether in disability payments, old age and survivors' insurance, emergency food supplements, unemployment insurance, or general poverty relief, the United States has stumbled rather than marched toward the social welfare state.

According to the classic explanation of how social welfare programs developed, the federalist tradition in the United States precluded the growth of much of a social safety net until the New Deal programs of the early 1930s—most particularly those inaugurated with the Social Security Act in 1935. Those programs, particularly old age and survivors' insurance, disability insurance, and state-administered unemployment insurance, were thrown to a restive population demanding significant change in the role which government would play in its life. The deprivations of the Great Depression had forced millions of working Americans to reassess their basic contract with America: one which stipulated that in exchange for hard work and individual initiative, they would live a reasonable middle-class life and achieve consistent upward mobility. Now these millions, led by activist farm and labor organizations, had realized that the system was fundamentally broken, and could only be fixed by broad government intervention in commerce, employment, insurance, and markets.

This classic description of the growth of American welfare makes two further claims. The first is that social insurance was demanded most vociferously by organized farm and labor groups, who under the pressures of a developing industrial society continued to safeguard the programs in succeeding decades, even as they were repeatedly attacked by social conservatives and laissez-faire market theorists. The second is that once the programs were implemented, Americans quickly cleaved to them and supported both their continued existence and their constant growth. In this historical account, the new social welfare protections created under President Kennedy's "New Frontier" and President Johnson's "Great Society" agendas were natural responses to a continued demand for expanding social welfare programs. Medicare, and to a lesser extent Medicaid, were simply Social Security applied to the medical sphere.

But several prominent scholars dispute these notions. The sociologist and social historian Theda Skocpol persuasively argues that industrialization did not lead to bureaucratic centralization. The half-century gap between the first wave of industrial development in the decades after the Civil War and the enactment of New Deal reforms is too wide to be bridged by this weak hypothesis.[6] Buttressing Skocpol, the political scientist Charles Noble argues that despite the popular image of a unified working class, labor has always organized more along racial and ethnic than class demarcations, and thus has always exhibited tepid support for government-sponsored social welfare programs, if not outright hostility. He notes that American workers tended "not to vote their economic interests, as did workers in most other capitalist democracies, but their cultural identities instead."[7]

But more damning to the classic vision of an ever-progressing American welfare state is Skocpol's innovative study of the rise and decline of the Civil War pension system in America. Skocpol argues that through Civil War pensions, America had already achieved an extensive national welfare system by the 1890s, during which time over a third of elderly American men received government assistance. And yet, even as progressive fervor reached its height in the decade between 1911 and 1920, the nation refused to renew this pension system, or develop a replacement system to ease the plight of the elderly and destitute. Of all the many progressive legislative goals envisioned during that decade, the only policies finding their way into law were those addressing industrial accidents, enacted by forty-two states.[8]

In fact, Skocpol argues, programs to alleviate poverty in the United

States became "feminized" over the ensuing decades, as women organized and fought for a tighter social safety net for children, widows, and single and abandoned mothers. This movement, exemplified by the creation of the U.S. Children's Bureau in 1912 and the passage of the Sheppard-Towner Act in 1921, reflected a "maternalist welfare effort," in Skocpol's terms, in which the nation committed itself to safeguarding the keepers of moral rectitude and familial structure.[9] Although Sheppard-Towner was allowed to lapse after seven years, during the time it was in force the government had distributed millions of pamphlets, conducted hundreds of health conferences, and funded tens of thousands of home visits, improving the lot of up to half of all babies born during that period.[10]

Succeeding years have only reinforced the feminine nature of both poverty and efforts to alleviate poverty in the United States. The poor have disproportionately been single mothers since the beginning of the twentieth century, and this group has only grown in its dominance of the poor rolls since 1959. Indeed, various studies of the past two decades indicate that the best single prediction of poverty is unwed motherhood at too young an age, and that a mother's chance of being impoverished is cut by almost half if she can wed before or while raising children.[11] In light of this, social welfare policy has been skewed toward protecting mothers and children since the onset of the New Deal programs. Aid to Families with Dependent Children (AFDC, colloquially "welfare"), the government's best-known poverty alleviation program, effectively precluded any able-bodied man, with or without children, from being classified as poor after 1935, and thirty years later the original Medicaid eligibility standards perpetuated this pattern. Americans seemed, and seem, most comfortable limiting both the definition of poverty and efforts to alleviate it to those deserving women who struggle to raise children as they fight for economic survival. Two-parent families and childless men need not apply.

American Exceptionalism

But why has America, alone among the industrialized nations, been so reluctant to embrace a broader social safety net? Different scholars answer the question differently. Noble offers a three-pronged explanation, according to which decentralized governmental institutions, an anemic labor base, and a unified business sector all combine to make radical reform all but impossible in American government. Unions, which at their apex never managed to attract more than one fourth of the American work force to their ranks, were never able to overcome the schisms created by differing immigrant ethnic groups and northwardly migrating African Americans. Thus to make themselves attractive to the broadest member base possible, they tended to eschew radical political positions (such as demanding broad social insurance reform) in favor of incremental improvement of their members' lots. In this mold, unions worked not toward national health insurance but toward providing better private policies for their individual members.[12]

Noble also postulates that the decentralized nature of American political institutions, as well as the winner-takes-all election process of congressional seats, has forced politicians with radical agendas to the margins. In a two-party system, both parties work toward moderation to attract a broad base, even as the elected members of those parties confront structural barriers to any comprehensive social reform.[13] Politicians elected in such a system cleave to pork-barrel politics rather than broad redistributive efforts. At the same time, the federal system of devolved legislative power encourages businesses to relocate to the most business-friendly (and frequently labor-unfriendly) states. The combined effect is to squelch debate on fundamental reforms and pressure legislative bodies to appease business and the political mainstream of the population.[14]

Skocpol offers not so much an explanation of American exceptionalism as a vigorous claim for its existence. Americans were never acclimated to a government-sponsored social safety net in the manner in which Europeans were, and the broadest program that the nation was able to adopt (before 1965) was low-level mandatory retirement insurance. In contrast to the almost plebeian "dole" in England, the United States had "welfare," which always carried with it pejorative undertones. "It refers," writes Skocpol, "to unearned public assistance benefits, possibly undeserved and certainly demeaning, to be avoided if at all possible by all 'independent,' self-respecting citizens."[15] Nevertheless, Skocpol argues, many traditional arguments, particularly those which focus on a unique national "character," are unpersuasive.

The truth is some amalgam of these arguments. The United States has remained uniquely open to immigration for most of its history, has facilitated access to land and capital for the credit-unworthy, and has leveraged technology and capital-intensive production techniques in the presence of constant labor shortages. Together these three characteristics of American life have led most Americans, most of the time, to believe that government is best when kept small, and that people ought to be held responsible for their own failings. In a land of abundant land, capital, know-how, and opportunity, people should be allowed to rise, and fall, as far as they deserve.

Medical Charity

Exceptionalism in social welfare in the United States has been mirrored in aberrant health policy. The United States, whether by fate, design, or strange luck, remains the only industrialized nation in the world which relies on the private sector to distribute health care, and health insurance.[16] Although debated fiercely and frequently, the dozens of comprehensive health reform bills submitted to Congress since 1912 have virtually all come to naught. The latest such measure, the Clinton health bill of 1993, was so costly in political capital for President Clinton's administration that it all but immobilized other domestic legislation for the remainder of his first term.

The political scientist Jacob Hacker struggles to understand the reasons for the uniqueness of the American health care system. Besides its dovetailing with the larger social welfare system, he cites the powerful interest groups created once most industrial workers began to receive health insurance from their employers.[17] Unions, pleased with the generous benefit packages already garnered by their members, viewed national health reform as detrimental to their members' interests, while employers, pleased with the stability of the arrangement, eschewed federal or state involvement with a system which seemed to work. Moreover, as private insurance companies grew to accommodate the huge demand for their health products, they created a powerful lobbying force, capable of winning the public to their side.[18]

Accompanying this unique profile of a health care system, or nonsystem, is the most porous charity health care network in the world. Again the United States is alone among the world's industrial nations in having a substantial number of uninsured citizens, most of whom fall into a "gap," too wealthy to qualify for Medicaid yet too poor to afford private health insurance. Alone among those nations, the United States maintains a de facto separate tier of health care for the poor (other nations maintain a separate tier for the rich). And alone among those nations, the United States continues to maintain high rates of infant mortality—one of the single best indicators of how deeply basic medical care has penetrated into a population.

Despite these dire pronouncements, the position of the poor in the American health care system has markedly improved in the past four decades. Starting with the passage in 1965 of Title XIX of the Social Security Act (Medicaid), America's poor have increasingly availed themselves of modern medicine. Medicaid, although imperfect, has eased access, provided prophylaxis, and delivered procedures. Despite its underfunding and large eligibility gaps, Medicaid has brought the rates of poor people's interactions with private doctors and hospitals up to, and sometimes beyond, the rates posted by the middle class. And despite bizarrely inconsistent reimbursement rates among the various states, Medicaid has improved life expectancy for all of America's poor, regardless of residence.

This book is a study of why and how Medicaid came into being, and how it grew. It seeks to present the vagaries of the charity care system as they existed in the United States up to 1965, and the paths which the different components of that system then took. Three main themes recur throughout the story: the ambivalence with which Americans attempted to bring the poor into the mainstream health system; the inability of Americans to reach consensus on fundamental reform within that system; and the debate surrounding broader welfare reform which paralleled and coincided with the debate over welfare medicine. Several smaller themes appear from time to time, sometimes running tangentially to the broader themes and sometimes flowing directly from them. They include the running debate over federalism in the design of poor-care programs, the tensions between the states over designing their poor-care systems, and the unpredictable relationships between the many poor-care programs, Medicare, and private insurers. Further complicating the story are the inconsistent stances on these issues taken by organized labor, the medical profession, and professional poor-care advocates.

The story is complicated because several narratives concerning poor care progressed concurrently. For example, even as American welfare policy changed dramatically in the 1990s, so too did understanding in the private sector of cost controls in health insurance. Furthermore, a usually obstinate medical profession abruptly moderated its opposition to government-sponsored payment reform in the late 1990s as a result of declining professional control wrought by managed care.

The evolution of poor care over the past half century, although a distinct story, is closely intertwined with broader developments in the health care delivery system, as well as debates over the still larger social welfare system. This book places that story within the context of those two other stories, while examining the internal debates and decisions made in poor care during that time. There is no easy thematic summary of the story. Ambivalence pervades, as do multiple small failures and large successes.

Thank you to various family members—my wife Rozlyn, brothers and sisters-in-law Andrew, Karen, Samuel, and Anne, and my mother Diana, for indulging my fiction of the writing life. None of them are quite sure of exactly how I earn a living, but so long as the kids are fed and the roof shingled, they seem content to let well enough alone. On a more practical note, thank you to various friends and relations who have hosted me in my research travels—Steve and Dale Sonnenberg in Austin, Michael and Janice Rosenberg in Chicago, and Noah and Andrea Jussim in Los Angeles. Suzanne Smith-Jablonsky assisted me in tracking down obscure journal articles, and saved my eyesight by doing virtually all of my microfilm work for me. Valerie Milholland shepherded the manuscript through the acquisitions and review process at Duke University Press, where Fred Kameny edited it. The project was supported by travel grants from Seton Hall University's faculty research fund and from the foundations associated with the Lyndon Johnson and George Bush presidential libraries. A huge note of thanks to Barbara Ward and the entire interlibrary loan staff of Seton Hall's Walsh Library, who tracked down over one hundred loan requests without complaint.

This book is dedicated to the memory of my father, Milton Engel, who died in August 2002. A kind and generous man who often romanticized the academic life, my father supported me unconditionally through the early years of my career, taking it on faith that scholarship had value in and of itself, regardless of its marginal place in society. To paraphrase the Hebrew, his memory is a constant blessing.

1

Antecedents: Poverty and Early
Poverty Care Programs

Health and Health Care in the
United States in the Early 1960s

By 1964 America was in the throes of its "golden days" of medicine.[1] Death rates due to infection, heart disease, and stroke had fallen rapidly since the 1940s, and even such intractable problems as cancer and severe mental illness were viewed as potentially treatable by an optimistic medical community. Tranquilizers without severe side effects were promising to salve the tension and anomie inherent in a competitive society, and nascent hormone therapies offered the promise of new treatments for congenital abnormalities and growth deficiencies. New surgical techniques were being developed to transplant organs, reattach limbs, and excise brain tumors. *Life* magazine wrote at the time, "With ingenious substitutes for human organs and bold experiments in transplants, man becomes master mechanic, on himself."[2] The promise of scientific medicine, as envisioned by medical soothsayers such as Abraham Flexner, William Osler, and Harvey Cushing in the early decades of the century, was being fulfilled.

Medicine had grown tremendously in the two decades since the end of the Second World War. By 1964 health care exceeded the nation's transportation sector both in its number of employees and in raw revenues generated, which at $33 billion were triple their level in 1949, representing almost 6 percent of gross national product and ranking health care sixth or seventh among the nation's industries (depending on accounting techniques). Investment in the nation's hospital infrastructure alone was well over $20 billion. Over the previous five years, 1,700 hospital construction projects had been approved, adding 72,000 beds to hospitals and health clinics. The nation's biomedical research budget had grown from $88 million in 1947 to $1.6 *billion* in 1964, an increase of nearly twentyfold.[3]

The increase in medical efficacy had saved the nation millions of dollars in lost labor and productivity. The federal government estimated that the annual cost of malaria to the thirteen southern states had dropped from the pre-war level of half a billion dollars to $50,000. Similarly, the Public Health Service recorded a decline in the incidence of polio from 1,000 cases a week to fewer than a dozen. Inoculation programs and pharmaceutical regimens had halved the man-hours lost to industry over the past decade, and reductions in sickness and accident payments ranged from 25 to 60 percent. "Health is our best investment," the surgeon general, Luther Terry, proclaimed to an audience in Detroit that May. "Thus we will increasingly charge the debits of premature death, prolonged disability, and high costs of care to the assets of improved health, greater economic efficiency, and enjoyment of life."[4]

The miracle of modern health care did not come cheap. The combined cost of physician and hospital services, prescription drugs, medical devices, research, and convalescence was over $170 per year per capita. A fourth of this was paid for by government—particularly research costs, medical care for the elderly poor, and hospitalization costs for the mentally ill—but three fourths of it was born by private individuals, corporate employers, and unions. For some services, such as hospital care, government paid for a bit more, while for other services, such as primary physician care, the burden fell more to the private sector, but the result in any event was the need for a substantial commitment by private citizens to fund their own care through cash payments, insurance premiums, wage reductions, or membership fees in prepaid health plans. While this health care balance between government and private citizen had existed for decades, the increasing efficiency of medicine made the opportunity cost of forfeiting private care greater, while the increasing cost of providing medical care made the cash sacrifice of obtaining it more acute.[5]

More than any other sector of health care, hospital care had grown in importance and cost, from 18 percent of the nation's health expenditures in 1929 to 33 percent by 1962, while almost all other health expenditures had declined as fractions of total health care expenditures. New surgical techniques, breakthroughs in trauma care, wound stabilization, transplants, and new life-sustaining therapies for chronic patients demanded financial commitments far greater than what most hospitals could hope to raise through traditional sources of philanthropy and government largesse. Philanthropy had declined to 3 percent of the nation's hospital budget, and state and federal hospital subsidy programs could make up less than a third of the remainder; 67 percent of all funds spent on hospitalization, whether for capital investment or operating reimbursement, needed to come directly from patient billings, and this share was growing.[6]

Hospital costs, unlike physician costs, were highly volatile for any given individual. While in any one year the majority of Americans would spend no money at all on hospital costs, for those who did the bill could run to thousands of dollars. The hospital bill for a significant surgical procedure such as a transplant or removal of a brain tumor exceeded the annual income of most American families. To distribute the risk of a catastrophic hospital bill over many years, or even over an entire lifetime, an increasing number of Americans had turned to private hospital insurance (and to physician insurance as well) in the decades after the Second World War. Insurance allowed for more predictable financial planning as well as a distribution of catastrophic risk over an entire labor force or community. And because a high proportion of all hospital insurance was provided by employers in the 1960s, its cost was psychologically easier to bear, as most American workers believed that more generous fringe benefits did not bring about a commensurate reduction in salary.

Private hospital insurance had existed in the United States since the late 1920s (when the first mutual Blue Cross plans were established) but had not become popular until the war years, when companies began looking for alternative forms of compensation to lure qualified workers during the tight wartime labor markets. When GIs returned from the fighting, American companies had enthusiastically expanded their insurance offerings, pleased with the benefit's lure to the most dependable and sought-after workers—stable family men. In the decade and a half after the war's end, the portion of Americans holding some type of hospital insurance policy grew from 22 to 74 percent—the fastest penetration of any type of financial instrument in the nation's history.[7] By 1965 over 80 percent of Americans in the prime of their working lives (ages 35 to 65) were covered, and over 70 percent of all children were covered as well. The single group with the lowest incidence of coverage, the elderly, still claimed a 63 percent coverage rate, and the poorest of the elderly, those least likely to be covered under a corporate pension plan and least able to afford private coverage, had benefited from the recently passed Kerr-Mills legislation, which offered medical subsidies for the impoverished aged.[8]

Studies conducted in the 1950s and 1960s indicated that hospital insurance coverage resulted in significantly better access to care and more successful outcomes from illness and trauma. As far back as 1952, the President's Commission on the Health Needs of the Nation reported that uninsured Americans entered the hospital in significantly higher numbers than insured Americans did, and once admitted stayed for substantially longer periods. Those covered by the most comprehensive policies, such as those of the Kaiser Foundation, the Group Health Association in Washington, and the Group Health Cooperative in Seattle, posted hospital admission rates of 80 to 90 per 1,000 per year, as compared to the general population's rate of 110 admissions per 1,000. Members of the cooperative plan stayed in the hospital an average of 6.4 days, while the general population stayed for 10.6. While Blue Cross patients were admitted at a slightly higher rate (122 per thousand), their lengths of stay were much closer to those of the cooperative plan members—7.4 days per admission. As a result, cooperative plan members stayed in the hospital for fewer than 600 days per thousand members per year, while the general population stayed for 1,165. Enrollees in the Blue Cross plan were in between, with 888 days per thousand per year.[9] While all these numbers had risen modestly by 1961, the magnitude of the discrepancy remained.

As hospital insurance became more important to Americans in planning for and financing their health care, those who lacked insurance lagged behind their fellow citizens in their ability to gain access to the best physicians and hospitals and to maintain their state of health. In 1932 the Committee on the Costs of Medical Care (CCMC) had reported that access to quality medical care was highly correlated with income, but the truly poor had always managed to find alternative means of gaining entry to the system. Public hospitals and clinics, pro bono service by doctors and dentists, and community-based philanthropy had historically minimized the disparity in access to health care between rich and poor. (The CCMC had found, oddly, that the very poorest group of Americans used doctors and hospitals as frequently as the wealthiest group, because of the availability of charity care. For all other groups, income dictated medical purchasing.) But the rise of hospital insurance undermined the existing mechanisms for equalizing access to medical care. By 1965 the discrepancies were obvious and stark. While only 13 percent of households with an annual income of $5,000 or more lacked hospital insurance, almost 40 percent of households earning under $5,000 so lacked. And for children of the poor, the situation was worse. In a nation in which over 80 percent of the actively employed had hospital insurance by 1965, only 22 percent of children living in households with an annual income under $3,000 had the same.[10] "Will the health system touch all, and not just the solvent and initiative-takers?," asked the public health scholar Charlotte Muller that spring.[11] Given the already described health advantages associated with hospital coverage, the wealth gap in health insurance loomed ominously over a nation which was becoming more concerned with social inequity and the persistence of endemic poverty.

The Poor

Who were the poor in 1965? One common sociological index was that families or households had "inadequate income" if their current earnings left them unable to meet at least 90 percent of their basic budget requirements (food, housing, clothing, health care, transportation). By this criterion 20 percent of American households were poor. But the line was hazy, and needed to be adjusted for regional cost-of-living differences, habits of living, unique expenses, and household standards. Another approach was to look at median family income. The median after-tax family income in 1965 was $5,906, of which $5,390 was spent on current consumption; 12 percent of households had incomes under $2,000, and another 8.5 percent had incomes between $2,000 and $3,000, leaving just over a fifth of American families below the poverty line of $3,000 set somewhat arbitrarily by the U.S. Department of Labor. A third approach was based on family food expenses, which the Department of Agriculture suggested should consume no more than a third of household income. By this measure, again, about a fifth of American households lived in poverty.[12] According to still another measure, the poor were the one sixth of American households which owed no income tax in 1963 because their household income fell below the mandated standard deduction—$1,325 for a mother and child, $2,675 for a married couple with two children. Among the elderly, half of those living alone lived on less than $1,000 a year, although their expenses (apart from medical care) were considerably less than those for the rest of the population, while among children, seventeen million (one in four) lived in families with inadequate income.[13]

Lack of income translated directly into lower use of medical care, even while ensuring higher rates of both acute and chronic illness. A person living in a family with under $2,000 in income, for example, could expect to lose twenty-eight days of productivity a year to illness, while one from a household earning over $7,000 would lose only thirteen. Yet at the same time, the member of the lower-income group would consult a physician only five times a year, while the one from the higher-income family would consult one six times. Differences in dental care were even wider: nearly 80 percent of people in the poorer group failed to visit a dentist in any given year (as opposed to 40 percent from the wealthier group), and when a poor person finally did go to the dentist, the visit resulted in an extraction 37 percent of the time (versus 10 percent for the wealthier group). Young bodies ordinarily recuperated on their own, and this minimized the consequences of inadequate care to some degree, but for the elderly poor the inability to consult a physician truly undermined the quality of life. A senior citizen from the poorer group, for example, would experience 50 percent more days of immobility and loss of functioning due to illness than would his counterpart in the wealthier group. And since loss of functioning, at all ages, translated into lost work days and diminished wages, the tendency of the poor to get sicker exacerbated their poverty. "These poor people who get sick and who go to the hospital are statistics," wrote the assistant secretary of health, education and welfare Wilbur Cohen. "But, they live among us; and their misery, buried in the statistics, is very real."[14]

Not only did poverty and illness tend to reinforce each other—the poor got sicker, the sick got poorer—but medical breakthroughs in the postwar years paradoxically made the problem worse. Where once all people, regardless of income, could count on a certain equity in the distribution of physical fortitude (in the nineteenth century infant mortality rates were actually higher among the wealthy in Europe, who would subject themselves to pernicious obstetrical techniques and unhealthy fashions), now money could buy better health. New drugs were capable of curing (rather than merely alleviating pain), and their very existence challenged prevailing notions of social equity. "I am 80 years old and for ten years I have been living on a bare nothing, two meals a day, one egg, a soup, because I want to be independent," a witness testified at a congressional hearing in 1959. "I have pernicious anemia, $9.95 for a little bottle of liquid shots, wholesale, I couldn't pay for it."[15] Illness and poverty were inseparable, and becoming more so. Traditional hallmarks of poverty, such as lack of education and adequate nutrition, unhealthy and unhygienic home environments, and poor social and psychological support structures, increasingly seemed like failures of the medical system rather than social pathologies. Governor Nelson Rockefeller of New York emphasized the bond between these two great social challenges when he reminded an assembled audience in 1965 that one of every six American adults was unable to hold employment or engage in the quotidian activities of life because of chronic disease or handicap, mental retardation, senescence, or alcoholism. Certainly access to private insurance did not cure all these ills, but it invariably salved and assuaged, speeded recovery, and retarded demise.[16]

The Genesis of Charity Care

Although formal charitable institutions did not appear in the United States en masse until after the Civil War, Americans of modest means living in farming villages and small towns could rely on informal community commitment for staples, shelter, and rudimentary medical care during difficult times, while America's few urban dwellers could turn to the almshouse, or even the prison, if desperate. Mass immigration after the potato famine in Ireland in the late 1840s, and then again after the political insurgencies and ensuing economic depressions in central Europe a decade later, shifted the American population from rural to urban and the work force from agricultural to industrial, and resulted in demand for more structured charitable institutions. Informal bonds of kin, church, and neighbor which functioned well in rural New England and tidewater Virginia were woefully inadequate in the Atlantic and Great Lakes industrial cities, which experienced explosive growth in mid-century. Many American cities quadrupled in population between 1830 and 1865; by the end of the Civil War, New York City claimed a population of nearly a million, Philadelphia of half a million, and the relatively new metropolises of Chicago, Buffalo, Cleveland, Cincinnati, and St. Louis of well over 100,000 each. Cities of this size, teeming with immigrants often isolated from family and *landsman*, required a more systematic approach to charity care.[17]

The sectarian, nonprofit, community hospital emerged to fill this role. Although civic leaders had been establishing private hospitals since the mid-eighteenth century, there were only 150 of these institutions by 1873. Almost exclusively Episcopalian in affiliation, these prestigious early arrivals—Pennsylvania Hospital, New York Hospital, Massachusetts General Hospital, and St. Luke's in New York among them—existed as much to serve the physician community as to serve the sick. Few people of means, or even of middle-class status, would consider obtaining care in the wards. No better equipped than the average middle-class living room for sick care, these early hospitals sheltered those patients who were cursed with attenuated family connections or distant kin, and who required bed, food, rudimentary nursing care, religious counseling, and weekly visits by a local physician who could frequently diagnose but rarely intervene. The physician's services were given gratis; possessing hospital privileges was its own reward for the doctor—an imprimatur of community standing, medical accomplishment, and often financial success. While his hospital service might occasionally lead to the referral of a patient, more likely it was an opportunity for him to dispense his civic obligation, meet young doctors in training, and assert authority within the community.

By 1920 the United States had over six thousand private hospitals. Slavic and Jewish immigrants from Central and Eastern Europe, Catholics from Italy and Ireland, Lutherans from Germany and Scandinavia,

Scottish Presbyterians, Methodists, and northwardly migrating African Americans followed the Episcopalian example of community largesse. Each group, eager to care for its own, established hospitals in cities with a critical mass of coreligionists and sought funds, nurses, doctors, and board members from within its own sect. Hospitals continued to provide little more than room, board, and succor to their unfortunate tenants, and most patients continued to avoid them when possible. Open wards prevailed, medical care was minimal and rudimentary, and prognoses were usually pessimistic upon admission. Nevertheless, groups placed a high priority on building these institutions, providing a locus for the medical training of kith, and the wherewithal to preserve indigenous culture if admission should be necessary. While a sick German could theoretically go to any hospital with little chance of being turned away, it was only at the local German or Lutheran hospital that he could be assured of finding familiar food, German-speaking nurses and staff, appropriate clergy, compatriot physicians, and a familiar milieu in which to either convalesce or die. Jewish hospitals offered the added attraction of kosher food; at Catholic hospitals there was daily mass, communion, and omnipresent crucifixes.

From the beginning these sectarian institutions defined their missions quite specifically. They were to provide community service and charity care to those in need, but only those who met minimal community standards of worthiness.[18] The "deserving poor" was a protean term, but throughout the late Victorian era it generally defined those who had fallen on hard times despite moral rectitude. The abandoned mother, the war widow, the orphan—these were society's downtrodden who maintained the promise of salvation. By contrast, the drunkard and the sloth either had failed to achieve grace from the outset, or had forfeited it through depraved acts of self-pollution. Various communities parsed the groupings differently, but all accepted the division to some degree. The wards, of course, were intended to serve the former group.[19]

Those deemed worthy entered an institution driven as much spiritually as medically. Since the majority of patients would die before discharge, hospitals defined their purposes broadly as salvation and succor. Nurses lent comfort to the suffering; clergy strove for absolution and repentance. "Many have heard the good news of salvation for the first time while lying on their beds of suffering," wrote one hospital super-intendent in 1892.[20] Medical staffing was closed, insofar as a patient's private physicians could not follow him into the hospital. Care was instead turned over to a select group of hospital physicians who were frequently medical leaders in the community, and who donated one or two mornings a week to observe patients, make recommendations, study the afflicted, and issue orders. The hospital was mission-driven (in today's parlance), and both workers and patients were preselected to comply with its ulterior goals. Few with alternatives chose to cede control over their lives to such a tightly ordered place; the regimen was of too little benefit to justify the surrender of domestic comfort.

Communities rallied round the institutions, however, often bestowing upon them philanthropic aid unparalleled by any other community association. In many neighborhoods fund-raising dinners, dances, and events were yearly social highlights. Membership on the board of trustees was highly prestigious and sought-after, and often culminated a lifetime of community service and civic involvement. Wives' groups, women's auxiliaries, volunteer brigades, and fund-raising committees grew up around the hospitals, drawing broad participation and helping to bind immigrant and religious communities undergoing the pressures of assimilation. The hospital was often the most generously endowed institution in any community, and its edifice the most impressive (particularly after the building spree from 1910 to 1930). It was neither the church steeple nor the local priory school which overshadowed the modest architecture of many urban neighborhoods, but rather the domed or vaulted cupola crowning the new *beaux arts* hospital building.

Public Hospitals

For patients who failed to meet the criteria of hospital admission, American cities began to establish public or municipal hospitals toward the end of the nineteenth century. These hospitals, which drew on the examples of a few early arrivals such as Bellevue in New York, were tax-funded and lacked the spiritual dimension of the sectarian institutions. Across the Northeast and the Midwest, cities constructed great holding pens for the disestablished. City Hospital in Boston, Martland in Newark, General

Hospital in Washington, Cook County in Chicago, and Kings County in Brooklyn all evolved from the earlier example of the public almshouse, whose goal was primarily to maintain public order by removing vagrants, shelterless migrants, seamen, and travelers from the streets. These were people who lacked the community ties and upstanding reputation sought by the private hospitals, and for one reason or another lacked family and friends to care for them when they fell ill. Income was not a significant factor in deciding who went to which type of hospital. Rather, community ties and reputation were the tickets for admission or denial.

One significant difference between the two types of institutions was billing. Municipal hospitals were free, as one would expect of an institution modeled on the almshouse. By contrast, the private hospitals charged a bed fee, even if nominally so. The fees helped to offset operating costs, but perhaps more importantly they established a precedent for self-help even among the poorest patients. Nineteenth-century philanthropists were keenly aware of the dangers which charity posed to beneficiaries; paupers could easily slide into vice and criminality if allowed to abrogate responsibility to themselves and their dependants, and the eleemosynary urge of the benefactor needed to be carefully tempered by the moral requirements of the beneficiary. "If a man will not work, neither shall he eat," the social theorist C. R. Henderson wrote in 1896.[21] Students of scientific charity recognized the distinction between poverty and pauperism, the latter being a moral affliction as well as a financial condition, and one which required philanthropic vigilance to thwart. "In nearly all cases, he who continually asks aid becomes a craven, abject creature with a lust for gratuitous maintenance," the reformer R. Hunter warned in 1904.[22] The setting of mandatory hospital fees, however modest, prevented this inevitable decline.

After 1910 both the mission and the operations of sectarian hospitals shifted toward the clinical. The impulse underlying the shift was the growing effectiveness of therapeutics. Analgesic and antiseptic surgery, first discovered in the latter half of the nineteenth century, came into broader use. Techniques first pioneered at the nation's research hospitals such as Johns Hopkins, Massachusetts General, and Presbyterian were disseminated to the medical hinterland, as surgical residents graduated from the most prestigious programs and went forth to establish their own practices. A revolutionary diagnostic tool, the x-ray, brought many middle-class patients to hospitals to use a technology rarely found in private offices, while new obstetrical approaches including use of the forceps, general anesthesia ("twilight sleep"), and cauterization promised safer and less painful deliveries. For the first time, many Americans began to view the hospital as not so much a spiritual venue but a medical one—the domain of the priest and minister had become the doctor's workshop.

Demographic changes accelerated this transformation. A wartime economy prompted greater internal migration within the United States, meaning that a substantial number of middle-class burghers lived distant from extended family. An expanding manufacturing sector and an increase in the money supply created economic growth and ended the decades-long deflation which had begun in the 1870s. More Americans had more money, but fewer community ties, on which to draw during a time of illness, and the existing sectarian hospitals became a natural refuge for the moneyed sick. The sectarian hospitals in turn upgraded their facilities from open wards to semi-private and private rooms, in the hope of attracting wealthier patients who could shoulder a larger portion of the hospital's operating budget. The hospital became associated with cure rather than death, and an institution founded under the guise of community service and spiritual elevation adapted itself naturally to the principles of medical procedure and professionalism. One satisfied customer explained at the time, "I can go to St. Luke's and for $21 a week I can have a private room with board, medicines, medical and surgical attendance and a trained nurse constantly with me."[23] Hospitals reinforced this perception by taking out advertisements in newspapers and serials touting their sophisticated equipment, highly trained nurses, and aesthetic attractions, in the hope of further increasing the ranks of the moneyed hospitalized.

Such developments spelled a fundamental shift in mission for sectarian hospitals. Born as glorified poorhouses whose fundamental client was the community, they had become medical workshops whose most important clientele were the skilled doctors practicing in that community. Pleasing local doctors became paramount for both trustees and administrators, since it was through the medical staff that prestige and import were garnered and billings earned. Trustees liked having well-regarded doctors on the medical staff; their reputations enhanced the reputation of the institution, and ultimately the social influence of the trustee. Likewise, administrators were eager to please the medical staff with professional nurses, sophisticated equipment, and modern facilities, as a way of both appeasing their own bosses (the trustees) and expanding their own purview. A prestigious hospital was a wealthy hospital, for prestige designated pride of place and attracted ever more philanthropy. As is common, the rich got richer.

But commitment to charity care was lost in this transformation. Private patients were now expected to bear larger hospital bills, and potential patients unable (or unwilling) to do so were now more frequently referred to the local municipal hospital. The distinction between the deserving and the undeserving poor was lost; now there were simply those who could pay, and those who couldn't. Although private hospitals did continue to provide substantial amounts of uncompensated care, this was now seen as an ancillary goal of the hospital rather than the central goal in and of itself. Also attenuated was the close identification which sectarian hospitals had previously held with a specific church, immigrant group, or sect. A Lutheran might now choose to seek care at the local Presbyterian hospital, as medical impetus overrode social inertia. Although boards continued to be drawn almost exclusively from the founding community, they now saw their primary commitment as one toward medical excellence, with commitment to the community at large or to the specific ethnic group which had founded the institution as secondary. The ties disintegrated gradually over the following half-century, until by the 1990s Swedish and Methodist hospitals began to merge with little cultural conflict, formerly Episcopalian hospitals advertised themselves as nonsectarian, and Jewish hospitals closed their kosher kitchens because of lack of demand for kosher food. Scientific medicine had proven itself a more compelling organizational foundation than parochial identity.[24]

Physician Charity

Charity care never had the institutional structure of the sectarian hospital. Rather, most doctors took it upon themselves to care for patients who sought their help, regardless of ability to pay. By the end of the nineteenth century most American physicians used a sliding scale for billing, under which they charged wealthier patients more and poorer patients less. Physicians regularly negotiated payment schedules, dismissed unpaid bills, took payment in farm produce or service-in-kind, and for the most part acclimated themselves to a life of modest income. In a depression, modest incomes could decline to incongruously low levels. During the early 1930s, for example, over half of all physicians earned less than $3,800 per year, and a quarter earned less than $2,300. By contrast, entry-level streetcar workers earned on average $1,900, freight train conductors $3,750, and locomotive engineers $4,700.[25]

Americans tolerated what financial barriers existed to access because generally physicians could do so little. Medicine before effective antibiotics or aseptic surgery was more art than science, and a majority of Americans preferred homegrown remedies to allopathic treatment.[26] A poor man who lacked the means to consult a specialist would usually minimize the potential benefit lost and turn instead to bed rest, teas, patent medicine (often containing morphine, heroin, or alcohol), and time. Death was also a more common occurrence, as evidenced by a life expectancy which stood at less than fifty years at the turn of the century (as compared to almost eighty years a century later). Moreover, visits by physicians often seemed to exacerbate a patient's condition rather than help it. Although the age of heroic medicine had largely come to an end by the Civil War, Americans at the turn of the century remembered the purgatives, emetics, and bloodlettings of yesteryear, and feared their therapeutic descendants. While physicians were more subtle in their diagnoses in 1910 than they had been in 1850, their ability to intervene in the natural course of a disease was still minimal.[27]

The advent of more research-driven medicine, as indicated by the founding of the Johns Hopkins Medical School in 1892, created a gap in health status between those who could pay and those who couldn't. Specialists and surgeons who trained at the best medical schools and hospitals (and who subsequently established urban specialty practices closely affiliated with major private hospitals) really could do more than the poorly trained general practitioners and osteopaths who served the countryside, and they greatly surpassed in healing power the quacks and alternative healers whose province was the western frontier and the rural hinterland.[28] For the first time, money bought not only a more salubrious environment (the high ground, the country retreat, fresher milk, more efficient plumbing) but better medical care as well. Public health officials who inspected immigrant tenements in the 1920s were disturbed by the squalor (as usual), but also by the absence of physicians' services. School vaccination programs which became common during the second and third decade of the century were in part a recognition of the increasing cost of missed medical care. Fifty years earlier the disparity in care would have been inconsequential.[29]

The growing disparity in access to medical care between rich and poor was partly obscured by the large-scale adoption of medical insurance after 1945. Relatively inexpensive physician insurance guaranteed to the vast majority of working- and middle-class Americans the same access to physician care as the wealthiest American. By 1975 even unskilled, uneducated Americans often had comprehensive family coverage. For many low-wage workers, health insurance actually became more valuable than the accompanying salary, particularly in those families which harbored a member suffering from a chronic condition or requiring complicated surgery. The extraordinary expansion of medical and surgical competency throughout the postwar years thus was made available to most Americans, unlike other types of technological developments which had often benefited only the wealthiest few. This broadening of the insured classes meant catastrophe for the truly poor, who lacked insurance and thus could potentially miss the single greatest benefit which modern science had bestowed on humanity. The response to this social travesty, as many reformers understood as early as 1920, required the participation of government.

The Sheppard-Towner Act and Early State Efforts

Not surprisingly, the first federal effort directed at more broadly distributing medical care targeted children. The head of the U.S. Children's Bureau, Julia Lathrop, a close associate of Jane Addams and a longtime resident of Hull House in Chicago, sponsored studies of infant mortality after the First World War which demonstrated the wide scope of the problem. By 1920 the infant mortality rate in the United States was 100 per 1,000 live births, resulting in over 230,000 infant deaths per year, and the maternal mortality rate was 15,000 deaths per year, placing the United States fourteenth internationally, with no demonstrated improvement in either area since 1900. (By contrast, the top-rated nation, New Zealand, posted an infant mortality rate of only 48 per 1,000 in 1920.) More sobering yet was the evidence showing that much infant mortality was directly attributable to poor prenatal medical care, leading Dr. Louis Dublin to call the deaths the "chief public health problem of the present day."[30] Congress responded in 1919 with the Sheppard-Towner Act, providing $1 million in matching funds to the states to further infant and maternal health efforts through clinics, well-baby programs, educational outreach, and postnatal care.

The proposed Sheppard-Towner program drew vociferous debate. American physicians, generally opposed to state-mandated sickness insurance, bridled at the prospect of federal involvement in medical care delivery. Joined by conservative members of Congress, they vowed to fight what they called a "Bolshevist" measure, one that in their view had been drafted almost exclusively by the (childless) socialists who staffed the Children's Welfare Bureau. The *Illinois Medical Journal* exhorted its readers to oppose the legislation, which had been sponsored by "endocrine perverts, derailed menopausics, and a lot of other men and women who have been bitten by that fatal parasite, the *upliftus putrifaciens*."[31] Lobbying for the motion was the League of Women Voters, whose influential member Florence Kelly reminded Congress of the nation's 680 infant deaths a day: "Surely, we are not to take this seriously," she admonished. "We are told that this country is so poor and this Congress so harassed by things of greater importance than the deaths of a quarter of a million children a year . . . is this really what Congress believes?"[32] The bill passed in late 1921, and for the next eight years it helped reduce infant mortality rates from 76 to 65 per 1,000 and maternal deaths from 6.8 to 6.5 per 1,000. Deemed "one of the major programs of social reform in America" by its supporters, it never fully overcame popular ambivalence toward federally mandated charity care, even for society's most vulnerable.[33]

Although the federal government made sporadic efforts over the subsequent forty years to meet the needs of the impoverished ill, these efforts were mostly limited to specific groups during difficult economic times. The original Social Security Act of 1934, for example, allocated federal funds to subsidize state public health efforts, and the Works Progress Administration financed numerous hospital construction and sanitary engineering projects throughout the South during the Depression.[34] Also notable were the farm sickness cooperatives established by the Farm Security Administration in the 1930s. These medical cooperatives brought primary physician care to thousands of impoverished farm families. Alas, as the wartime economy drew physicians to undermanned urban markets, and generally reduced unemployment to tolerable levels, political commitment to the programs declined, and so ultimately did the programs themselves.[35]

During the 1940s and 1950s states and municipalities began to assume the role of charity care guarantors. States had played some role in charity care since the mid-nineteenth century through their administration of psychiatric and tuberculosis hospitals, which often ended up harboring the generally disenfranchised as well as the targeted patient populations. None, however, took an active role in providing basic clinical care to the poor much before the 1950s. Providers of such care, when they existed, were charitable foundations, "community chests," and Catholic well-baby clinics. Municipalities devoted themselves almost exclusively to in-patient hospital care—a situation which invited abuse of municipal hospital emergency rooms by patients eager for primary medical care but unable to afford that offered by the private sector.

In the postwar years a few municipalities did commit themselves to creating medical clinics that provided free outpatient care for all residents who met certain maximum income standards. The clinics employed physicians on either a salary or capitated basis, and many also subsidized prescription medications, eyeglasses, medical devices, and psychotherapy. The racial breakdown of the programs' patients was notable. While there were many more poor whites than poor blacks in the United States in 1964, impoverished whites lived mostly in rural areas, while impoverished blacks were concentrated in the old industrial cities of the Northeast and Great Lakes states. Had charity care efforts been coordinated nationally by the federal government, this skewed distribution would have been inconsequential. But because the initial poverty care programs were state programs, and the states which inaugurated the programs were mostly industrial and heavily urbanized, the programs' patients from the outset were disproportionately black (and in a few areas Hispanic). Thus from the outset state-mandated charity care was influenced by the needs of minority populations, which in turn created a unified political constituency for the programs often absent in rural states. The most powerful advocates for charity care throughout the 1960s were black politicians (or white politicians with large black constituencies), who viewed charity care as disproportionately a black problem.

State charity care efforts in the 1950s, when they existed, were predominantly crippled children's programs, which had grown steadily since their inception in the 1930s. Aimed primarily at children with physical (mostly congenital) malformations, as well as epileptics and the mentally retarded, the programs served 375,000 children nationwide by 1960. The reach of the programs varied from state to state, however, and while policy analysts suggested that an optimum level of service was 120 children treated per 10,000 population, only three states reached this standard, and some states served fewer than 15 children per 10,000. A report by the Department of Health, Education and Welfare (HEW) in 1964 concluded that 480,000 additional children (beyond the 375,000 currently treated) could benefit from the programs were they adequately funded. Even then, the programs would only treat children with congenital defects, leaving the primary health needs of all other poor children unaddressed.[36]

Shortfalls in pediatric care, specifically, began to draw increased federal attention in the 1960s. A study of draft-age men revealed that 15 percent of them would fail to pass basic military medical examinations, and that three-fourths would have benefited from either earlier or more substantial medical treatment. Although school-age mortality had declined sharply over the previous half-century, chronic and congenital conditions continued to afflict the poor population. Certain chronic conditions, such as secondary syphilis, asthma, and emotional disorders, were actually increasing in prevalence in children and teenagers in the early 1960s, despite their treatability. Nearly a fifth of all school-aged children were judged emotionally maladjusted in one study by the American Public Health Association in 1961, while a large number had correctable heart disorders, cleft palates, speech deficiencies, and hearing and vision defects.[37] A White House commission in 1964 recommended that these deficiencies be corrected through more comprehensive school health services, screening projects, city clinics, and hospital outpatient programs. Other programs could follow.[38]

Beyond the unsurprising discovery that poor children fared worse in the nation's health profile, the White House commission found a more disturbing trend: health status to some degree resulted from the culture of poverty more than from the tangible deprivations of poverty itself. While more clinics and public hospitals could remedy some of the inequities, they alone would fail to rectify the problems of inappropriate diets, abusive family environments, community violence, and the general culture of ignorance which had always accompanied poverty. To many health planners in the 1960s, the declining health of the poor was inseparable from a broad litany of social pathologies which afflicted them, and which would all need to be addressed to create a more equitable society. While government funds could purchase more physician and nursing care, they could not bring pregnant women forth for prenatal care, or compel children to seek eye and ear testing, emotional counseling, or gynecological care. "The roots of the problems of many of these youngsters are in the early years of childhood in an environment of deprivation—emotionally, intellectually and economically," wrote the secretary of HEW, Anthony Celebrezze, to President Johnson in 1964.[39] If this was indeed true, a comprehensive charity care effort would need to attack the very roots of poverty.

A Culture of Poverty

Entrenched poverty was somewhat of a mystery to government planners by 1964. A steadily expanding economy with accompanying wage increases had somehow failed to reach a large portion of the population; in that year 38 million people, a fifth of the population, lived below the federal poverty threshold of $3,000 per year. While certain life choices or situations were clearly associated with poverty—lack of schooling, widowhood, premature parenthood, rural farm labor—social scholars began to suspect that a more profound difference separated the poor from everyone else. A culture of poverty, born of deeply rooted maladaptive life strategies, seemed to precede the tangible predictors of poverty for certain portions of the population, and this culture was frustratingly hard to break. "Citizens at these low income levels have a world of their own, neighborhoods of their own, and often a vocabulary of their own," wrote the public health expert George James in one study of the phenomenon. "Somehow or other, they have been 'centrifuged' out of the society in which we live and cut off from it."[40] Isolation wrought by poverty reinforced certain habits which could only exacerbate and perpetuate the cycle, leading to "cancerous pockets" within the wealthiest country in the world.[41]

One of the great questions which social theorists wrestled with in the early 1960s was the genesis of these pockets. Were the poor, through acts of extraordinary imprudence, responsible for their own situation, or were their life patterns merely a natural response to deprivation, racism, and childhood violence? The truth no doubt lay somewhere in between, but the general bias of welfare officials and poor-care advocates tended toward the former explanation in the early decades of the twentieth century. The 1953 edition of the *Encyclopedia of Social Sciences* held the poor to be "sinful, worthless, lazy, inebriate, or of low biologic stock," for example, a notion that drew on the nineteenth-century image of the pauper as living in a state of "degeneracy, drunkenness, vice, and corruption."[42] Because the primary responsibility for pauperism was assigned to the pauper himself, early charity workers would exploit welfare programs for opportunities to impart moral teachings to their beneficiaries. One welfare administrator would greet applicants with the following: "Do you know that you are throwing your family onto the county, and it will be a disgrace to you as long as you live? Now go home and see if you can't get along."[43] Only those supplicants who persisted after this reproof would receive the charity funds.

Most reformers were concerned with the danger of "pauperizing" someone who was temporarily down on his luck. They feared creating a cycle of dependence in which the pauper, upon receiving help, lost the will to support himself and his family, and became a lifelong ward of the state—a financial burden as well as a spiritual disgrace. Welfare was thus tied to humiliating conditions designed to impel the recipient back to work, whether through hard toil (breaking rocks, digging ditches, chopping wood) or the social stigma of the almshouse. Only the deserving poor—widows, crippled children, the mute, the deaf, and the blind—were exempt from such derogation and welcomed into public institutions and relief programs without comment. Able-bodied men and women were expected to work, no matter how onerous the conditions or meager the pay, or do without.

As a result of these attitudes, welfare recipients at mid-century were for the most part widows and their dependents. The widow had not left her husband of her own accord, nor been improvident enough to choose a man who would voluntarily leave her. Orphans comfortably fit this pattern as well, and so to a lesser extent did the blind, the deaf, and the crippled (although some surmised that these physical deformities reflected a fall from Christian grace). More problematic were dependent war veterans, first from the Civil War and then from the First World War, who drifted from city to city unable to hold work and maintain a family. Although they appeared able-bodied, because of their record of service social reformers were willing to spare them the moral opprobrium usually applied to vagabonds and drunkards. Still, they did not fit naturally with widows and orphans, and an appropriate charitable venue was elusive. The result was the soldiers' and sailors' homes established throughout the country at the turn of the century, which served to house and care for the veterans while distinguishing them from the true deserving poor who profited from mainstream welfare programs. The Veterans Administration hospitals created after the First World War met a similar need.

Attitudes began to change in the 1960s. The poor came to be seen by many liberal reformers as blameless victims, condemned to a life of poverty by forces quite beyond their own control. Rapid industrialization had left many rural residents ill-equipped to compete in a postwar economy, while generations of ignorance, disease, and discrimination had undermined their chances at leading a full life from the onset. Wilbur Cohen, assistant secretary of HEW, warned in 1963 that the "*causes* of poverty" and of economic dislocations needed to be attacked before poverty itself could be abolished, and a general shift in assumptions concerning family responsibility reinforced this thinking.[44] The "structuralist" conception of poverty dictated a different approach to welfare, for under this theory poverty was merely a symptom to be salved (while broader societal corrections were enacted) rather than a moral failing to be rectified. Neither theory was wholly satisfying to most Americans, who were offended at the idea of supporting those who could support themselves, yet reluctant to ignore the needs of the truly deprived. The social scientist Joel Handler described the dilemma: "Idleness, beggary, dirtiness, and other social characteristics commonly applied to the poor are outrages to the community. But starvation, neglect, delinquency, and death, particularly for children are also unacceptable."[45] Government at all levels struggled to respond to the challenge of poverty without violating public sensibilities.

Distribution of Poverty

Complicating this search for a cause was the skewed distribution of poverty. Race, age, education, region of origin, marital status, and gender were all highly correlated with the problem. Farm dwellers were substantially more likely than city dwellers to fall below the federal poverty line ($3,000 in 1964), and those without a high school degree substantially more likely than those with one. Large households were associated with poverty—the average poor household contained 4.1 residents to the non-poor household's 3.6—as were young children. As children aged, families gained wealth, resulting in a substantial wealth differential between households with toddlers and those with adolescents. A family of five with three small children, for example, had an expected income of $6,900, while a family with three children over eighteen had an expected income of $12,600.

Most pronounced were the racial discrepancies. Nonwhites (mostly African Americans) were more than twice as likely as whites to live in poverty, and nonwhite children four times as likely as white children. Thus the 14 percent of America's children who were nonwhite accounted for 38 percent of all children living in poverty, and 60 percent of all African American children lived in households below the federal poverty threshold. This was partially attributable to lower education levels among blacks, and partially to racial barriers in employment. But part of this discrepancy was due as well to the substantial (and increasing) gap between blacks and whites in the prevalence of single-parent households. By 1964 only two thirds of black children lived with both parents, whereas over 90 percent of white children did. This fact alone accounted for a substantial portion of black child poverty, as black children living in single-family households suffered even more than their white counterparts from the absence of a second parent. Altogether, the single most damaging threat to a family's economic security was the absence of a father earning a reasonable wage over an extended period, and black families met this criterion nearly five times as frequently as white families did.[46]

Poverty rates also differed significantly between geographic regions. Families in the South were more than twice as likely as families in the rest of the country to be poor, regardless of race. White families from the South had nearly double the poverty rates of white families elsewhere, and while most female-headed families were poor wherever they lived, the phenomenon of the impoverished male-headed household was almost a uniquely southern occurrence. The elderly were far more likely to be poor if living in the South, and members of the working class were more likely to be as well. Southern children collected roughly their proportional share of poverty benefits, but this may have been due to underenrollment in charity programs by the rural children who typified southern poverty. There was also a notably high rate of poverty among families in which the male head of household held year-round employment, owing largely to the lower wage scales which pervaded southern agriculture and the lack of industrial employment opportunities.

Nonwhites in the South fared even worse. Although blacks nationwide earned less than whites, the disparity was greatest in the South, where black wage earners made less than half the income of white earners. This was partly due to the high proportion of black workers on farms in the region (a situation which had been somewhat ameliorated by the large outmigration of black workers to northern cities in the 1940s and 1950s), but it was due as well to persistent segregation in southern schools and universities, lack of access to alternative educational resources, and racially discriminatory hiring practices in the large industrial firms. Southerners in general, and southern blacks in particular, exemplified the insular culture of poverty which welfare planners found most daunting.

Conquering such poverty, if one cleaved to structural explanations, would require profound changes in attitudes toward education, family, and race.[47]

Health Effects of Poverty

Poverty meant poor health for reasons besides simple inability to pay medical bills. Poor patients who ultimately sought hospital care, for example, usually from a public municipal hospital or a private hospital committed to charity care, arrived at the hospital much sicker then their nonpoor counterparts. Although the poor had fewer hospital admissions per capita than the nonpoor, they stayed almost twice as long upon admission and had higher rates of readmission for the same illness. Black patients, given their higher rates of poverty, had longer hospital stays than white patients, averaging 9.8 days instead of 5.6 days.[48] These patients had waited while acute infections festered and correctable conditions deteriorated before seeking help, either in hope of avoiding physicians' bills or through simple ignorance and lack of medical sophistication. The predictable result was sicker, more expensive patients, with depressed treatment outcomes.

Illness reinforced poverty, while poverty reinforced illness. Illustrating the "avalanche phenomenon," the public health physician George James described the working-class stroke patient who increasingly became socially isolated during his convalescence, as well as depressed and partially physically disabled: "As he removes himself from the mainstream of life, he reduces the feedback from society that would ordinarily tend to keep him oriented . . . soon we may find the individual far less active than he needs to be, far less in touch with the world and, after the circle has turned a few more times, sometimes totally immobile."[49] Moreover, the permanently poor were less acculturated to medical intervention than the general population. The social scientist Edward Suchman investigated the relationship between ethnocentrism and medical orientation in the early 1960s and found that different ethnic groups, be they mainstream Protestant, Jewish, Puerto Rican, African American, or Irish, had varying levels of allegiance to their own ethnic group, and these allegiances were correlated with positive attitudes toward physician care. Controlling for income, Protestants and Jews had the most positive attitudes toward doctors and the medical establishment, while blacks and Puerto Ricans had the least positive.[50] While rising incomes lessened some of these ethnic differences, strongly held social biases were difficult to uproot.

As usual, blacks suffered most from generally negative attitudes toward mainstream medicine. Already disadvantaged by geographical isolation (in the South), lack of education, unstable families, and discrimination, blacks suffered further from the racist attitudes often held by physicians. The civil activist Michael Schwerner (later murdered while working on a voter registration drive) cited one black boy's reluctance to go to the doctor because "he did not like going in the back door."[51] A shortage of black physicians only made matters worse: while blacks accounted for over 10 percent of the population in the United States, they accounted for less than 2 percent of physicians, and this percentage had actually declined in the years since the end of the Second World War. The nation had only two traditionally black medical schools (Howard and Meharry), which together could graduate only 150 doctors yearly. The remainder needed to train in the white medical schools, and their numbers had fallen from 236 graduates in 1955 to 164 in 1962. But as the (historically black) National Medical Association began recruitment drives to induce more young blacks to enter medicine, it found a severe shortage of qualified black college graduates willing to undergo the rigorous training. The removal of racial barriers which followed the desegregation decisions of the 1950s could not quickly alleviate the effects of decades of poverty, inferior schools, and racial discrimination. "Our young people in primary and secondary schools should be made to realize that there are many opportunities open and waiting for them if they would work hard, excel, and push ahead," wrote Edward Cooper, a black physician from Philadelphia, in 1964.[52]

War on Poverty

Traditional responses to poverty, whether local community chest programs, church-organized shelters and charity drives, or the state-sponsored Aid to Dependent Children (later shifted to the federal government and renamed Aid to Families with Dependent Children), accepted the pathological view of poverty. Potential beneficiaries needed to be judged individually, on their own moral accountability, and urged to mend their ways and lead more functional (and morally sound) lives, in exchange for public largesse. The original Social Security program tacitly endorsed this view of poverty when inaugurated in 1935 by requiring certain employment prerequisites to qualify for benefits through either old-age, disability, or unemployment benefits. But as a more structural view of poverty began to replace the traditional Christian-oriented view, efforts to alleviate poverty began to shift. Social Security eligibility requirements declined, until the relationship between "premiums" paid into the funds and benefits drawn out became only tenuously related. (By 1960 over a third of the benefits drawn out of the system had not been paid for through the beneficiaries' own payroll taxes.)[53] And welfare advocates in the 1960s began to argue more and more forcefully for a large-scale attack on the structural origins of poverty, ignoring whether those who would eventually benefit were morally worthy.

This "war on poverty," as it was dubbed by the Johnson administration, drew the support of liberal social scientists. The Swedish economist Gunnar Myrdal, author of the infamous report on race relations *An American Dilemma* (1944), called for a "Marshall Plan" to eradicate poverty in the nation in 1964: "This is a moral imperative. The unemployed, the underemployed and the now unemployables are also America's biggest wastage of economic resources," he wrote in *Harper's* in 1964.[54] The economist John Kenneth Galbraith more explicitly called for vast investments in education, training, medical and mental care, housing, counseling, urban recreation facilities, and slum abatement. "Poverty can be made to disappear," he wrote. "It won't be accomplished simply by stepping up the growth rate any more than it will be accomplished by incantation or ritualistic washing of the feet."[55] For both of these theorists, and for the many lesser-known scholars who followed their lead, the psychological profile of the poor was of trivial consideration in determining the etiology of poverty. Remove social barriers—inadequate resources and facilities, indebtedness, racism—and the poverty itself would wither away. Since the removal of the barriers was largely a financial matter, the solution was simply to spend more: a relatively easy task for the world's wealthiest nation. Poverty could fall as easily as infectious disease.

Shifting perceptions of poverty invited a broader government role in providing charity care too. The traditional public health providers—clinics, sectarian and municipal hospitals, private physicians engaged in pro bono work—had proven themselves inadequate to the task of making America's poor healthy. Under the traditional, pathology-based explanation of poverty, the poor had ultimately themselves to blame for their maligned state, and thus the ability of agencies to rectify disparities between the poor and the nonpoor must always be limited. But under the new, structuralist explanations of poverty, government could no longer make a credible case for deferring more substantial involvement in poor care. With the stroke of a pen, Congress (and various state legislatures) could equalize the health status of all Americans, regardless of income or education.

2

Precursors to Medicare and Medicaid

Early Federal Efforts in Health Services

The federal government had been involved in safeguarding the public's health, and in providing a limited array of clinical services, since shortly after its founding. The U.S. Public Health Service (PHS) was founded as the Marine Hospital Service in 1798 to care for sick and disabled merchant seamen. In the nineteenth century the PHS broadly expanded its purview to include quarantines, port closures, food and drink inspections, and limited sanitary engineering projects (most of which were undertaken by state and municipal health departments). In the early twentieth century the service further expanded to supervise immunization programs aimed at contagions and parasites throughout the rural South, often in conjunction with nonprofit foundations such as the Rockefeller Sanitary Commission. Still later, the PHS took to investigating outbreaks of diseases, coordinating epidemiological record keeping, and overseeing the nation's biomedical research efforts through the National Institutes of Health.

Absent from these functions was the general provision of clinical and hospital services. As one of the nation's five uniformed service divisions (along with the Army, Air Force, Navy, and Marines), the PHS theoretically answered directly to the president through the leadership of the surgeon general, and could be mobilized to battle disease outbreaks and health crises; in reality the service's primary task was more one of coordinating efforts by local public health authorities. Although by the mid-twentieth century its efforts were broad and omnipresent, their effects were barely felt by most Americans, who associated health care with either private sector actors and institutions or municipal health departments.[1] For general poor care, Americans needed to look elsewhere within the government.

Popular support for government-provided (or government-subsidized) sickness insurance waxed and waned episodically throughout the twentieth century, reaching its heights during the years before the First World War, the early years of Franklin Roosevelt's administration, the early 1940s, and 1948. During each of these "peaks" of interest in some sort of socialized medical system or government insurance program, legislative leaders in Washington and various state capitals introduced bills providing for different levels of government-funded medical care. Some bills called for matching federal grants to states, some for an all-out government takeover of the medical system, and some for simple tax subsidies to allow the poor to purchase private insurance. Although none of the more ambitious bills passed, each bout of legislative wrestling resulted in some sort of expansion of government-provided charity care: the Sheppard-Towner Act in the 1920s, the public health provisions of the Social Security Act in the 1930s, and the Hill-Burton hospital construction act of the 1940s (as well as an expansion of the National Institutes of Health). Notably, all these efforts shied away from the general provision of *clinical* care. Research, construction, public health works, and infant immunization were politically palatable; government doctors were less so.[2]

Each time the national health care issue arose during these years, interest groups fell into predictable niches. Organized medicine (particularly specialists and urban practitioners) would oppose the legislation, as would politically conservative groups such as the Veterans of Foreign Wars, the American Legion, and the Daughters of the American Revolution. More progressive political groups typically favored the legislation, as did organized labor, public health and poverty advocates, and scholars of health economics and health policy. The majority of the population, however, remained ambivalent. During the most extreme economic times (notably the 1930s), the proposals gained favor with moderate Americans, but this support was quickly withdrawn when economic deprivation ceased. Some observers of the American political scene suggested that the American populace was being brainwashed by a highly effective publicity campaign led by physicians, but this was probably untrue. Progressive labor groups such as the AFL and CIO refrained from endorsing government-mandated insurance, as their employees found that employer-provided insurance was usually more than adequate. And even the most homogeneously liberal blocs, such as foundation officials, professional reformers, and liberal legislators, began to withdraw their support from a program of government insurance as employer-provided coverage expanded. By 1952 the matter was notably absent from the American political debate, and candidates ceased highlighting it as a campaign issue.

By the mid-1950s a growing number of middle-class Americans had private insurance through either an employer contract or private purchase, and most states felt that the poor were being adequately cared for through public hospitals, community clinics, and private hospital charity care programs. These last, the most important element within the charity care spectrum, were essentially subsidized by the whole community, as hospitals shifted the cost of their charity care to paying patients, who were then reimbursed through nonprofit Blue Cross plans. Thus everybody paid for poor care, whether through higher individual premiums than they would have paid had they purchased insurance coverage at an experience-rated premium, through higher prices in manufactured goods, or through diminished salaries. Few people minded. The cost of health care was still relatively small—less than 4 percent of gross domestic product—and large companies were comfortable subsidizing public charity care through their artificially inflated health insurance premiums. The system seemed relatively stable.

If there was a single group which appeared to lack adequate medical coverage in 1955 it wasn't the poor but rather the elderly, or more precisely the elderly poor. Although the Social Security old-age benefits had lifted the majority of America's elderly above the federal poverty threshold, they remained the poorest single group of Americans, and usually the one with the greatest medical need. Chronic illness or complex surgery could quickly impoverish an elderly patient living on Social Security or a modest company pension, and medical calamities often hit at the precise point when many patients lost private medical policies which had been linked to work. While a few elderly were adequately wealthy to care for themselves, or had corporate pensions which included health plans, many others found themselves incapable of paying the increasing cost of medical and hospital care just as they began to draw on it the most. Because the elderly were numerous and voted in disproportionately high numbers, the problem of medical care for the elderly became more prominent in federal planning.

The primary question for legislators and policy experts in debating elderly care was one of inclusiveness: Should legislation encompass the needs of all elderly, or merely those who could prove themselves impoverished? The question was important, for the legislative response would create a template for future forays into the federal provision of clinical services (or payment for services). If legislative efforts were confined to the elderly poor, the federal government would be merely enlarging the established precedent of poverty relief—an area in which it had been involved since the 1930s. However, if it attempted a program to care for all elderly, without a means test, it would be establishing a precedent of providing government medical care for broad swaths of the population. While compelling arguments could be made that the elderly would never be appropriately covered by private health insurance, as they were retired and had modest pensions and incomes, disposing of a means test meant risking the wrath of those interest groups—organized medicine, the American Legion, conservative political groups—which had historically resisted an enlarged federal role in health care. Legislators interested in the issue needed to weigh the political price of each option.[3]

In 1957 several longtime advocates of national health insurance, including the self-described "reformers" I. S. Falk, Wilbur Cohen, and Robert Ball, and the labor leaders Nelson Cruikshank and Andrew Biemiller, persuaded Representative Aime Forand (D., R.I.) to sponsor a bill providing sixty days of hospitalization coverage and sixty days of nursing home coverage to all Americans over sixty-five years old who qualified for Social Security. By tying the bill to the Social Security program, its sponsors presented it as an expansion of the Social Security benefits which were already well accepted by American voters. The bill was in fact a natural stepchild to the various Wagner-Murray-Dingell national health insurance proposals which had been introduced throughout the 1940s, ultimately to no avail. Falk and Cohen, staffers in the research bureau of the Federal Security Agency (predecessor to the Social Security Administration), had worked closely on the bills, and Cruikshank had garnered the support of organized labor for most of those previous efforts. For these health reformers, providing hospital coverage to the elderly was a potential break in the defenses of opponents to national health insurance legislation, particularly if the new benefits could be closely associated with the popular Social Security old-age program.[4]

One impetus to the program was the growing realization that according to simple underwriting formulae, the elderly could never be carried on private insurance. Blue Cross, like all insurers, added value by distributing risk, and the activity was grounded on the randomness of occurrences with adverse effects. Should a high-risk group attempt to purchase health insurance, premiums would rise for all, including low-risk beneficiaries. Low-risk persons would quickly realize that the premiums they were paying were far in excess of the true risk profile they presented, and opt out of the system accordingly. Only two options remained to keep the system solvent if it were to include the growing number of elderly: either all Americans could be mandated to purchase insurance, individually or through their employers, or the government (state or federal) could subsidize the cost for the elderly. Left on their own, markets must ultimately exclude the elderly from coverage, or charge them prohibitively high rates.

The Forand Bill resonated with many Americans. A growing number of the elderly, as well as children of the elderly, had begun to realize the fundamental paradox of purchasing health insurance for a high-risk group. When medical care had been cheap (or ineffective), the paradox could easily be remedied through a cash system, but as the cost of catastrophic care escalated, most Americans found that direct payment to providers was too financially onerous. Private pensions and insurance markets were showing their natural limits in covering this population, and a large portion of the American population was willing to consider the substantial legislative action embodied in the Forand Bill.[5]

The usual opponents of national health insurance opposed the bill vociferously, led most stridently by organized physician groups and the insurance industry. Reflecting on the debates years later, Wilbur Cohen, who became secretary of health, education and welfare in Lyndon Johnson's administration, wrote, "It is difficult for many younger people today to realize how harsh many of the criticisms and arguments against these health proposals were."[6] Countering the physicians were union groups that worried about their diminishing ability to negotiate health benefits for their retiring members and feared ever-increasing hospital rates. The president of the United Auto Workers, Walter Reuther, testified for the Forand Bill in committee, demanding redress for the "most glaring deficiency in health security today."[7] Both physicians' groups and representatives of the insurance industry argued that the bill would be an "opening wedge" for further incursions of government into health care provision, and warned of the need to stave off action that they regarded as socialist: "Does it not seem inconsistent that we should be fighting Communism in Geneva while introducing legislation supporting it in Washington?," demanded Dr. Frederick Swartz, president of the American Society of Internal Medicine, in testimony to the committee.[8] While the bill failed in committee in both 1957 and 1959, it garnered more attention than many proponents had expected, and encouraged liberal members of Congress and their supporting advocacy groups to make further attempts (albeit with altered strategies) in the following years.

Whence came physicians' opposition to federal aid for elderly care? Partly the response had simply become innate: forty years of opposing all federal insurance proposals had heightened the skepticism with which most doctors scrutinized arguments for broader governmental roles in medical care. They feared loss of control, loss of professional autonomy, and diminishing quality should the federal government become the provider of medical services, or the principal insurer. But for some doctors, who presented a more sophisticated and enlightened response to legislative medical care proposals, the Forand Bill was too facile and too hastily conceived to merit support. For one thing, it lacked any provisions to fund physician care (as opposed to hospital care), and thus would unnecessarily drive elderly patients to inpatient treatment, which would be covered, and away from outpatient treatment, which would not. Second, the bill too closely resembled a modified welfare proposal, extending benefits without examining in any depth the fundamental needs of the growing health care system. "The problem deeply involves the practice of medicine, the quality of care, and the organization of medical care services," wrote the physician Osler Peterson. Before billions of dollars were dumped into America's hospitals, he suggested, proposals should be considered for more closely controlling rising hospital costs and coordinating physicians and hospital care.[9]

The Kerr-Mills Bill

The failure of the Forand Bill invited efforts at the alternative route to meeting the elderly health care challenge: a targeted program for the impoverished elderly which included a means test. Such a program was incorporated into a bill drafted in 1959 and introduced in 1960 by Representative Wilbur Mills (D., Ark.) and Senator Robert Kerr (D., Okla.). Mills was, in Wilbur Cohen's estimation, the only member of Congress who really understood the Social Security system, and as chairman of the House Ways and Means Committee he had special charge over the financing of all the government's entitlement programs.[10] Although both Mills and Kerr opposed a federal takeover of all elderly health payments, they each supported an elderly poor care program. For Mills, such a program was consistent with his commitment to alleviating poverty and would earn him political backing from the great number of impoverished elderly in his Arkansas constituency. Kerr too would be able to claim sponsorship of a program which would disproportionately benefit his constituents, who were both older and poorer than the rest of the population, while at the same time forestalling Republican efforts to introduce an elderly care program which would funnel funds through private insurance firms.

Kerr-Mills established a program of matching federal grants to the states (graduated from 50 to 80 percent, depending on the per capita wealth of the state) to fund a program of Medical Assistance to the Aged (MAA) which would be appended to the Social Security Act as Title XVI. In contrast to the Forand Bill, MAA was predicated on a means test for qualification. Like the Old Age Assistance (OAA) program which had existed since the 1930s, the program would target only a small portion of the elderly; unlike that program, however, MAA would exclusively provide medical benefits (hospital and physician costs), with more inclusive standards of eligibility. The bill far more closely resembled a welfare program than a national health insurance program. The means test attached a certain stigma to the program, which would be funded out of general tax revenues, and recipients of the program's benefits would be designated "beneficiaries" as opposed to "participants" or "members." Opponents of socialized medical care who had lived comfortably with the Social Security Program's OAA provisions for three decades could hardly oppose this modest extension of benefits.

Physicians and insurance executives, as usual, opposed the program, claiming that most of the elderly were also opposed and that in any event the problem of elderly poor care was overstated. The president-elect of the American Medical Association, Leonard Bismark, referred to a study by Emory University which concluded that over 60 percent of elderly respondents had more than $7,500 in cash on hand, while the president of the Health Insurance Association of America, H. Lewis Reitz, reminded an audience that "health care for the aged is particularly subject to emotionalism," and that great strides had been made over the previous ten years in providing medical care to the elderly poor.[11] The president of the Blue Cross Association, Walter McNerney, similarly emphasized at the annual convention of the American Hospital Association that any successful poverty care program must ultimately strengthen, not undermine, the private insurance markets; in his view there was no evidence that the elderly were in a state "of great unmet need," although he admitted that they might be in "an anomalous economic purchasing position."[12] That this "anomalous" situation was characterized by abject poverty was left unsaid. Contrasting these claims were those made by a board member of the American Public Welfare Association, Charles Schottland, who told the House Ways and Means Committee the following year that fewer than 20 percent of the elderly claimed income of over $2,000 per year, and 5 percent received less than $1,000. "It must be obvious," he testified, "that for the vast majority of the aged the payment of medical bills by the individual is out of the question."[13]

One powerful constituent group which favored the program but had hitherto remained silent on issues of health payment reform was the American Hospital Association (AHA). The nation's nonprofit hospitals had received neither benefit nor harm from the rise of private insurance through the 1940s and 1950s, and thus far had succeeded in shifting the costs of the poor and elderly to private payers without excessive opposition. But many hospital executives recognized the precariousness of the system as hospital costs continued to rise. Thus far large employers had not complained much about excessively high premiums for employee health benefits. The American economy had grown quickly in the decades after the Second World War, and with European industry still rebuilding from the war American firms enjoyed an artificially large share of worldwide orders for manufactured goods. But hospital administrators feared the day when corporations would begin to more carefully audit their expenses and question the bloated Blue Cross premiums which were being siphoned off into poor care. With most state governments unwilling or unable to substantially expand their own uncompensated care programs, a federal commitment to elderly poor care (if not elderly care in general) was necessary for the long-term fiscal solvency of many hospitals. Few hospital boards in 1960 were prepared to start refusing admission to elderly charity cases; many patients had no municipal alternatives to turn to, and even those who did were quick to report on the crowded conditions and low-quality care often found in municipal institutions. Thus the Kerr-Mills program, the AHA executive Robin Buerki reported, was "entirely consonant with the Association's philosophy."[14]

After the passage of Kerr-Mills in 1960, states on the whole were quick to establish MAA programs reimbursable by the federal government. By 1962 forty-three states and territories reported expanding their coverage of the elderly poor, through either existing OAA programs or the newly established MAA programs. Sixteen states had already established MAA bureaus, and six more were in the process of doing so. The number of recipients of MAA funds reached 102,000 by 1962, and 129,000 the following year. While states varied in their eligibility requirements (within the constraints of the federal guidelines), all states were in the process of expanding eligibility and welcoming an increasing number of the elderly into the programs. One AHA member, Thomas Hale, reported to assembled delegates in 1963 that four additional states were in the process of seeking approval for their programs, and that ten more were in the process of designing their own. Despite still existing problems in reimbursement levels and eligibility requirements, progress was being made in the "very important program," and further state action could be expected.[15]

Despite these early successes, the MAA program had obvious flaws. Eligibility standards varied from state to state, and often entailed a byzantine set of standards and requirements which thwarted applications from patients who clearly fell under the purview of the original legislation. States required different levels of family contributions to the beneficiary's medical care, and offered different reimbursement payments to hospitals regardless of contribution rates. As a result, spending per beneficiary varied widely, from $353 per recipient in Pennsylvania to $16 in Maryland, with an average of $207 in 1961. Compounding these discrepancies were varying deductibles, co-payments, payment ceilings, and customary rate schedules, all of which undermined the program's overarching goal of a unified elderly charity care program. Instead, fifty separate programs were developing with only mild similarities, as mandated by federal regulations on benefit packages and eligibility.

Of particular concern to hospitals was the growing delay between billing and reimbursement. The AHA expressed concern over this matter at its convention in 1962 but admitted befuddlement at its cause. Were the state program offices responsible for the growing lapses in reimbursement, or was the problem at the federal level? Regardless, the delays caused private hospitals to accept Kerr-Mills patients with some trepidation, and ultimately undermined the program's original intention of expanding access to private hospital services for the elderly poor. Albert Snoke, a delegate from Connecticut, charged at the convention that his state's policy of charging $100 deductibles to MAA patients was a cynical ploy to shift state commitments to private hospitals: "[The patients] can't pay this $100 deductible, so it becomes a subsidy that the institutions must pay."[16] As delays increased and reimbursement rates declined relative to the prevailing rates of private insurers, Kerr-Mills patients began to be seen as glorified charity patients, rather than private paying patients with government-subsidized insurance policies. Ultimately many hospitals stopped accepting Kerr-Mills patients altogether, and shunted them off to the public hospitals. Writing of the MAA program in 1965, the public health researcher Charlotte Muller noted that "skimpy budgets, inadequate payment to hospitals and physicians, lack of supervision of quality, and lack of coordination between programs cannot fail to affect what is received."[17] Similar limitations on the national Medicaid program enacted in the following year resulted in a comparable shift of charity patients to public hospitals: a pattern not rectified until the widespread adoption of managed-care hospital reimbursement in the late 1990s.

Other federal medical care programs were also considered, and in some cases adopted. In 1963 Congress passed the Community Mental Health Centers Act, which provided federal construction funds to states so that they could build comprehensive community mental health centers to care for mentally ill patients who were then being released from the nation's large psychiatric hospitals. The program implemented the recommendations of *Action for Mental Heath*, the final report of a joint commission established by Congress in 1955 to investigate the state of the nation's severely mentally ill and design alternative treatments. The report had recommended large-scale deinstitutionalization, coupled with broad use of anti-psychotic medication and the new community mental health centers, to bring the formerly institutionalized back into their communities. Although the program was strongly backed by the Kennedy administration and viewed by many as a model program of federal involvement in charity care, in fact it continued the federal government's long tradition of eschewing direct provision of clinical services. The initial legislation paid only for the centers' construction, leaving staffing to the states and localities. And although limited staffing provisions were included in subsequent bills, most state governments ultimately found the staffing needs of the centers too expensive to fund adequately, and the program failed to obtain many of its originally envisioned goals.[18]

A far more ambitious program was proposed by Representative Cecil King (D., Calif.) and Senator Clinton Anderson (D., N.M.) in 1961 to provide hospital coverage for all Americans sixty-five or older, regardless of financial need. The King-Anderson bill made no pretense of being charity care, and instead frankly acknowledged the systemic challenges facing the elderly as they attempted to purchase health insurance through private markets. Lacking a means test, the bill was also the first legislative effort at government health insurance since the failed Wagner-Murray-Dingell bills of the 1940s (with the exception of the limited Forand Bill), and thus faced opposition from the same groups. The landscape had changed somewhat, however. Whereas the Wagner-Murray-Dingell bills had attempted to provide government-sponsored insurance for everyone, King-Anderson was aimed exclusively at the elderly. And whereas in the 1940s Americans were still somewhat suspicious of an insurance product aimed at hospital and physician coverage, by 1961 the products were widely used and quite popular. Two of the major challenges which early federal efforts at health insurance had faced—lack of understanding of the basic product, and an ambivalent American populace—had been removed. The elderly were no longer ambivalent about the need for some sort of help (recognizing their diminished chances at purchasing private health insurance), and Americans mostly embraced the idea of third-party payment.

The King-Anderson bill used the Social Security old-age eligibility guidelines to define the beneficiary group for the new program, and funded the added benefits through an increased payroll tax (meaning that the program would be funded disproportionately by working-class and middle-class taxpayers). The secretary of HEW, Abraham Ribicoff, urged Congress to consider the question of elderly care in a new light: "The issue is not whether to pay these costs. The only issue is how to pay them," he testified to the House Ways and Means Committee.[19] The AMA opposed the measure, fearing an undermining of its authority and autonomy as the government gradually made inroads into medical payment mechanisms. "We oppose this bill vigorously," testified the AMA spokesman Edward Annis. "Under H.R. 4222, Government will decide for the patient what services should be provided and by whom and then assume the responsibility of paying for the services involved."[20] The King-Anderson bill failed in committee, but it opened debate on the broader issue of an insurance program for the elderly which would recognize the substantial challenges imposed on the elderly by the choice between purchasing private insurance and financing their own medical care. It also fundamentally separated the issue of elderly care from that of charity care, and recognized the elderly as a specific, nonimpoverished group which nonetheless merited special consideration from the government in obtaining medical care.[21]

By 1961, after just one year of the Kerr-Mills program, the total government allotment toward medical care topped $7 billion—more than double the investment of a decade previous—although the federal government's portion of total health spending in the United States had remained flat at about 43 percent. Virtually the entire expansion of federal funding of medical care had thus been accounted for by the overall increase in the nation's health care enterprise, and with the exception of a few elderly poor who benefited from Kerr-Mills, America's poor still relied almost exclusively for their care on the efforts of municipal and county programs and hospitals, as well as on charitable work by private physicians.[22] Real growth in federal health care programs had taken place, but mostly in military and veterans' programs, and in research, whose budget had grown from $8 million in 1947 to almost $1.5 billion by mid-decade. Various programs passed in the early 1960s served to aid migrant and agricultural workers in obtaining clinical services, but the federal government had consciously refused to enact a substantial program of poor care, whether through central control or matching grants, whether provided in the private sector or through government clinics. In a strongly worded memorandum to the White House in 1964, Wilbur Cohen emphasized that future initiatives must continue to expand health coverage for the elderly, the disabled, and children of low-income families ("areas in which we have not even begun to meet our responsibilities," he wrote).[23] The poor in America were still relying on a patchwork of community clinics, hospital-provided charity care, pro bono care from physicians, and as much out-of-pocket payment as they could manage. The result, predictably, was an ever-widening gap between the health profile of the poor and that of the rest of the population.

Rural Health

"Like poverty, rural living is a relative condition," wrote the public health researcher Robert Strauss in 1965. While demographers might argue about the exact nature of rural living, certainly by any measure it entailed lower levels of employment in the manufacturing sector, with an accompanying depressed wage structure endemic to farm life. Rural Americans in 1965 were undereducated, underemployed, and underserved by physicians and hospitals. Poor health and poor educational opportunities created a special type of insular poverty which recreated the impermeability of the urban ghetto, albeit in a far more widely dispersed way. "For those who are caught in the lowest social class [in rural areas]," Strauss wrote, "the increased premium placed on education and training for jobs in almost every industry or activity is resulting in some conditions more suggestive of a caste than a class society."[24]

Inhabitants of rural areas faced several unique challenges which decreased the likelihood that they could obtain adequate health care in 1960. Dispersed as the rural population was, it could rarely attract well-trained specialists, who required a large critical mass of people to fill their practices. For the same reason, rural residents had a difficult time supporting private hospitals, which required a minimum number of people in a "catchment area" to fill their wards and amortize their capital costs. Then too the population, being poorer than the national norm without benefit of corporate health benefits or union health plans, was disproportionately forced to purchase medical care with cash (or agricultural products or services), and in bad times could offer little more than promissory notes and negotiated payment schedules. The result of these conditions, not surprisingly, was a disproportionately low prevalence of both primary-care and specialty physician practices, few and poorly equipped hospitals, and an aging professional population. In southern Appalachia in 1965, for example, one of the poorest of the nation's rural regions, more than half of all counties had no public health medical officer of any kind, about a third shared a medical officer with an adjacent county, and only about 15 percent had their own. Almost 40 percent of all practicing private physicians in the region were over sixty-five (as compared to 12.5 percent of urban physicians). Fewer than half of all counties had their own hospitals, and even fewer would have had them but for the Hill-Burton federal hospital construction program, which had been steadily providing funds for rural hospital construction since 1946. Because rural physicians were generally overworked and underpaid, their opportunities for advanced training were limited, and most had skills which would have been considered obsolete in urban areas. A typical general practitioner in Appalachia in the mid-1960s saw forty patients a day, posting a yearly average of over ten thousand patient visits. Limited nursing and hospital support, and a nonexistent specialty infrastructure, dictated that the working conditions would not improve on their own.

Rural residents exacerbated their own medical situation by posting birth rates substantially above the national average. Harlan County, Kentucky, for example, led all counties in the United States in 1960 with a fertility rate of 869 per 100,000, compared with 576 for the state and 563 for the nation. While this was admittedly an extreme, rural birth rates remained stubbornly high well into the postwar decades. As a result, obstetrical and pediatric work took up a disproportionate share of most general practitioners' time, leaving even fewer medical resources to treat the other ailments and injuries of rural life. Strauss wrote of the challenges of rural life: "All these problems are magnified by the conditions of poverty; contaminated water; inadequate sewage disposal; crowded living space unprotected from heat, cold, insects, vermin or rodents; inadequate clothing, especially shoes; nutritional deficiencies; meager education, and physical and cultural isolation from the concepts and resources of modern hygiene and health care."[25]

The Johnson administration was aware of the special challenges which rural poverty posed to the provision of health care, but in its first few years it had little response beyond reaffirming the PHS commitment to rural programs and endorsing isolated federal poverty alleviation programs. In West Virginia, for example, the federal government had taken over a series of hospitals formerly run by the United Mine Workers Welfare and Retirement Fund after the fund abandoned the units in 1962. Within two years the hospitals were nearly bankrupt, despite a substantial infusion of federal funds. "Without these facilities, totaling 1,024 hospital beds," wrote Governor Edward Breathitt of Kentucky to President Johnson in December 1964, "adequate medical care in these areas would become virtually nonexistent, even if the population could afford to pay for care."[26] The president responded merely that he would take all possible actions to preserve the hospital system, without offering details.[27]

Neither the administration nor Congress had a workable plan for general charity care in the United States, nor had either considered the needs of any special groups beyond the elderly poor. Needy patients in rural areas, bereft of the philanthropic institutions scattered throughout poor city neighborhoods, were forced to rely on the meager staffing resources of PHS medical officers and a dwindling number of aging private physicians. Although the Hill-Burton construction program had eased the hospital bed shortage over the previous two decades, on the whole the medical situation remained dire.

3

War on Poverty and the Genesis of Medicaid

Policy Planning in the Mid-1960s

The Johnson administration in 1965 faced an array of issues surrounding the provision of health services. Most pressing was whether elderly and poor care planning could be conducted in isolation or needed to be considered within the context of reforming the whole health care delivery system. In either event, the role for community advocates, nondoctors, and neighborhood clinics would need to be considered, as would the roles of community mental health centers and public health officers. "How to offer services, how to do it easily, humanely, and with the minimum . . . of slippage (the loss of a patient between diagnosis and the host of health and social treatments), should be high among our immediate goals," wrote the physician Leonard Duhl in 1965.[1]

In the two years since Lyndon Johnson had assumed the presidency, broader provision of medical care had risen near the top of his domestic agenda. Along with civil rights and antipoverty programs, medical care for the elderly and poor was an area in which he assumed he could leave one of his most substantial legacies. White House policy meetings from the early years of Johnson's term included discussion of health reform in a plethora of guises, from rural and urban programs to community health centers, specialized "ghetto medicine" programs, mobile health vans, education programs, and an expansion of health manpower. Novel financing mechanisms were considered, as were new narcotics-control programs, nutrition outreach, efforts at improving basic hygiene and sanitation among the nation's poor, prescription drug subsidies, and improved data collection.[2]

In light of the compelling need for planning, Johnson appointed several commissions throughout his presidency charged with studying the larger health system and making strategic recommendations to reorganize and reconfigure the relationships between hospitals, doctors, ancillary clinical personnel, medical schools, public health authorities, and community clinics. One such early body, the National Commission on Community Health Services, produced a report entitled "Health Is a Community Affair" for the president in 1966, urging volunteerism and "action planning" in addition to the usual calls for broader provision of medical services for all underserved groups. What exactly constituted action planning was left unsaid, but the call exemplified the optimism of the health planners and community activists called to participate in the heady early days of the administration.[3]

Spurring the torrent of health reform zeal was a general recognition that America's health was being compromised, not so much by lack of effective therapeutics and accurate diagnostic tests but for want of political commitment. Any American who could get himself to a doctor regularly could take advantage of the antibiotic revolution and the breakthrough developments in hygiene, diagnosis, and prophylactic care. Certain cures were cheap: a course of penicillin was a fraction of a day's wages for working-class Americans, and the cost of adequate prenatal nutrition even less. Rather, the greatest barrier to optimal health for all Americans was want of physicians and dentists, cash, and private health insurance. A stunning statistic emerging from the military draft in the Second World War was that among inmates of orphanages in North Carolina—a generally impoverished group, albeit one given access to regular preventive medical care—only 1.4 percent had been rejected from the military, compared with 56.8 percent for North Carolinians as a whole.[4] This indicated to health planners that the greatest need in medicine lay not in research or revolutionary new procedures but in broadening access to the knowledge and skills already existent. The question for Johnson was how best to accomplish that.

Medicare

The most promising path politically to broadening access to medical care lay in the approach established in the Kerr-Mills program—expanding access for the elderly through a tax-funded government payment program. The elderly were an appealing beneficiary group, not least because they were a large and growing political constituency, but one which drew sympathy from the nonelderly as well. They had proven themselves beyond the reach of private insurance programs because of their skewed medical risk profile, and they stood to benefit greatly from newly developed procedures and medical interventions. Further reinforcing the argument for such a program was the redistributive precedent established by the Social Security Old Age, Survivor's, and Disability Insurance program (OASDI). Social Security was one of the most popular government programs in the country, immune from criticism by even the most libertarian members of Congress.

The Kerr-Mills program had proven itself successful in broadening access to medical care among the impoverished elderly without inviting serious political opposition, but much had been left undone. The failed King-Anderson bill in 1962 had attempted to rectify the shortfalls of the original program, and the efforts of its sponsors received a boost from President Kennedy's proposal in 1963 to establish a national health insurance program for the aged. King and Anderson, in conjunction with the administration, resubmitted their proposal the following winter, and the legislation meandered through House and Senate committees over the summer of 1964. Although the attempt died in conference committee, King and Anderson again resubmitted their proposal in January 1965, as H.R. 1 and S. 1.[5] After being reworked over the following seven months the legislation came to encompass two old-age health insurance programs, the first a quasi-mandatory program of hospital insurance for all OASDI beneficiaries funded through a special payroll tax (distinct from the general income tax), and the second a voluntary (though heavily subsidized) program of old-age physician insurance paid for by individual beneficiaries. Both programs included sizable deductibles and copayments, exclusions, lifetime maximums on hospital stays, and the like. Notably, both programs excluded payment mandates for prescription drugs. The two programs were signed into law by President Johnson on 30 July 1965 as Public Law 89-97, the new Title XVIII of the Social Security Act, and collectively dubbed "Medicare."[6] In signing the bill, the president called it "the most important measure in the history of social legislation in the United States."[7]

The main opposition to Medicare had come from physicians' groups, primarily the American Medical Association and its state affiliates. Although doctors would ultimately benefit mightily from the generous remuneration stipulated in the law, at the outset they feared that national health insurance for the elderly (which Medicare essentially was) would open the door for national health insurance for everyone. As far back as 1956, when staff members in the Eisenhower administration had begun to cautiously explore the possible establishment of an expanded care program within existing Social Security programs, the AMA had asserted that it "vigorously opposed" the proposed changes, as they were "needless, wasteful, dangerous, and contrary to the established policy of gradual Federal withdrawal from local public assistance programs."[8]

Doctors' fears were mostly unjustified, however. Although a few administration officials hoped that Medicare would be a precursor to general national health insurance, the general administration policy was articulated by Wilbur Cohen, assistant secretary of HEW, who emphasized "absolute" opposition to socialized medicine even as he championed Medicare. Cohen perceived, as did most of Johnson's health planners, that the elderly had unique health needs which could never be appropriately addressed by the private sector, and thus required specific government remedy. The existing Kerr-Mills program (which the AMA supported) was plainly inadequate for many of those needs, and thus needed to be expanded. The expansion did not need to be limitless, however. "I am a middle-of-the-road person," Cohen told an audience in 1965. "The proposal for hospital insurance through social security is a middle-of-the-road approach."[9] This road to appeasement was well articulated by a Treasury aide, Seymour Harris, who suggested how the administration might reply to its AMA critics: that "once the most vulnerable group is provided with medical care, namely the old, the chances of national health insurance would be greatly reduced."[10] Nonetheless, the Scripps-Howard newspapers' lead headline for 20 June 1966 was "AMA Sees Wilbur Cohen as 'Enemy No. One.' "[11]

Medicaid

Buried in the Social Security amendments of 1965 was an additional program aimed at providing medical care (both hospital and physician care) to the poor, blind, and disabled, to be codified as Title XIX of the Social Security Act. Known as Medicaid, the program was largely the brainchild of Cohen, who had been slowly gestating the idea for it since he observed the state of Rhode Island in 1942 attempt (and ultimately fail) to purchase medical care for certain welfare recipients with existing federal public assistance funds. As early as 1950 Cohen had been able to facilitate passage of a model amendment to the Social Security Act (P.L. 734) to allow states to provide medical assistance with part of their federal welfare payments, and thus in a "minuscule manner" had inaugurated an era of federal aid in medical financing. There things lay until a fortuitous confluence of events in 1961, which included John Kennedy's assuming the presidency and Wilbur Mills's taking charge of the Ways and Means Committee. The two men, both strong advocates of expanding access to health care, pushed Cohen to develop a more substantial program of medical aid.[12] Opportunity for passage of the program presented itself after Democratic landslide victories in both the White House and Congress in 1964. Mills used the opportunity to propose federal hospital insurance, federal physician insurance, and a joint federal-state program of poor care, the programs together constituting a "three-layer cake."[13]

The resulting assemblage of charity programs differed markedly from its more glamorous old-age cousin. For one, it did not amount to a unified federal program of aid, but rather committed federal matching funds to any state which might wish to create a charity program on its own. Second, the programs would be limited to recipients who met established guidelines of existing federal welfare programs (mainly Aid to Families with Dependent Children, or AFDC, as well as aid programs for the blind and permanently disabled), meaning that a certain number of the needy would be excluded, regardless of their ability (or inability) to afford necessary medical care. And last, the amendment stipulated that eligibility management would be housed within existing state welfare departments, meaning that most government officials and legislators would view the program primarily as welfare, not medical care. Congress furthered this perception by naming the intended beneficiaries "recipients." By contrast, designated beneficiaries of the Medicare program were referred to as "beneficiaries," which was the usual term describing holders of private insurance policies.

Such distinctions drew criticism from the start. Advocates for the poor protested the stigma which would accompany enrollment in the program, and children's advocacy groups noted that a large number of minors would continue to go uncared for under the program. AFDC requirements excluded any family in which a father was present and working, regardless of the meagerness of his income; thus children of a working father who earned wages at or just above the poverty level would be ineligible for Medicaid. Moreover, a large number of children from families which were just making ends meet without public assistance were known to lack primary medical care, and these children would be locked out of the proposed program as well. One study of school-aged children in Cook County, Illinois, in 1960, for example, found that over 52 percent of schoolchildren had had neither physical examinations, nor eye tests, nor hearing tests during the previous year. Similarly, the Ways and Means Committee's own investigation of child health in 1964 had found that half of all children in the United States under the age of fifteen had never been to a dentist.[14] "We regret the decision that health care for children will still come, in most part, through the persistent 'poor-law' philosophy of providing vital public assistance means tests," stated the Citizens' Committee for Children of New York in 1965.[15]

At its inception, Medicaid received scant attention from public, press, and government planners. Overshadowed by the much vaster Medicare program, and described as a mere expansion of existing welfare programs, the proposal drew little opposition from organized medicine, and not much support from Johnson's staff. At least one historian has suggested that the amendment was so hastily drafted by HEW staffers because they were confident that either Johnson or Vice President Hubert Humphrey would win the White House in 1968 and quickly propose a national health insurance program which would supersede any charity care program previously passed.[16] Most protest leveled at the program emanated from child welfare and poverty advocacy groups (who focused on its rather strict eligibility requirements), and from physicians and hospital administrators who warned against the inflationary pressures that the program would place on the health system. The president of the AMA, Donovan Ward, testified in 1965 that "there is no effective method or methods which will keep the costs of the program under control," while the associate director of the AHA, Kenneth Williamson, wrote, "It is a new day in health affairs. Things are not the same either for hospitals or physicians or the public. Things will never be the same again."[17] Both men would be proven correct almost immediately, as state budgets rose quickly to accommodate the financial strains of the new program.

The program, as passed, mandated that states which decided to establish Medicaid programs needed to include AFDC families, the disabled, and the blind among the recipients, and could opt to include the elderly indigent as well (who might not be able to afford Medicare's co-payments and deductibles). Eligible recipients would receive inpatient and outpatient care, laboratory and imaging services, and, notably, nursing home care and prescription drugs. Cost sharing was effectively prohibited, as were deductibles and co-payments. The federal government would contribute 55 percent of the reimbursable costs to states that had a per capita income at the national average or higher, and up to 83 percent of reimbursable costs for the poorest states. The program would commence on 1 January 1966.

Several lesser poverty care programs were either created or expanded along with Titles XVIII and XIX of the Social Security Act in 1965. Annual funding for the Maternal and Child Health Program, part of the original Social Security Act of 1934, was to be gradually expanded over a six-year period from $40 million to $60 million by 1970. States would receive new funds for mental retardation planning, as well as training grants for professionals working with crippled children. The previous exclusion of mental and tubercular patients from the old-age assistance and medical assistance programs (now superseded by Medicare and Medicaid) would be lifted, and certain limits of earnings by children and disabled persons would be allowed without jeopardizing eligibility for the two main programs. All these changes were minor, however, compared to both the scope and philosophical import of the newly created Medicare and Medicaid programs.

The most contentious issue emanating form the original Medicaid legislation was eligibility. Conservative members of Congress, fearing the program's ultimate cost, lobbied to set income eligibility limits as low as possible, thus excluding all but the extremely poor. The administration desired higher income limits as a means to extend the program to the greatest number of needy children. The ultimate figure decided upon, 133 percent of the federal poverty level, angered administration officials who noted that it excluded a substantial number of Americans considered poor enough by their states to qualify for cash assistance, and thus presumably too poor to pay their own medical bills. The secretary of HEW, John Gardner, testified to the Senate Finance Committee that the proposed limitations would "destroy the concept of medical indigence in a number of states."[18] In Indiana, for example, a family of four would receive cash assistance (through existing federal welfare programs) if its monthly income was less than $271, but could not qualify for Medicaid unless its income fell below $137. Likewise in Texas, the cash assistance monthly threshold was $163, but that for Medicaid only $124. Such a discrepancy could only hurt many people whom the program was intended to help, while promoting fraudulent applications, the hiding of income, and undeclared parental assistance to children born out of wedlock. The White House assistant Douglass Cater postulated that an appropriate remedy would be to require a *minimal* average income level for Medicaid qualification, thus forcing states to supplement incomes that fell below it.[19]

Early Responses

States moved quickly to establish Medicaid programs upon the passage of the bill; within two years twenty-six states were participating, and within five years all but Arizona had implemented some sort of program which met the program's standards.[20] The first challenge facing program administrators was finding potential recipients and enrolling them. While the promise of free medical care might seem unequivocally appealing, such was not necessarily the case. The poor in America in 1965 did receive care, although with less frequency (and at a lower level of quality) than the middle class and the wealthy. Bringing the poor into the new program would entail wooing them from whichever source they were currently using to receive care, and persuading them that the new state-federal amalgam could treat them with greater ease and convenience, and with higher quality, than the public clinics, municipal hospitals, and charitable physicians and nurses which currently treated them. Complicating the challenge was that a small minority of patients receiving treatment from these sources would be ineligible for care under the Medicaid program, placing program officers in the uncomfortable position of sorting out the eligibles from the ineligibles.

Moving a large number of patients from established treatment locales into the private medical system would create tremendous financial and organizational pressures for all institutions involved. One study in New York, for example, found that just over 90 percent of all patients treated at the outpatient clinics of the city's public hospitals would be eligible for treatment under the state's new Medicaid program.[21] The city thus needed to consider closing some or most of the clinics, but the precise number would be influenced by the number of patients now treated in the clinics who migrated to Medicaid.

But simply enrolling in Medicaid would not guarantee care. Private providers and institutions would need to agree to care for the new enrollees, and planners were not certain that these providers existed, or would emerge. The poor usually lived in poor neighborhoods, isolated from the general population, and these neighborhoods were underserved by private doctors and hospitals. In addition the poor disproportionately lacked private automobiles, and could not depend on public transportation to reliably transport them to suburban practices and hospitals. These physical barriers to care posed a real challenge to implementing the program.

Certain cultural characteristics of poverty also loomed as a barrier to the program's success. Multiple studies had shown not only that poverty was associated with undertreatment, but that living in an impoverished area (whether poor or not) exacerbated this tendency. That is, the insular culture of the ghetto was negatively correlated with preventive medical care, even for those residents who had private insurance. In part this could be explained by a lack of health education in impoverished areas, and a paucity of role models: ghetto residents had few examples of friends and relatives who habitually visited private physicians and dentists.[22] Another contributing factor was the higher-than-average rate of family dysfunction in poor areas—divorced and never-married persons made regular use of medical and dental care at lower rates than their married counterparts, and the same was true for their children.[23]

These problems led many social planners to criticize the approach of Medicaid, even before it was passed into law. In the opinion of many, the program was fundamentally deficient in that it tucked medical care for the poor into the general portfolio of poverty programs, without looking more broadly at the existing design and coordination of medical and hospital systems. Eveline Burns, for example, a well-known professor of social work at Columbia University, acknowledged the potential profundity of the new law's impact ("This law will go down in history as the most important piece of social legislation enacted in this century after the original Social Security Act," she wrote in 1966), while criticizing its basic conservatism.[24] In Burns's opinion, that the program was predicated on indemnifying providers merely perpetuated the fee-for-service system of medical care, which turned medicine from a calling and social good into a quasi-business.

Community Health

The idea of community health drew the attention of an increasing number of public health professionals, medical planners, social scientists, and government officials through the years surrounding the passage of Medicaid. A National Commission on Community Health Services issued a study report in early 1966 urging the nation to not only train additional health personnel but make them sensitive to the needs of the specific communities in which they would be practicing. In 1966 William Willard, a professor of medicine at the University of Kentucky, called for planning which was "community-wide" and structured to provide continuity and "not be a one-shot effort, forgotten by all concerned in due time."[25] The call was reiterated by the director of the Office of Community Action Programs within the Office of Economic Opportunity (OEO),

Theodore Berry, who called for a "massive commitment" to "imaginative and innovative solutions" that would provide medical care for all.[26]

The planners who criticized Medicaid envisioned a program which would both treat and empower, employing community residents in neighborhood health centers which would meet the unique needs and idiosyncrasies of the local population. The planners blamed the past failures of poverty programs (including charity care programs) on their insensitivity to the unique needs of the poor. To Lisbeth Bamberger, for example, administrator of the Community Action Program of the OEO, "the belief that needed changes must take place in the attitudes and behavior of the poor, rather than in the programs of the agencies that serve the poor" had been one of the "major deterrents" to developing more effective charity care programs in the past,[27] while other public health scholars called upon the nation's health planners to recognize the "neighborhood-based worker as a new and important member of the public health team."[28] Such critics looked to the turn-of-the century settlement houses in New York and Chicago as constructive examples of innovation in service delivery; the workers had frequently lived in the same neighborhood as those whom they served, and insofar as was possible had employed them to staff the programs of the houses. The public health officials Herbert Domke and Gladys Coffey wrote that antipoverty planners must apprehend what settlement house workers had learned long ago: "to get a job done, we must work with people in their homes and neighborhoods . . . to be more effective, our programs must be translated into their terms."[29]

At its base, the new skepticism refused to hold the poor accountable for their own lot. Poverty, in this view, was an inevitable byproduct of a misconstrued social order which failed to distribute land, goods, services, resources, and opportunities equitably. Because of the autonomy and independence which came with financial wherewithal, the poor could make more constructive life choices to fit their specific needs than could the bureaucrats, philanthropists, and professional planners who aspired to serve them. Giving aid without giving the requisite autonomy and control would inevitably lead to failure—the poor would benefit from the program in the short term but eventually regress to their previous state in the face of insurmountable social and professional discrimination. Old-fashioned charity medical care could only exacerbate the revolving-door effect of social welfare programs by temporarily raising living standards, but ultimately returning the poor to poverty when political support for the program ended. Community action programs, neighborhood health centers, community clinics, and local empowerment zones were the institutions on which these social visionaries rested their hopes, all of which would integrate community members into their boards and staff: to serve while at the same time uplifting. When community action programs were formed, one staff member at OEO wrote, it meant that "for the first time, the community has recognized that the poor do not create their own poverty."[30]

The planners of Medicaid had not looked to the settlement houses as a design template, however, but rather to the nation's Blue Cross and Blue Shield programs. Noting the substantial discrepancy between the health status of rich and poor, they had assumed that the most compelling explanatory variable was access to private insurance. Numerous studies had demonstrated the association between private insurance and the use of medical services.[31] Consequently, the organizing principle behind the Medicaid legislation had been to replicate, as far as possible, the experience of private insurance for the poor. Given a subsidized insurance policy, the poor could then use the same sophisticated medical care system which had so benefited the rest of the population, and thus raise their own health outcomes to national norms. The plan had the added advantage of leaving untouched the basic organizational scheme of American medicine: it required no new construction or hiring (except of the administrators) and left the provision of medical and hospital services in the private sector where it was firmly ensconced. While the Medicaid program might not profoundly change patterns of poverty in the United States, it stood a good chance of bringing basic medical services to many people who had not previously received them.

War on Poverty

The enactment of Medicaid (and to a lesser extent Medicare) was part of a grand series of legislative initiatives undertaken by the Johnson administration, collectively named the "War on Poverty." Perhaps best exemplified by the Economic Opportunity Act of 1964, the program responded to a growing public awareness in the early 1960s of the depth and magnitude of poverty in America, as well as to a sort of jingoistic optimism which gave many planners and activists the confidence that poverty could be conquered given the proper leadership and commitment. The president himself felt that the moment was propitious for a grand public effort for the social good. "The people were ready for action," he wrote in his memoirs years later, "and when I looked inside myself, I believed that I could provide the third ingredient—the disposition to lead."[32] Charles Noble writes, "Johnson constantly raised the stakes, setting more ambitious goals, and arguing for a far more active role for the federal government."[33] Equally important was Johnson's continued influence with Congress, and his ability to tie his legislative agenda to Kennedy's unfinished New Frontier program.

The receptiveness of Congress to the war on poverty in some ways coincided with Johnson's "honeymoon" period, but it also reflected a general public sympathy to antipoverty efforts. Michael Harrington's book *The Other America* (1962) and Harry Caudill's *Night Comes to the Cumberlands* (1962) had brought the harshness of contemporary poverty to the attention of millions of Americans, while several government reports on poverty (notably Robert Lampman's "The Problem of Poverty in America," which became part of the 1964 *Economic Report to the President*) persuaded many Americans that the time had come to readdress the persistence of poverty in the country. "The poor inhabit a world scarcely recognizable, and rarely recognized by the majority of Americans," wrote the President's Council of Economic Advisors in 1964.[34] National periodicals ran numerous stories on poverty and poverty alleviation in those years as well, including "It Can Be Done: Conquering Poverty in the U.S. by 1976" by the Yale economist James Tobin (in the *New Republic)* and "What Poverty Does to the Mind" by the Harvard psychiatrist Robert Coles (in the *Nation*). "No mind can ignore an ill body," Coles wrote, "—one that is feverish, paralyzed, crippled, injured, pain-ridden, undernourished, infected with worms, covered with sores, or denied the signaling and informative function of its senses."[35] Government statisticians estimated that 33 to 35 million Americans were living beneath the poverty line in 1962, even after an extraordinary seventeen years of postwar economic growth.[36]

Johnson responded by enthusiastically endorsing a $1.5 billion proposal of his economic council for alleviating poverty, while making the issue the centerpiece of his first State of the Union Address in early 1964. "This administration today, here and now, declares unconditional war on poverty in America," he told Congress. "It will not be a short or easy struggle, no single weapon or strategy will suffice, but we shall not rest until that war is won. The richest nation on earth can afford to win it. We cannot afford to lose it."[37]

The war on poverty was mostly laid out in the Economic Opportunity Act, notably titles I, II, and VI. Title I created various youth programs, including a national job corps aimed at unemployed young men, as well as work training and work-study programs. Title II provided federal funds to finance community action programs, vaguely defined as anti-poverty programs which would draw on the local resources (both capital and human) of impoverished areas, and could be aimed at improving education, health, employment, vocational training, and housing. Title III (ultimately removed) established farm improvement grants, and had been included, among other reasons, to win over reluctant southern legislators who might otherwise balk at such a vast commitment of federal funds to a disproportionately black population. Title VI established the OEO, which would run myriad poverty alleviation programs through its regional offices, including the National Voluntary Service Corps (VISTA) as well as the neighborhood health centers. The president signed the act into law on 24 August 1964 and promptly installed the director of the Peace Corps, Sargent Shriver, as the first head of the OEO.

The war on poverty, while consisting of numerous programs and legislative funding mandates enacted over several years beginning in 1964, took three major tacks: new or expanded training and educational opportunities for citizens hitherto cut off from them; removal of racially discriminatory barriers to employment and education (notably through the Civil Rights Act); and provision of basic necessities to poor communities such as health care, increased cash allocations, food, housing, and social services. The three-pronged approach drew on research indicating that the poor were disproportionately undereducated, undertrained, sick, ignorant, and isolated.[38] As previous poverty alleviation programs had in many instances failed to rectify these problems, the solution for planners in the mid-1960s was to make future programs more accessible, more culturally attuned to the target population, and more sensitive to the stated needs of the population. This thrust explained the centrality of community action, community health clinics, and community youth centers, and also the most vociferous pronouncements of the era. "City Hall—and Washington—must be closer to the people they govern," Cohen wrote in one of his many calls to action.[39] And Johnson wrote in his memoirs, "Community participation would give focus to our efforts . . . The concept of community action became the first building block in our program to attack poverty."[40]

Given the primacy of this community orientation, Medicare and Medicaid were oddly inconsistent with the administration's approach to social betterment. Both were huge programs which essentially retained the private provision of health services, including the many social and cultural barriers which progressive planners claimed prevented the poor from improving their lot. For Medicare, a program aimed primarily at a group accustomed to purchasing services in the private sector, this was understandable. But Medicaid was specifically aimed at the most isolated people in an increasingly sophisticated and institution-driven society— the permanent and endemic poor, incapable of taking advantage of the many programs and opportunities which had previously been presented to them. In theory, a voucher program for hospital and physician services should fail for the precise reasons that many educational and training programs had failed: the inaccessibility of services, the cultural insensitivity of administrators, and implicit racism from authority figures. Of all the services required by the poor, medicine was the one in which the most intimidating and alien professionals disbursed their wares, and thus stood the greatest chance of failing those who most eschewed the new and the intimidating. Yet Medicaid was the antithesis of a community-oriented poverty alleviation program.

The explanation for this incongruity lay largely in the political reality of medical opposition to Medicaid (and Medicare). Johnson was well aware of most doctors' fears of government incursions in medical care, and he chose the path of least resistance in attempting to provide medical services to the poor: the well-trodden private sector. Fearing a boycott of Medicare and Medicaid by physicians, even if the legislation survived a congressional vote, Johnson lobbied almost as hard for the programs among physicians as he had among members of Congress. In one pivotal effort in 1965, he invited AMA leaders to the White House to impress upon them his great respect for the profession and his willingness to grant them such demands as they deemed necessary to preserve their professional autonomy. "I talked about how much the devotion of our family doctor had meant during my father's final illness," the president wrote years later. "I spoke of the unique strength and influence that doctors possess."[41] The strategy ultimately worked. Although the AMA briefly proposed its own Medicare alternative, "Eldercare," it ultimately supported all the Social Security amendments for elderly in 1965, and for the poor as well.

The political scientist Jacob Hacker, among others, has noted that Medicare and Medicaid were designed to fill gaps in the private insurance system, rather than to supersede that system. The very nature of insurance would inevitably limit access to those with statistically highest-risk profiles—the elderly and the poor (as well as those with a history of chronic illness)—and thus the government's quickest path to expanding coverage would be to fill precisely those holes and no more. Hacker writes that while Medicare forced the government to provide a substantial amount of health care payment, "it also conformed to the logic of private sector developments." Furthermore, Medicare ultimately served to thwart efforts at national health insurance, by strengthening the constituency for the existing system linked to private employers.[42]

An Orphaned Program

Given the strange compromise of its birth, Medicaid was somewhat of an orphan. Although part of the larger war on poverty, it was philosophically different from most other, community-oriented poverty programs of the Johnson years, and ultimately had to compete for administrative attention with the more glamorous (and favored) OEO programs, including Shriver's neighborhood health centers. The Medicaid vouchers were thus hamstrung from the beginning. Lacking support from the great lobbying force of the elder lobby, but standing outside the general thrust of the community action approach to poverty, Medicaid quickly suffered because of its origins in political compromise. Congressional conservatives hated funding a federal program concerned with what they deemed primarily a local and state responsibility, while committed liberals disliked the manner in which Medicaid preserved the traditional fee-for-service provision of health care, while failing to promote an increase in hospitals and doctors in poor areas. And health care visionaries, such as Wilbur Cohen, Isidore Falk, and Edward Kennedy, viewed the program as a mere stepping-stone to a comprehensive national health insurance program, which would ultimately supersede the ill-construed Medicare and Medicaid amendments of 1965. The program lacked committed political support from its inception.

Further complicating the integration of Medicaid into the war on poverty was the racial disparity in wealth in the nation. While the majority of poor Americans were white, blacks were disproportionately represented in their ranks. In the mid-1960s, 8 percent of white families in the United States were poor, compared with 33 percent of nonwhite families. For families in which the family head was over sixty-five, the figures were 20 percent and 47 percent. And in central cities, where over half of the poor lived, over a third of all families were nonwhite. Nationwide, the black poor were younger, poorer, and more deeply mired in a culture of poverty than their white counterparts.[43] These racial discrepancies meant that the war on poverty (and its associated programs) would disproportionately benefit black families, raising the suspicions of southern legislators. To be politically viable, the Economic Opportunity Act would need to aid the poor without seeming to hinder the middle class and wealthy, meaning that busing, scatter-site public housing, integrated health services, and forced distribution of community resources were all unacceptable. Services would need to be provided in an insulated setting rather than a heterogeneous one, and the ultimate stated goals of the program could not be socioeconomic integration. Nicholas Lemann wrote in the *Atlantic*: "The beauty of community development for a politician was that it allowed him to express concern about the ghettos without angering white neighborhoods."[44] While no liberal politician could publicly make such a statement, none could afford to ignore its basic truth either.

For Medicaid, this meant that white suburban doctors and hospitals could not be forced to accept black patients, and neither would the government force doctors to practice in inner-city neighborhoods where the need was greatest and the resources most scant. Blacks accounted for fewer than 2 percent of the nation's physicians in 1965, and their numbers had actually been *falling* for several years at all the nation's medical schools, save for the two historically black ones. Thus Medicaid, envisioned as a simple voucher system, faced the daunting task of providing medical care to a poor population which was disproportionately minority, without the tools of community action and neighborhood empowerment. Black clinics could scarcely operate in the absence of black physicians, and black hospitals had never been able to raise the requisite capital for first-rate facilities. While Medicaid would certainly help the poor and disadvantaged, from its start it was hobbled by professional antipathy, political compromise, and racial ambiguity.

Medicaid in the States:
Cost Overruns and Eligibility Limits

Nineteen states created Medicaid-eligible programs in the first year after Medicaid became effective on 1 January 1966. Wealthy states such as California and New York were at the forefront in starting their programs, but so were states of such varying means as Kentucky, Vermont, Virginia, Massachusetts, and Connecticut. Although all were bound to the basic requirements of eligibility, they varied on leniency for expanding eligibility limits, as well as on their service mix and their generosity of payment to providers. New York's program, by far the most expansive and generous, technically qualified nearly 40 percent of the state's residents for participation, compared with 13 percent in California and 7 percent in Massachusetts, and its reimbursement rates were substantially higher than those in other states.[45] Other states were more inclusive than federal law required in allowing specific groups of patients into their programs. Connecticut, for example, moved to cover persons over sixty-five in mental and tubercular institutions, Idaho created a special category for children under twenty-one, and Louisiana and Kentucky added x-ray services and various components of emergency room care, laboratory testing, and home care. Utah kept eligibility requirements fairly standard, but it increased maximum allowable hospital stays as well as reimbursement for psychiatric evaluations.

While each state organized its Medicaid program slightly differently, in general the new Medicaid programs enlarged previously existing charity care programs in the states rather than displace their antecedents entirely. Kentucky, for example, established the Kentucky Medical Care Program in 1961, but the program could cover only 5 percent of the state's residents given its funding limitations. By contrast, the Kentucky Medical Assistance Program, the state's Medicaid program established in 1966, was soon able to insure nearly 9 percent of the state's population, although an early report on the program suggested that as many as 17 percent of the state's residents could probably be defined as medically needy.[46] Likewise, the California Medicaid program built on the existing Public Assistance Medical Care program with the new "Cal-Med" (later switched to "Medi-Cal") program. Cal-Med reached far into California's poor population, covering full costs for families with incomes under $3,000 per year, and catastrophic and unusual costs for families with incomes substantially higher. Jesse Unruh, speaker of the California Assembly, described the new program as "not simply a program for the poor, but a protection for all against the economic catastrophe of illness."[47] The new program provided drugs, radium therapy, elective surgery, physical therapy, dental care, and other services for all recipients; the old one had provided these services only for children, or in some cases not at all.[48]

As predicted, the early state programs began to run over budget within two years of their start, with the two most generous programs—those of New York and California—encountering the problem first. By mid-1967 the Health and Welfare Agency (HWA) which ran Medi-Cal proposed a rollback of services in an effort to stem the unexpected costs. Services would be reduced to the five essential ones mandated by Title XIX— physician, hospital outpatient, hospital inpatient, laboratory and x-ray, and nursing home care—as well as a few add-ons such as emergency dental care, essential pharmaceuticals, and Part B Medicare premiums for the elderly poor. Gone were extended hospital stays, elective surgeries, outpatient psychiatric services, eye refractions, podiatry, orthotics, certain nongeneric drugs, and overly generous physician payments. Backed by the fiscally conservative governor Ronald Reagan, the legislature complied with the HWA's requests, despite court challenges from various medical and patients' advocacy groups. New York's program incurred similar debts quite early in attempting to fund a generous catalogue of benefits as well as the highest physician reimbursement rates in the country. Physicians sought to attract Medicaid patients, as they found that the program reimbursed at higher levels than private payers, and hospitals too welcomed the boon of cash payments for what would previously have been dismissed as uncollectible debts. The *Syracuse Post-Standard* called the program "insane, fiscal irresponsibility, socialism, New York's Gigantic Giveaway," and the legislature began to investigate incidents of fraud.[49]

Overall, however, the first two years of the Medicaid program were successful. Most states either implemented, or planned to implement, a Medicaid-eligible program, and in every state where a program was begun, health statistics recorded declining rates of untreated infection, hernia, dental decay, heart murmur, skin disease, epilepsy, and eye and ear disorders. Physicians' and hospital groups generally dropped their opposition as soon as they realized that the programs would not weaken their financial position, and in many cases would strengthen them. The single flaw which exhibited itself most obviously in many of the programs in the first two years was a paucity of patients; many who could qualify simply refused to sign up, creating a new challenge for state welfare departments used to defending themselves against fraudulent applicants. Agency administrators considered publicity campaigns, increased social work budgets, and aggressive outreach to case workers as possible means of bringing in the qualified but reluctant, while governors and budget directors generally rejoiced at this unforeseen development. Planners worried most about the children being denied care, while others questioned the very idea of a means test for qualification. Governor Nelson Rockefeller of New York, for one, defended the low penetration rate of his state's program, explaining that his state's previous charity care programs had only registered 25 percent of the eligible recipients, but planners went unconvinced.

Opposition by Doctors and Hospitals

All early Medicaid plans had two great obstacles to overcome: the recalcitrance of physicians and the skepticism of private hospitals. Health care's marquee profession and central institution were both reluctant collaborators with Medicare and Medicaid, having resisted nearly all federal incursions into health care over the previous half-century. The AMA had almost single-handedly halted the Wagner-Murray-Dingell health insurance proposals in the 1940s and claimed primary responsibility for defeating Representative Claude Pepper (D., Fla.), a frequent advocate of these proposals and others, in a Senate primary in 1948. For the AMA, all federal health care proposals were suspect, regardless of any pecuniary gains that its members might be predicted to reap. Their suspicion was grounded in the fear that any program could provide a stepping-stone to more expansive government health care, perhaps a national health insurance system along European (or Canadian) lines, or worse yet a national health system on the British model in which doctors surrendered their practices to the government. Medicine under such a system would ultimately prove more highly controlled and scientifically adulterated (so the belief went), not to mention impecunious. For a profession peopled by proud stalwarts and independent entrepreneurs, the idea was intolerable.

For these reasons, the AMA had consistently opposed the elderly care legislative measures proposed throughout the early 1960s, and had agreed to allow the passage of Titles XVIII and XIX only after wringing broad concessions from the Johnson administration. The AMA's president, James Appel, for example, had telegrammed the presidential aid Douglass Cater in the summer of 1965 urging delay on the pending Medicare bill, arguing that it had "far-reaching implications for health care in the United States," and that "more study and national dialogue" were necessary.[50] And Wilbur Cohen, the administration's point man in dealing with physicians, warned Cater at the same time that it was "essential" for doctors to play an "important role" in implementing any new program.[51]

Bowing to the pressure, the final bill placated doctors by guaranteeing that patients would have complete discretion in choosing a doctor under Medicare, that no federal officer or authority could "exercise any supervision or control over the practice of medicine or the manner in which medical services are provided," that no doctor would be compelled to participate in the program, and that any doctor participating in the program would draw payment through Blue Shield (which would act as the government's fiscal intermediary) rather than directly from the newly created Health Care Financing Agency. Last and most important, physicians would be reimbursed customary and prevailing charges for all services rendered.

Medicaid faced less vocal opposition than Medicare, as the program did not really exist at the federal level but was only a coordinating umbrella for the many state plans which would soon be developed. Moreover Medicaid, as envisioned, would be much more limited in scope than Medicare, and would fill a niche which doctors had long recognized merited some level of government participation, be it at the municipal, state, or federal level. Nonetheless, doctors claimed that Medicaid would replace a comfortable patchwork system of charitable agencies with a catalogue of rigid guidelines concerning eligibility, services, and quality. And even though states would be required to reimburse doctors at customary rates, and no doctors would be required to participate in the program, physicians feared, as they did with Medicare, that the provisions enacted in 1965 would be only a first step to a more broadly envisioned socialized medical care system. Even after many Medicaid programs were securely implemented and all but displaced the old community clinics, some doctors questioned the added utility wrought by federal controls. In theory, for example, Medicaid was supposed to give all poor persons access to a private physician, but James Boland of the Massachusetts health department questioned whether this access was really more desirable than public clinics. "Our evidence, casual at best," he wrote to the *New England Journal of Medicine*, "is that in low income neighborhoods, clinics and health centers frequently give better medical care than that provided by an aging and dwindling stock of neighborhood physicians."[52]

One reason why so many doctors were concerned about the new

Medicaid program was its unknown effect on private hospitals, even for those doctors who did not necessarily plan on treating a large number of Medicaid patients. One of the goals of Medicaid was to provide the same quality of medical care for the poor as for the rich, and this meant granting access to the same private hospitals which most of the nation used, as opposed to the municipal hospitals disproportionately used by the poor. But private physicians, long accustomed to hospitals which catered primarily to the needs of their medical staffs rather than those of the *community*, feared losing control of their workshops. A large number of poor inpatients would create different demands on the nursing staff, on the hospital budget, and on hospital administrators, as they struggled to cope with the unique demands of the poor and previously under-treated. Already in the early 1960s hospitals were beginning to implement programs of community education, preventive medicine, and satellite outpatient services, and all these programs drew resources away from the central inpatient functions most highly valued by the medical staff. Additionally, expanding the medical staff to include physicians who primarily saw poor, Medicaid-eligible patients would change the dynamic of the staff, and indeed the culture of the hospital. Young, liberal physicians, many of them committed to academic medicine, family practice, and public health, would use their increased influence to reorient hospitals from physician workshops to community health centers.

Hospital administrators responded to these pressures with political deftness. While generally supportive of Medicare and Medicaid, which they viewed as a potential financial boon, they feared any loss in their own autonomy once federal payment guidelines began to be implemented. "The Hospital community has tremendous responsibility for making every effort to ensure the successful operation of this program," Horace Cardwell, chairman of an AHA committee, opined about Medicare in 1965.[53] Yet in the following year the AHA's board adopted a resolution stating that although constituent hospitals would care for Medicare beneficiaries in a professional and humane manner, it was their "responsibility and intent" to ensure that "in taking care of the Medicare beneficiaries, there is no damage done to the viability, to the strength, and to the continued improvement of the voluntary health and hospital system."[54] Medicaid presented problems both greater and lesser than those presented by Medicare. While the program would be smaller, and ultimately less consequential for private hospitals, it would probably be funded at lower levels (given the relative poverty of most state governments compared to the federal government), and would open hospital doors to whole new groups of patients which had previously sought care elsewhere.

The hospital community responded by establishing the Committee on Health Care for the Disadvantaged in 1968, charged with drafting proposals to maximize hospital revenues from private patients while also increasing service to the community. The committee recommended that hospitals attempt to serve Medicaid patients insofar as was fiscally possible, while helping to "erase the causative factors" of illness, through improved housing, education, transportation, and community outreach. At the same time, the committee acknowledged that disregarding the long-term costs of programs to the poor would be "unwise and unacceptable," regardless of the desirability of the programs.[55] In reality, this meant that hospitals stabilized the most desperate patients while referring many Medicaid recipients to the local public hospitals. Some hospitals refused to participate in Medicaid entirely, provoking at least one class-action lawsuit against ten hospitals in New Orleans which had been partially financed with Hill-Burton funds but refused to serve Medicaid patients.

For the states struggling to establish their Medicaid programs through the late 1960s, the reluctance of doctors and private hospitals to fundamentally alter their practices to accommodate the new patients meant that the programs could achieve only incomplete success. For a program whose stated vision was the supersession of a two-tiered health system, the upper tier was proving stubbornly unwilling to adapt. Part of the problem was inadequate funding, as Medicaid reimbursement rates quickly fell behind the customary charges paid by both Medicare and the private sector. This much could be deduced by observing those exceptional states (such as New York) which reimbursed doctors at near competitive rates, and posted much higher rates of Medicaid penetration into predominantly private-payer physician practices. But equally challenging was the cultural gap between the new and old patients. Medicaid patients were poor, and poor people were different in their life habits. Poor people were less healthy, less cooperative, less pleasant to deal with, and less attractive. Private doctors and hospitals feared alienating their long-standing patients by having these new patients sit in their waiting rooms, or recuperate in their wards. For institutions and individuals who had long prided themselves on their autonomy and independence, the new patients threatened to dilute their identity and mission.

4

Hard-to-Reach Groups

Among the failures of Medicaid in its early years was its inability to reach certain populations of poor people who were unable, or unwilling, to use the nation's health care resources despite now having the financial means to do so. Whether defined by geographic locale (inner-city and rural), race and ethnicity (blacks and Hispanics), or age (minors), these populations faced a variety of challenges which exceeded the ability of Medicaid to ameliorate them. Because they were denied physical access to proximate physician practices or hospitals, or cultural access to comfort with modern medicine, or the wherewithal and transportation by which to get themselves to health care facilities, these populations proved difficult to reach. State and municipal governments, and eventually Congress, instigated programs in the late 1960s to compensate for the shortcomings of Medicaid, and in some cases these were successful. Nonetheless cultures of poverty, or of alienation, or of indifference, continued to force these groups to the margins of the nation's health system, even amid the improvements wrought by Medicaid.

Urban Medicine and Public Hospitals

Many of the communities most in need of increased funding for charity care were located in the inner areas of America's major cities. Increasingly inhabited by blacks and Puerto Ricans, these urban "ghettos" were proving to be oddly isolated from middle-class culture, even as they were physically close to it. Although most Americans (and certainly all city planners and administrators) were aware of the phenomenon of white flight by 1965, few policy experts had clear solutions to the problem.

Health care in inner cities had declined precipitously since the Second World War in both quantity and quality, as private physicians followed the middle class to the suburbs and induced private hospitals to follow the population shift a few years later. In 1940, for example, the city of Baltimore had 950 physicians for 850,000 residents, while by the mid-1960s the number had declined to 300 for a population of 920,000, creating a physician-to-population ratio of 33 per 100,000. Similarly, the physician to population ratio in Los Angeles by 1965 had declined to 127 per 100,000, in Chicago to 126 per 100,000, and in the two poorest health districts in the Bronx to 3 per 100,000. By contrast, most middle-class and suburban areas maintained ratios of more than 200 physicians per 100,000, and sometimes more than 300.[1]

The inner-city poor, as a result, faced not only the usual financial barriers to medical care which were endemic to poverty but resource barriers as well, leading at least one medical observer to note that when only one doctor was available to care for six thousand people, the "major prescription" for medical care was "waiting."[2] Urban residents did their best to obtain medical care when and how they could get it, aggressively taking advantage of the many charity programs available in urban areas before 1965, such as community clinics, outpatient clinics in public hospitals, and emergency rooms in public hospitals. The last option, exercised with growing frequency by the poor through the 1950s and 1960s, forced the emergency rooms of public hospitals to become the family physicians of many local residents, a task for which they were poorly adapted. Long waits, harassed nurses, and inexperienced medical interns and residents all served to frustrate the poor in their quest for care, drain the public hospitals of resources better spent on inpatient care, and demoralize a young medical staff which had expected better training opportunities. The health services researchers M. Alfred Haynes and Michael R. McGarvey observed of the urban health care network: "If some genius of a devil had expended his best efforts in contriving some situation which would achieve the maximum dissatisfaction for all concerned, he could not have achieved more spectacular results."[3]

Initially, the enactment of Medicaid provided no panacea for these areas. Many local residents would not qualify for the programs, of those who did qualify many would not seek to enroll, and of those who sought to enroll many would find scant or nonexistent professional and institutional providers from which to seek care. Cities, counties, and states responded by continuing many of the poverty care programs already in operation, even as they added Medicaid, while at the same time formulating strategic plans to better integrate the new program into the social safety net. By 1968 Baltimore provided charity care through at least twelve programs, including the state's Medicaid program, Medicare, the state psychiatric hospitals, city clinics, a large municipal hospital, the veterans administration, a state-funded tuberculosis hospital, neighborhood health clinics funded by OEO, model cities programs, community mental health centers, and Health Services to Needy Children. These programs were each administered by a different agency at either the municipal, county, state, or federal level, and they were coordinated hardly at all.

Medicaid quickly became the largest single source of funds for impoverished urban areas, but income from the other funding agencies continued to be crucial. In response, cities established planning committees in the years after Medicaid was inaugurated, charged with creating strategic plans for charity health care which would coordinate hospital and clinical services with neighborhood health centers, private physicians, and municipal hospitals, and generally try to replicate the experience of private medical care in the public arena. Planners in Chicago, for example, envisioned a "three echelon" system of care composed of primary-care nurses' aides and paraprofessionals, who would attempt to mimic the role of the family physician in the lives of most middle-class families; neighborhood health centers; and private and public hospitals. Ideally the poor would be dispersed among the many private hospitals in the Chicago area, rather than continue to seek the majority of their care at the public Cook County Hospital, which treated 30 percent of all charity care patients for the region.[4]

New York City, the nation's largest and most complex metropolis with the largest pool of Medicaid recipients, and controlling no fewer than thirteen public hospitals, developed what was probably the most comprehensive community health plan of any city. The challenge was vast. Nearly half of all residents received their health care from the city in 1967 (whether through municipal providers or municipally administered payment programs), and city planners uniformly agreed that the quality of care was inconsistent and typically lower than that provided to private patients.[5] The city responded by establishing a single Health Services Administration to coordinate all charity care provided through city agencies and programs. Gone would be the persistent problem of welfare patients obtaining primary care from city hospital emergency rooms (expensive and ineffective), as well as discharged patients unable to obtain postoperative care in city rehabilitation facilities. Rather, through a newly incorporated, nonprofit Health Services Corporation, the city would construct primary-care community clinics throughout the neighborhoods and boroughs which would function as the main entrance to the health care system, and would provide both triage and case management in addition to primary and preventive medical care.

An immediate result of the new Medicaid programs was a rapid decline in inpatient populations at public hospitals. The number of city hospital beds nationwide declined from 51,000 in 1960 to 44,000 in 1970, even as the number of voluntary hospital beds rose in that decade from 141,000 to 175,000. Public hospitals, which accounted for nearly a third of all hospital beds in the country in 1950, would drop to little more than an eighth in 1980, mostly as a result of the combined purchasing power placed in the hands of the relatively poor participants in both the Medicaid and Medicare programs.[6] Many municipal administrators viewed the declining patient populations in public hospitals more as a threat to their bureaucratic livelihood than as a promise of improved hospital services for poor patients. For city hospital administrators and boards, the siphoning off of welfare patients to private hospitals threatened their positions and influence, as well as undermining their general vision of appropriate poor care. James Fitzgerald, for example, chairman of the San Mateo County Board of Supervisors, viewed with alarm the low occupancy rate in County Hospital in 1968 for increasing its costs per patient. Responding to a suggestion of converting the hospital to a private institution, however, he derided the idea as an "easy way out" which would be an abrogation of the county's commitment to its poor residents.

Many public hospital planners argued in the late 1960s for a "partnership" between the public hospitals and Medicaid, but on the whole they failed to recognize that the new program would lead to a diminished role for their institutions in providing charity care.[7] Witnessing a hemorrhage of their erstwhile public charges to the private sector, they resolved to improve the quality of their own offerings in an effort to compete in the free marketplace of medical services. This was a battle they were destined to lose, for private hospitals were actually getting stronger as a result of Medicare and Medicaid, not weaker. Huge infusions of cash accompanied the masses of elderly patients, Medicare policies in tow, who flocked from the public hospitals to the private hospitals, and even the previously small population of charity care patients who had always been treated in the private hospitals now brought with them their (modest) Medicaid vouchers rather than seeking care for free. Private hospitals responded to this bounty by investing heavily in building projects, sophisticated equipment, staffing, and ancillary services. Even as hospital philanthropy declined in these years, Medicare subsidies more than compensated for the shortfall, as hospitals repeatedly elevated the quality of their services and passed on the costs to private insurers and Medicare.[8] One result of the changing hospital landscape was severe inflation throughout the health care sector, caused by thousands of administrative decisions to purchase programs and staff which previously had been deferred. Writing of his conversations with hospital administrators throughout the country in the late 1960s, the journalist Godfrey Hodgson recorded a commonly made statement: "I have a little list of things I want to do for the hospital. When Medicare came along, I could start checking them off." More to the point was the trenchant observation of a professor of medicine at Tufts University: "Medicare has proved a better mechanism for insuring the providers than the patients."[9]

Overall, Medicaid's immediate effect on cities and city hospitals was both more and less than might have been expected. On the one hand, many welfare recipients—those who both qualified for the new program and were willing to take advantage of it—found themselves with an array of new provider options, ranging from private physicians, to private hospitals, to necessary preventive care, to a dependable source of financing nursing home care for aging parents. At the same time, city boards, mayors, and hospital advisory bodies recognized the potential magnitude of the changes being brought about by Medicaid, and they gathered themselves into specialized planning entities to chart out new directions for municipal health services in the new health care world.[10] Yet both the opportunities available to the poor and the plans drafted by the visionaries fell short of the promised utopia. Poor urban residents, chits in hand, sought private care only to find a dearth of private physicians and hospitals in easily accessible locales. Planning commissions insisted on cleaving to a nineteenth-century vision of the essential role of public hospitals, even while looking to "community," "coordination," and "caring" as the templates for a post-Medicaid world. The resulting mélange was an imperfect solution to the needs of impoverished city residents, a compromised result not easily rectified.

Rural Care

Even worse than the health conditions among the urban poor were those among the rural poor, particularly children. A study of infant and child health status in rural Kentucky in the mid-1960s exposed a litany of horrors, including triple the rates found in middle-class populations for ear and eye disorders, respiratory obstructions, skin afflictions, untreated epilepsy, and intestinal parasites (found in more than 50 percent of schoolchildren's stool samples in one study). Untreated rheumatism, diabetes, goiter, and congestive heart failure prevailed at almost nineteenth-century levels.[11] Dental care was nonexistent; at an early age children displayed skin ulcerations, tooth decay, open sores, boils, abscesses, impetigo, rat bites, trichinosis, and hookworm. Similarly, a report sponsored by the Field Foundation on child health in Mississippi exposed conditions which almost defied credibility. One investigator observed children's medical and nutritional conditions and described his findings thus: "In child after child we saw: evidence of vitamin and mineral deficiencies; serious, untreated skin infections and ulcerations; eye and ear diseases, also unattended bone disease secondary to poor food intake; the prevalence of bacterial and parasitic disease, as well as severe anemia . . . We saw children afflicted with chronic diarrhea, chronic sores, chronic (untreated) leg and arm injuries and deformities."[12]

As bad as medical conditions were in rural areas, social and nutritional conditions were even worse, with families living in tar-paper shacks bereft of electricity, clean water, screens, or sewage disposal. Children in such families survived on diets wholly deficient in the most minimal nutritional requirements, consisting almost entirely of starch— "grits, bread, Kool-Aid." Many of these families had not bothered to apply for food stamps, or if they had applied they had been turned down. Children subsisted on one meal a day, often provided by impoverished neighbors who had marginally more than the child's own family. "They are living under such primitive conditions," a commission reported, "that we found it hard to believe we were examining American children of the twentieth century."[13]

Such diminished health conditions begged for an explanation beyond mere poverty, and theories abounded. As far back as 1940, Earl Koos, in his classic study of rural health *The Health of Regionville*, found that attitudes toward health and medical care in a rural village in upstate New York reflected local cultural norms far more than prevailing medical or scientific knowledge. Poor residents of rural areas were even more isolated from broader social mores than poor residents of urban areas were, and this isolation exhibited itself in indifference toward adverse health symptoms and suspicion of professional health care providers. While this "cultural lag" diminished with rising income, it still persisted stubbornly in rural enclaves long after economic conditions began to improve.[14]

Expanding on Koos's theory, public health officials trying to understand rural poverty in the mid-1960s struggled to explain away the "fallacy of the empty vessels": the notion that ignorance of hygienic habits represented a void which could easily be filled with modern hygienic principles. Rather, rural residents maintained strong beliefs about health and medicine which would need to be aggressively displaced by new attitudes if their health status was to be improved.[15] This had been well demonstrated in England after the inauguration of the National Health Service in the late 1940s, when it was believed that the health of all citizens would rise with the lowering of economic barriers to health care. In fact, the educated and well-to-do showed themselves far more likely to take advantage of the free National Health clinics and resources than the poor, ignorant, and isolated.[16]

This phenomenon was among many labeled "medical alienation" by some researchers. Alienation prevented poor people from seeking the help available to them because of a general fear of, or skepticism toward, authority figures. Under the alienation theory, welfare medicine needed to do more than simply remove financial barriers to health care; it needed to remove social and emotional barriers as well. This was the thinking underlying the community health movement, and theory dictated that rural health efforts must follow similar guidelines. One study of rural counties in North Carolina showed that families which scored higher for "alienation-powerlessness" were more likely to visit a public clinic than to use public money to see a private physician, even controlling for proximity and negative experience with physicians.[17] Significantly, poor blacks in the area were even more likely than poor whites to experience the alienation effect, and to avoid medical situations which challenged their sense of comfort and safety. They favored solo practice physicians who disproportionately did not belong to the local medical society. Waiting rooms at these practices were often crowded with farmers and family members who treated the long waits as a chance to be sociable—there was "an air of companionship among those waiting their turns," the researchers observed. Payment was in cash (if at all), diagnoses were often made without the aid of available tests, and records were poorly kept. While simple proximity and pervasive Jim Crow restrictions contributed to the segregation, the alienation effect dictated that even those blacks able to travel to more competent physicians were willing to settle for a lower level of care in a more comfortable milieu.[18] The Mississippi commission agreed with this assessment even as it concluded that welfare and food programs were administered by authorities who used them "selectively, politically, and with obvious racial considerations in mind."[19]

Medicaid programs implemented in rural states in 1966 and 1967 struggled to offset these difficult challenges. Even more than states with urban poverty, states with predominantly rural poverty (particularly in Appalachia) sought to coordinate the new services provided through Medicaid funds with existing programs of public health nursing, vocational rehabilitation, crippled children's programs, mental health centers, and tuberculosis commissions. States such as West Virginia, Kentucky, the Carolinas, Tennessee, and Arkansas saw the need for community health services as acutely as their industrial counterparts did. For these states, Medicaid could not possibly supersede existing programs, since a voucher program presupposed the existence of adequate private health care providers, whether individual or institutional. Rather, Medicaid would be yet one more tool in an arsenal long aimed at alleviating the worst of rural poverty. Use of the new tool would need to be made in accordance with "health cultures," requiring (in the words of one expert on rural care) "distinguishing between the psychosocial processes of acceptance and adoption in cultural change."[20]

As a result, rural states more than urban ones concentrated on increasing medical manpower and strengthening community outreach, even as they implemented their Medicaid programs in the years immediately following the passage of Title XIX. In addition, they were more likely to try integrating community health center grants (funded through the OEO) with their nascent Medicaid programs, which were often underfunded and lacked the political commitment of programs found in the wealthier states. "If the present trend continues," a pair of analysts wrote about Virginia, "that state will have no physicians in a rural area within 15 years."[21] Some states started community clinic demonstration projects at the exact moment when the implementation of Medicaid programs might have been expected to slowly obviate the need for having the clinics at all, while others chose that moment to invest in county hospitals and rural clinics run by the state health department. Kentucky, for example, began a large program of investment in its Appalachian Regional Hospital system (a small, rural hospital system originally established by the United Mine Workers' Fund) at the exact time that many urban public hospitals were facing declining admissions due to Medicare and Medicaid.[22]

The great weakness in rural programs of regionalization, community orientation, and clinic building was the demise of the rural physician. Clinics could not coexist with private doctors, nor could public hospitals fail to undermine the admission privileges of the practitioners. The only people who expressed awareness of this trend, however, were rural practitioners themselves. The AMA, long controlled principally by urban specialists, was largely insensitive to the plight of rural doctors, and public health officials and state health planners minimized their potential roles. In aspiring to create community health centers and regional rural health authorities, these authorities effectively stymied the original intent of Medicaid. Rural doctors, overworked and underappreciated, expressed disgust and fatalism at the "ivory tower socialism" exemplified by central planning, and feared for their independence and livelihood. One irate doctor in West Texas complained, "They, the Ivory-Tower socialists, have usurped my rights, they have raped the future of my children and have compelled me to accept an involuntary course. I must specialize or be stricken from the ranks. I must submit to conglomeration or cease to exist at all. No longer will I be a person of whom one can say 'He is my doctor.' I will be a limited technician, an automaton."[23]

The problems specific to rural areas—social isolation, a medical cultural gap, and lack of medical resources—were the problems of urban ghettos writ large. As in urban areas blacks fared poorly, but unlike in urban areas they struggled alongside a sizable contingent of impoverished whites. There was a different relationship, however, between the Medicaid programs and alternate avenues for charity care. Poor rural states never conceived of the new Medicaid programs as a marquee approach to alleviating poverty, nor could they realistically view a program predicated on private sector vouchers as a meaningful replacement for charity medicine. In addition, the meager state funds available for Medicaid meant that the federal match would be low, even when adjusted for the poor-state bonus built into the legislation, and thus the programs could not be generous enough to make a substantial difference in the lives of the rural poor. While each state's Medicaid program differed slightly in its details of eligibility and benefits, most rural states comported their programs to these common needs, and sought alternate services and funds accordingly.

Medical Care for Poor Blacks

Black Americans drew special attention from health planners in the mid-1960s. Living in the shadow of slavery and nearly a hundred years of legal discrimination in the Jim Crow South, blacks exhibited rates of poverty and social dysfunction substantially higher than those of all other Americans, including recent immigrants, Hispanics, and Native Americans. Although by 1965 only 50 percent of all blacks lived in the South (down from 90 percent at the turn of the century), most found themselves nearly as socially isolated in their new urban homes as they had been in Dixie. The vast majority of blacks who had left the South over the previous forty years now lived in poor inner-city neighborhoods, generally in major metropolises. Six cities alone—New York, Chicago, Philadelphia, Detroit, Washington, and Los Angeles—harbored over a fifth of all blacks in the country, leading one social scientist to observe that such concentrations of a racial minority heightened the "visibility" of Negroes in the public policy debate while straining urban resources and services.[24]

Black Americans trailed white Americans by a wide margin in virtually every category of social achievement in 1965. Blacks over the age of fourteen claimed a median of 9.7 years of education, versus 12 for whites. (In the South the disparity was even greater: 8.1 years for blacks, 12 years for whites.) Half of black men (and one fourth of black women) had less than six years of school, compared with 9 percent and 6 percent of whites. And while only a few adults of either race had attended college, blacks again lagged alarmingly, with only 5 percent of adult black men and 9 percent of black women having spent any time in college (versus 16 percent for white men and 20 percent for white women). Even these numbers made the situation seem better than it was, as most blacks were educated in entirely or predominantly black schools (de jure in the South, de facto in the rest of the country), which usually had fewer resources and less well trained teachers. Nearly all black college students attended historically black colleges, where they studied, in disproportionate numbers, agriculture sciences, home economics, education, and nursing—all fields which led to lower-paying jobs upon graduation.[25]

Lower levels of education among blacks predictably depressed incomes and elevated poverty levels. By 1967, 13.4 percent of all Americans lived beneath the federal poverty level, but over 35 percent of black Americans did so (although this had been reduced from 55 percent ten years previous). For female-headed households the story was even worse: 28 percent of white female-led households lived below the poverty level, but over 60 percent of black female-led households did so.[26] The Social Security Administration maintained some of the best income data in the nation in the 1960s, demanding basic income and asset data of all qualified Social Security recipients (which included nearly all Americans over sixty-five). These data illustrated that disparities between whites and blacks were substantial. Over 70 percent of black men, for example, and 90 percent of black women applying for Social Security benefits in the late 1960s had a personal monthly income of under $150, while for white men and women the comparable figures were 40 percent and 75 percent. The difference was partially related to differing types of employment (blacks disproportionately worked on farms), but even for employees in similar occupations disparities remained. Among all retirees from private industry, for example, white men were more than twice as likely as black men to have private pensions, and white women were *eight* times as likely as black women to have pensions. Both black men and black women who had worked in the private industrial sector had disproportionately held low-wage, nonunion positions—custodians, cooks, gardeners—while white men had more often held unionized line positions, or else managerial positions. The few white women who had labored in industry had worked disproportionately in marketing and management, both of which typically provided pensions and other fringe benefits.[27]

High rates of poverty among blacks led directly to poor health and poor health conditions. Black babies in 1960 were far more likely than their white counterparts to have been born at home and attended to by midwives, and in the South this pattern was observable even in white and black families with the same income. In one study in Selma, Alabama, in 1963, for example, where there were almost identical numbers of white and black families living in poverty, fewer than 1 percent of white babies were born out of the hospital, compared with over 70 percent of black babies.[28] Black mothers were disproportionately denied adequate prenatal and nutritional counseling, and as a result their babies were born smaller than average, with a substantially higher incidence of respiratory disorders and mental retardation. Once born, black children failed to receive general pediatric care, immunizations, reasonable nutrition, or annual physicals at adequate rates, and they overwhelmingly lived in substandard housing, in families with substandard incomes, and in neighborhoods with high crime rates. Ultimately blacks would die younger, maintaining their proportional share of the population in the United States only through substantially higher birth rates.[29] Life in the ghetto was described by one nurse as "a life that knows crowded housing and little privacy, fetid odors, and many bugs; where the streets are filled with drifting and sometimes angry males and young mothers of many young children."[30]

One rarely mentioned corollary to poor black health was poor black scholastic performance. Public health researchers were well aware by 1967 not only that black children were falling behind in school, but that even those with the same levels of education as white children posted lower test grades and IQ scores. One study of eighth-grade schoolchildren in New York City showed black children with a mean IQ of 87.7 and white children with a mean of 100.1 (a difference of more than one standard deviation). At the same time, a study of eighteen hundred black schoolchildren in the South yielded a mean score of 80.7, which the American Association of Mental Deficiency rated as "borderline retarded." The gap was actually widening through the 1950s and 1960s, leading participants at a conference on Negro health at Howard University to identify "inferior intellectual functioning" as among the more prevalent health problems facing the black population. While part of the explanation for the differing scores no doubt lay in poorer schools, biased testing instruments, and a generally less literate culture, much of it could be attributed to poor health care. One participant at Howard noted that the disparities were not due to any genetic difference but rather to "socioeconomic and environmental deficiencies," such as inadequate housing, health care, employment, police protection, and incomes.[31]

But as much as the black condition was dictated by racism, or the legacy of slavery and racism, blacks were at least partly responsible for their own plight. Rates of social breakdown had actually increased over the previous twenty years, even as many blacks had migrated to the North, where schools and facilities could not be legally segregated and industrial jobs could be had at elevated wages (albeit not so elevated as for whites). Church attendance and college attendance had declined, while out-of-wedlock births and juvenile crime had increased. Black community leaders—ministers, physicians, teachers—were flummoxed by the growing dissolution of their communities, and to some degree they turned away from the gathering chaos. Newer immigrant groups, with incomes initially lower than those of black workers, were quickly overtaking their more established compatriots in income, education, and health status, and maintaining cleaner, safer neighborhoods with a more orderly community life. A handful of black doctors began to recognize that internal community attitudes were contributing to declining health and social order as much as societal prejudice was, and that a substantial federal program would be required to educate black Americans to the point of their being able to take advantage of Medicaid, Head Start, and other social welfare programs. A professor of medicine at Howard, Paul Cornely, warned in 1968, "Unless this is done with dispatch, our communities, particularly the urban centers, will continue to grow into black jungles of unmanageable proportions."[32]

The idea of a "black" approach to social service delivery took hold among certain physicians, public health nurses, and other medical care providers, who began to suspect that the problem of ill-health in the black community was at least partly due to a culture gap.[33] "These health problems spring from a social context with a culture that is foreign to most of us," admonished a visiting nurse from Detroit, Nancy Milio.[34] The solution was to offer medical services in a uniquely black "style" which could be both nonthreatening and comprehensible in the alien milieu, but how such a style should be developed was not readily apparent. The radical psychiatrist Leonard Lawrence wrote that a black professional trained in a predominantly white milieu had already been tainted, for he had been taught to "learn white," and indoctrinated in theory which had been developed for treating whites. "He, in effect, is asked to deny his heritage," Lawrence wrote.[35] The black studies scholar Nathan Hare suggested that under the extant system of medical education, black doctors were "whitened" during the course of their training, losing their cultural identity and their willingness to ally themselves with black nationalism.[36] And the radical black psychiatrist Price Cobbs wrote in 1968 that a black therapist could not be effective until he "begins to grapple with his own feelings about being black, ineffective, and victimized in a powerful white nation."[37] The natural solution, in the opinion of these critics, was a wholly separate track in which black professionals were trained in black environments to treat only black patients.

Although the solution to the problem was not obvious, unique (and disparate) medical cultures did exist. Blacks perceived their health differently from whites, regardless of income or education, and sought medical care at different times, for different reasons, and in different forms. One study in 1968 found that financial barriers were not significant in determining whether pregnant black women sought prenatal care. Rather, young black women failed to seek the care because in general they did not believe in its efficacy or importance in the same way as white women.[38] Their beliefs were wrong, however, as evidenced by the higher rates among blacks of prenatal complications, low birth weight, and infant mortality. The solution to this troublesome problem clearly involved education, outreach, and training, and probably the use of black social workers, nurses, and doctors to deliver the message. But what exactly the message should be, and specifically how it should be delivered, remained unknown.

Contributing to the problem was the declining number of black doctors. The majority of black physicians since the 1920s had received their medical training at one of the nation's two historically black medical colleges—Howard and Meharry. The nation's ninety-five other medical schools (the precise number fluctuated through the decades) graduated only fifteen to twenty black physicians annually. Almost all the white medical schools had preset quotas for black students, and through the 1950s one third of the schools admitted no black students at all. (The last medical schools to admit blacks did not do so until 1968.) By 1965 this dearth of training opportunities resulted in only six thousand practicing black physicians in the country, or barely 40 for every 100,000 black persons. By contrast, the ratio of white doctors to the white population at large was nearly 200 per 100,000. Black physicians constituted 2 percent of all the nation's doctors, a number grossly at odds with the nearly 12 percent of the general population made up by blacks.

In theory, this situation was supposed to be improving by 1965. Nearly all white medical schools had dropped their formal black quotas, and many had begun actively soliciting qualified black students. The results were hardly encouraging, however. Many well-intentioned medical schools quickly realized that there were not enough black undergraduates to fill substantial portions of medical school classes, and colleges in turn were having a difficult time recruiting enough qualified black high school graduates. Although many élite private colleges began actively recruiting blacks in the mid-1960s and were somewhat successful, they were unable to attract blacks in proportion to their presence in the population at large. Edward Cooper, the chairman of the talent recruitment council of the (historically black) National Medical Association, noted in a speech in 1965 that although Princeton, Harvard, and the Seven Sisters colleges were now actively recruiting blacks, the numbers were still dismal. Princeton, for example, had managed to recruit thirteen black freshmen in 1965 (compared to its previous years' two or three), but this was in an entering class of a thousand. The Seven Sisters did little better, together managing to recruit only fifty-five black students—well under 2 percent of their aggregate entering classes. "The essential problem is the shortage of Negro applicants," Cooper said. "Efforts of school people in steering toward Princeton qualified Negro applicants will be appreciated."[39]

Shortages of well-educated black students throughout the education system could hardly be rectified by aggressive recruiting at the medical school level, and indeed efforts to boost blacks to 12 percent of the medical school population by 1975 failed miserably.[40] By 1970 blacks constituted less than 6 percent of *undergraduate* students, and as their quality appeared to be declining they were becoming less competitive, on average, when they applied to medical school.[41] Black medical school applicants had posted almost a 75 percent acceptance rate in 1950, yet by 1974 that rate had declined to 57 percent. Certainly the number of black doctors was up, but it was nowhere near the goal of proportional parity. The proportion of black medical students ultimately peaked in 1975 at 7.5 percent, and thereupon declined to 6.5 percent, where it remains today. Moreover, by the 1980s the few black medical schools (whose ranks now included Morehouse and the Charles Drew Postgraduate School of Medicine) continued to train the majority of black doctors, usually in less academically competitive surroundings by less research-oriented faculty. In 1985, of the nation's 1,117 black medical students, 922 (82.5 percent) were enrolled at historically black medical colleges.[42]

The scarcity of black doctors might not have been such a problem had not a very large number of all black Americans, particularly poor black Americans, sought care from them. Racial prejudice appeared to cut both ways: white doctors frequently shunned black patients (although this was at least partly because they were poorer than whites), but black patients would also eschew white medical care. As a result, blacks in general and poor blacks in particular faced a chronic and worsening shortage of competent care providers. Exacerbating the matter were pervasive shortages in all health professions, including nurses, pharmacists, health aides, and mental health professionals. The shortage of black dentists was so acute by 1968 that Paul Cornely of Howard University Medical School described the black dentist as "a vanishing American."[43] And for many of these professions (excluding doctors), black growth in the profession was minimal or nonexistent. The number of black dentists actually declined during the 1960s, from 4 percent of all American dentists to 2 percent. At Howard University Dental School, the primary source of the nation's black dentists for decades, only 70 of 375 applicants in 1968 were black, leading to the anomalous situation of a majority-white class at a historically black professional school.

The shortage of black health care providers appeared intractable to all but the most optimistic policy planners in 1965, and only the most arrogant could credibly claim to know the answer. Money, as always, could help, but only up to a point. And another possible response, inducing white physicians and dentists to serve in poor black areas, contradicted the reality of cultural norms as well as the ideological movement toward community-based medicine. It could only be a stopgap at any rate, for white doctors would inevitably desert the community as soon as their required stint ended. The long-term goal was either more black providers or a society which had moved wholly beyond segregation in a profound and lasting manner. Few were optimistic about either alternative.

Child Health

The inability of Medicaid to provide adequate care for urban and rural citizens as well as large portions of the black community was most apparent in pediatric care. Children's health had always disproportionately drawn public empathy and political action, and by 1967 the issue once again demanded response. A fifth (14.8 million) of all children in the country lived in poverty, and thus constituted the single largest age group of all poor Americans. Children under eighteen accounted for 43 percent of all Americans living in poverty, and the percentage had been growing since Social Security had begun lifting most elderly out of the poorest category in 1935. This impoverished state was correlated with inadequate health care, which in turn produced incongruously high levels of infant mortality, neonatal medical problems, mental retardation, and chronic developmental problems. While Medicaid had begun to correct some of these health problems, many were yet unaddressed. George Silver, a professor of public health at Yale, wrote in a White House report in 1967 that all of the nation's child health programs taken together fell "far short of providing adequate health care" for poor and handicapped children, and the president of the American Academy of Pediatrics, James Hughes, stated that same year, "I think it unnecessary to review the incontrovertible evidence that large numbers of American children are receiving little or no health supervision."[44]

By 1967, two years after Medicaid was begun, only 40 percent of all childhood chronic conditions (including congenital malformations, vision and hearing problems, psychiatric problems, heart abnormalities, and asthma) were being treated in low-income areas, and only a third of handicapped children requiring help from a crippled children's program received the help that they qualified for. Dental care, as usual, was in even greater demand. Nearly 80 percent of poor children received no dental care, while the comparable rate for wealthier children was only 20 percent. Regional variations were substantial. In the South, for example, nearly 60 percent of all children, regardless of income, received no dental care in a given year, while in the Northeast the proportion was only 33.9 percent.

Initial recommendations to alleviate these problems were conservative and tentative. A program analysis group at the White House which investigated the problem in 1966 and 1967 suggested budgeting extra funds for maternal and child health centers, family planning programs, treatment of chronic conditions, research on childhood diseases, and fluoridation.[45] Such tepid actions, costing less than $100 million, would be inadequate. True improvement of child health would require a substantial investment in medical manpower, prenatal and neonatal health care, pediatric and dental clinics, nutrition programs, and Medicaid funding. The federal commitment to elderly health care in 1967, for example, totaled over $200 per person, while the figure for poor children was only $10. While the elderly in general required more health care than children did, a twenty-fold differential in spending was inconsistent with needs. That Medicaid was funded at different levels in the different states only exacerbated the isolating effects of poverty and the skewed distribution of pediatric poor care. The public health professor Lester Breslow derided the whole system in a speech in 1968 for its "bizarre fluctuation of eligibility and benefits" and "wild estimations of cost."[46]

One of the strangest (and most destructive) symptoms of poverty in the world's wealthiest country was the continued existence of pockets of malnutrition, particularly among children. In addition to the usual listlessness and enervation associated with starvation, malnutrition in infants and young children depleted red blood cell counts, compromised the body's immune system, and caused irreparable harm to the central nervous system.[47] Various studies of malnourished infants conducted at the time pointed to long-term diminution of learning capacity, retarded problem-solving ability, and maladapted interpersonal skills.[48] Yet despite the availability of various federal and state programs, including WIC, AFDC, and Supplemental Security Income (SSI), many poor families were simply unable to purchase adequate amounts of food. By 1967 over 60 percent of poor families were undernourished, and were spending less than $4 per person per week for food—$1.25 less than the cost of the USDA low-cost food plan for the South. In fact, over three fourths of the 27 million Americans living in poverty were not receiving federal food program benefits in 1968, and anywhere from two to four million of those disqualified from receiving food aid were children. Furthermore, of the five million needy children under the age of six, fewer than one million were receiving food aid through Head Start or day care centers.[49]

Further exacerbating the problems of infant and pediatric health in 1967 was that many patients with *private* insurance found adequate prenatal and postnatal care beyond their means. As most indemnity insurance plans were geared toward acute-care hospital stays, they reimbursed incompletely for preventive outpatient care, including prenatal checkups. (Women enrolled in prepaid group plans tended to have more comprehensive prenatal coverage in the 1960s, but they were in the minority.) Consequently, privately insured patients found that only 63 percent of their pregnancy-related expenses were covered. Wealthy women paid the balance out of pocket to purchase comprehensive prenatal care, but working-class women found the costs difficult or impossible to incur and yet were ineligible for Medicaid. Undertreatment of pregnant women threatened the future health of their infants because of exposure to environmental pollution, inadequate prenatal nutrition, alcohol use, untreated high blood pressure and diabetes, and treatable contagious diseases such as German measles and syphilis.

Kiddycare

The persistence of pediatric malnutrition, along with the flaws in Medicaid and other charity health care programs aimed at children, induced the Johnson administration to begin planning a new and substantial program of poor care in 1967. Labeled the Child Health Insurance Program (CHIP, or colloquially "Kiddycare"), the program aimed to provide comprehensive care for every pregnant women and newborn infant in the country, regardless of eligibility status for existing poor care programs. It would cover all physician and diagnostic services, pharmaceuticals, laboratory expenses, and counseling (in addition to hospital stays) related to pregnancy, birth, and infancy for over 95 percent of the nation's births, with no deductible, and have a "capitation" provision for obstetric care to minimize costs. The remaining 5 percent could potentially be covered by an increased state buy-in to the existing Medicaid program that would cover the medically indigent. The program was to be financed by an increase of 0.7 percent in the Social Security payroll tax rate.[50]

Alongside the CHIP program, White House staff also developed a health manpower program in 1967 to begin alleviating the chronic shortage of physicians, dentists, nurses, pharmacists, and mental health counselors. Intended to increase the number of health workers trained annually by almost 100,000, the program aimed to exploit programs already in place such as the Job Corps, the Neighborhood Youth Corps, the Adult Work Training program, and the Professions Educational Assistance and Nurse Training Acts. In addition, inactive nurses and other retired or semiretired health professionals could be resuscitated through "refresher" training programs, while six thousand unemployed workers could be trained as home health aides and nurse's assistants through the OEO.[51]

While the health manpower proposal met with near unanimous approval, Kiddycare did not. The plan took the United States a step closer to the national insurance program so feared by organized medicine, political conservatives, and much of the American electorate. Moreover, evidence suggested that alternative approaches to prenatal and postnatal medical care could be equally effective while being substantially less disruptive. The White House budget director Charles Schultze, for example, argued adamantly against the program, noting that the additional payroll tax would bring federal payroll taxes to 11.8 percent by the mid-1970s: a growing (and possibly intolerable) burden on the American taxpayer. Also, many Americans would oppose a putative "social insurance" program from which they could never benefit once they were past childbearing years (making the program, in effect, an entitlement program). Medicare and Social Security, by contrast, were popular insofar as nearly everyone who paid in ultimately drew out, often much more than the value of the initial contribution.[52]

The more immediate argument against Kiddycare, however, was that it was just not necessary. Elevated rates of infant mortality in the United States, the most widely available indicator of inadequate prenatal and pediatric care, did not stem from general lack of care but rather from isolated care gaps. Infant mortality was largely a problem of poor, nonwhite mothers, particularly those still in their teens or having more than three children. Most of the cases were confined to 2 percent of all the counties in the United States, and if the infant mortality rate in these counties could be reduced to 18 per 1,000 live births, the nation's infant mortality rate would be within acceptable limits. Moreover, of the four million pregnant women who would be covered by the proposed program in any given year, three million were already receiving adequate prenatal care—the nation, in Schultze's words, would be "spending $3 on those who don't need help to get $1 to those who do."[53] The situation thus called for a sharply targeted program rather than a general program covering all mothers.

A more cost-effective approach to the problem, it was argued, would be to expand the growing fleet of Neighborhood Health Centers (sponsored by the OEO) and Maternal and Infant Care Centers (sponsored by HEW), and turn funding responsibility over to Medicaid. A concurrent increase in the federal match to all states would help as well. Last, investment in pediatric and obstetric training programs with loan forgiveness for young physicians who chose these professions could further reduce infant mortality. Ultimately, the law of supply and demand must prevail, and newly minted obstetricians, frozen out of attractive suburban locales, would be forced to establish offices in poorer urban neighborhoods and rural areas. All this together would cost less than a fifth of CHIP.

The program as ultimately proposed, the Child Health Act of 1968, followed a modified CHIP proposal, with federal investment in Medicaid to be used for up to 75 percent of Title V (maternal and child health) provisions. With yearly budget increases of up to $400 million by 1974, the program would cover 75 percent of the costs, while requiring of the states that they target populations of impoverished mothers, children, and pregnant women while continuing to maintain their own programs in those areas. (Planners feared that state agencies would use federal funds to replace state funds for the same programs.) In addition, the program would increase funding for Head Start, mental retardation clinics, crippled children's programs, manpower training, physical fitness, and research. Implicit in the proposal was the understanding that the bounds of clinical understanding were no longer the primary limitations on medical care. President Johnson told the Congress, "Success in a laboratory, however brilliant, is not complete if barriers of poverty, ignorance or prejudice block it from reaching the man who needs it, or the child who wastes away without it."[54] CHIP was meant to overcome these barriers.

"Hard-to-reach" groups presented themselves to health planners in the late 1960s as proof that increasing access to health services required more than just money. Although each presented unique challenges, inner-city dwellers, the rural poor, black Americans, and children all defied the ability of Medicaid to place impoverished citizens at the doors of physicians' offices and hospitals. Part of the problem was one of physical proximity—the first two groups dwelled disproportionately in areas in which private doctors' offices and private hospitals did not exist in adequate numbers to serve the populations, and blacks frequently felt uncomfortable, or were made to feel uncomfortable, in getting care outside the scarce black physicians' practices. Children of these groups faced the same problems of dislocation, but even more so given the paucity of competent pediatric care.

Perhaps even more vexing were the cultural barriers which seemed to prevent members of these groups from gaining access to care. Whether through suspicion of, ignorance of, or simple indifference to modern scientific medicine, members of these groups felt uncomfortable walking into private physicians' offices and private hospitals to obtain care, even when money was no longer the principal barrier. A combination of education and community-based health centers seemed to be a partial answer, but planners disagreed about the ultimate solution. A quick fix was unavailable in the late 1960s, although for some time to come both the federal and state governments would tinker with programs designed to ameliorate the problem.

5

Redefining Health

Redefining Health and Planning for Change

The late 1960s were characterized by ever-expanding definitions of health and health care, placing increased burdens on charity care programs to deliver more comprehensive services. Departing from the narrow, pathogenic model of disease which had prevailed since the late nineteenth century, the World Health Organization (WHO) had presented its own definition of health earlier in the decade: "the state of complete physical, mental and social well-being, and not merely the absence of disease or infirmity."[1] In the course of a few years, this expansive definition became the norm for health planners and reform-minded doctors. One physician, L. J. Duhl, wrote in 1969 that health was a "state of competence—of emotional, mental and physical strength enabling [man] to set goals, investigate alternatives, make decisions and instigate action to control his environment,"[2] while another, Herbert Abrams, wrote in the following year: "We have been disease-oriented and health-disoriented."[3] Liberal politicians cleaved to the new vision as well, with U.S. Senator Edmund Muskie (D., Me.) advising government health planners to "treat the whole society" rather than merely the illness,[4] and the health commissioner of New York City, George James, concluding in 1965 that poverty was "the third leading cause of death in New York City."[5]

In appealing to social malaise as the province of health care providers, health care critics were harkening back to a vision of medical care which predated the disease model by several centuries. The eminent pathologist Rudolf Virchow had concluded in 1848 that physicians were "the natural attorneys for the poor, and social problems fall to a large extent within their jurisdiction," and modern critics resurrected this view.[6] Herbert Abrams, for example, professor in the department of community medicine at the University of Arizona, began to look beyond the standard environmental toxins afflicting the poor, and added unemployment, underemployment, poor housing, excessive accident hazards, and demoralization to the mix. In this sense, poverty itself entered the accepted purview of the physician, and political activism became a tool of medicine on a par with antibiotics, surgery, and vaccinations. "Slums cannot be eliminated," wrote the public health officer Elliot Segal in 1968. "They are a public health problem in the same sense as polio or venereal disease. They can at best be controlled—but with strong preventive measures."[7]

Closely associated with this expanded view of health was a vision of health care as a right rather than a commodity. Physicians, political leaders, and social scientists began to promulgate this rights-based ideal in the late 1960s, despite logistical barriers to its realization. "Medical care in the form of personal health services is now accepted as a universal civic right rather than a private luxury or a philanthropic gesture," wrote Kerr White, a professor of medicine at Johns Hopkins, in 1966.[8] Two physicians from Brooklyn, Seymour Glick and Gerald Thomson, wrote a few years later, "Regrettably, the practical application of the right to health care has lagged behind that of the right to free education and other 'rights,'"[9] and President Johnson himself declared in a speech: "Good health services are the right of every citizen, not the privilege of a few."[10]

Such rights-based talk was illusory and self-defeating, however. Physicians fiercely defended their professional autonomy and were loath to redefine themselves as public servants, while states were reluctant to offer the full judicial protections accorded to more traditional civil rights. At least one skeptical physician in Cleveland held his ground in the midst of the rights movement, whose spokesmen he derided as naïve and fatuous. "It appears that someone has coined a catchy phrase," wrote Peter Poulos Jr. in 1970, "that now, by virtue of its being repeated over and over again, has assumed somewhat of a Sacred Cow position and because it is repeated so many times, it is being held as being a basic truth."[11]

Accompanying the expanding definition of health was an expanding vision of public health. "Sanitary engineering," as the profession was known through the nineteenth century, had its roots in the control of infectious disease, originally in the closely packed neighborhoods of immigrant slums, and later in the parasite-ridden fields of rural America. Even before Koch and Pasteur promulgated their pathogenic theories of disease in the late nineteenth century, public health officials understood that a clean-smelling city was for the most part a healthy city, and thus targeted their early efforts at removing standing water and other sources of miasma. The first sanitarians applied their expertise in antebellum American cities by safeguarding drinking water, grading streets, constructing sewers, and removing offal, manure, and decaying animals from public places. Later efforts aimed to elevate the quality of food by inspecting restaurants, taverns, dairies, and butchers, while early-twentieth-century efforts included eradicating parasites in the rural South and aggressively treating venereal disease. Throughout, public health officials posted quarantines, closed ports when epidemic disease threatened, and monitored natality and mortality statistics.[12]

The accomplishments of public health efforts were (and continue to be) profound. Modern public health efforts raised life expectancy in the United States by nearly 50 percent in the first half of the twentieth century, from 45 years to 65—an accomplishment unparalleled in the history of medicine. By contrast, the entire antibiotic and technological revolution in medicine since the Second World War has added only an additional decade to the lives of most Americans. The single factor most responsible today for the discrepancy in lifespan between nonindustrialized nations (where life expectancy hovers around 35 years) and industrialized nations like the United States (where it is 70 to 80 years) is not the existence of a modern health care system but of a basic public health infrastructure. Thus the major efforts by the United Nations and the World Health Organization to dig latrines, eradicate malaria and schistosomiasis, monitor food supplies, and offer hygiene education to pregnant women—the payoffs from such efforts are potentially grander than those promised by modern hospitals or specialty-trained physicians.

By 1960, however, public health was facing a professional crisis. Infectious disease, the bailiwick of the public health establishment, had ceased to be a major concern for most Americans. This was due in part to the successes of public health campaigns throughout the previous hundred years in controlling water-borne bacteria, in part to aggressive immunization programs which had brought many childhood diseases under control, and in part to the advent of effective antibiotics. Together these developments stripped the profession of the role it had filled since its inception, and created for it the need to either redefine itself or wither into obsolescence. The profession chose survival, and deemed the mitigation of social ills (and environmental hazards) its next goal. Across the nation in the 1960s, public health agencies established divisions which focused on domestic violence, child neglect, drug abuse, teenage pregnancy, and accidents. Criminal violence itself came to be considered a health problem (rather than a law enforcement problem), and alcoholism was redefined as a disease rather than a vice. The shift comported nicely with the expanding political definition of health, and brought public health officers into the midst of health planning, the organization of community clinics, and manpower training.

By 1966 scholars from many disciplines were publishing overtly political pleas for health reform. The water resource specialist Dwight Metzler, for example, wrote in the public health flagship organ, the *American Journal of Public Health*, that he was "outraged" at the five thousand maternal deaths due annually to botched abortions, and called for community "sparkplugs" to ignite civic activism and combat child abuse and inadequate health care.[13] The public health social worker Celia Deschin issued a call for recognizing the "interrelatedness of medical and social problems."[14] Similarly, Vice President Hubert Humphrey enumerated environmental change as one of the prongs of attack in health reform, writing passionately in 1968: "The urban poor live in surroundings where smog hangs heavy, where refuse collects in the streets, where rats run, where plumbing fails."[15] The equation was simple: public health must turn its attention from polio and typhus to poverty and the dissolution of communities. The problems weren't new—social workers had been addressing them for over half a century—but their recategorization as medical and public health challenges was.

Perhaps the most eloquent and influential spokesman for this revised vision of public health was Milton Terris, professor of preventive medicine at New York Medical College and longtime advocate for more community-based delivery of medical care. Terris argued ardently for the same goals as many other public health progressives—more neighborhood clinics, more prenatal care for the poor, better school immunization programs—but in addition he argued for government-sponsored smoking cessation and alcohol treatment programs, as well as better public housing and food programs. This approach was new, insofar as it sought to blur the traditional boundaries between social work and medicine. Whereas previous generations of sanitary engineers had viewed the pathogen as their nemesis and the population as merely the vector, Terris declared that all public health problems were social, and that ignoring this fact was an "evasion" of public health's responsibility.[16]

This new vision of health, health care, and public health, incorporating such diverse services and concerns as hospital care, neighborhood clinics, mental hygiene counseling, health education, public housing, consumer advocacy, food aid, and child care, required comprehensive planning to coordinate the myriad government and nonprofit agencies which would provide the necessary services. Congress responded with the Comprehensive Health Planning and Public Health Service Act of 1966 (P.L. 89-749), which distributed federal grants to state health planning agencies to coordinate manpower training programs, facilitate the construction of hospitals and clinics, and subsidize clinical public health services and school nurses. Like many service-oriented federal efforts, the program required each state to establish a health planning agency (which all did by 1967) and apply for funds which would be distributed based on state population and per capita income.

For health planners, the planning act was a welcome step on the path toward a federally coordinated, nationwide health system. Envisioning a sort of health improvement crusade, James Cavanaugh, special assistant to the U.S. surgeon general, wrote in 1967 that the nation must "marshal a wide array of health resources," including clinicians, public health engineers, and social service providers.[17] The surgeon general himself called for a "breakdown" of restrictive barriers between federal and local agencies in an effort to reorient the whole health planning axis within the health system.[18] The new law, in the view of the surgeon general, would be a "point of interlock" between programs in social welfare, urban and regional planning, and a "host of other health and health-related enterprises."[19]

The health planning act was more problematic than it appeared, however, for although good planning in general could hardly be disputed as an asset to effective government, it presupposed that government had any legitimate role in the range of health services for which it proposed to plan. The pro-planning group assumed that market-driven health care was simply no longer a viable, or at least not an ethical, option for distributing the nation's medical resources, yet well over 90 percent of all health care continued to be delivered in the private sector by 1967. Even Medicare and Medicaid did not fundamentally alter this picture, for while both programs committed greater governmental resources toward paying for medical care, neither would have any effect on *providing* medical care. Paradoxically, Medicaid was actually undermining the influence of government in the provision of medical care by giving the nation's poor patients access to private-sector physicians and hospitals which had hitherto been denied to them. Planners in favor of a more centralized model of health services delivery often played down the extent of capital investments in private hospitals, private health insurers, private physician offices, private pharmaceutical manufacturers, and private psychiatric clinics, which could only be expropriated by unprecedented governmental fiat. In the previous century only one large industrial nation, the United Kingdom, had effectively nationalized an existing private health system, and that nation was politically incomparable to the United States because of its uniquely powerful labor party. All other industrialized nations had incorporated state payment programs while maintaining the private provision of medical care, and had legislated binding planning programs into effect with differential success.

Somewhat at odds with federal and state planning efforts in the late 1960s was the continued emphasis on increasing medical manpower. Nearly all participants in the health care system, from clinicians to public health officers to health planners, agreed that medical personnel shortages were exacerbating flaws in Medicaid and preventing the effective delivery of medical care where it was needed. In November 1967 the National Advisory Commission on Health Manpower recommended that more government funding for training be provided in the near future—

enough to rectify the shortfall in the system estimated at 500,000 persons by the surgeon general, William Stewart.[20] Arguing against increasing available manpower, however, was the threat of health care inflation. Planners had noticed by the late 1960s that health care resources created their own demand, and that a greater number of doctors and hospital beds increased the total demand placed on the system. Centralized health planning exacerbated this spiral of demand, as prices could not be allowed to rise to an efficient level. The White House manpower commission appreciated this conundrum when it recommended that the president utilize any additional manpower in ways "to introduce economic incentives" for greater efficiency.[21] If current inflation rates continued unabated from 1967 to 1975, health care costs were projected to increase by 140 percent and hospital costs by 250 percent, as opposed to a predicted increase in the general cost of living of little more than 20 percent. Extra workers would only add to the bill, which was becoming increasingly unwieldy for cash-strapped state governments.

Community Health

The trend toward an expanding definition of health, coupled with a movement toward centralized health planning, produced the community health centers movement, which grew out of funding measures created in the Economic Opportunity Act of 1964. While the act had allowed for the creation of new avenues for providing health care, it was not until 1967 (after a report of the National Commission on Community Health Services) that the federal government began to make a substantial commitment to the program.[22] Starting with a handful of demonstration projects funded by the Office of Economic Opportunity (OEO), the U.S. Department of Health, Education and Welfare (HEW), various medical schools and municipalities, and private funding agencies, the program was scheduled to grow to eight hundred functioning health centers by 1975. While the number never reached even half that goal, a substantial number were built between 1965 and 1975.

The concept of community health centers merged smoothly with the social welfare optimism of the 1960s, as well as with the aspirations of reformers for both community empowerment and comprehensive planning. The centers would house the practices of primary-care physicians, pharmacies, laboratories, and facilities for nursing, outpatient surgery, and limited mental health services, bringing the whole panoply of primary-care health services within close proximity of all eligible patients in a given catchment area. These services could be closely coordinated by in-house administrators and case managers, ensuring that redundancy and service gaps were eliminated, and that unsophisticated poor patients would not be overwhelmed by the complexity of the health system as they sought care for their maladies. The National Commission on Community Health Services noted that under the present charity care system, patients stood a "good chance of getting lost in the maze," and recommended neighborhood health centers as the ideal remedy. Simple physical proximity to the target population increased the chance that the centers would provide care to any one patient, and their comprehensiveness brought the promise of better care for less sophisticated patients who were incapable of negotiating the system on their own behalf.[23]

More accessible and better-coordinated clinical services were only part of the allure of community health centers. The centers would also invite community participation by requiring that community leaders serve on their advisory boards, and would help train local residents in useful skills by hiring them for appropriate jobs and then training them adequately. Lisbeth Bamberger Schorr, a program development officer for OEO, noted that the centers' attributes included "intensive participation by and involvement of the population to be served."[24] Such participation could potentially empower communities to solve their own problems by using approaches best suited to the unique needs of each—approaches presumably unknown to outside professional managers, planners, and scholars.

Public health advocates too liked community centers for their melding of preventive medicine, clinical care, and hygiene education. Long the holy grail of public health leaders, the merging of medicine and prevention was seen by many as the inevitable end to which all health sciences would gravitate. Progressive-minded physicians, public health officers, nurses, mental health workers, and health educators all saw the community health centers as a reasonable vehicle not only for delivering charity care to poor areas but also for rejuvenating a lost vision of medicine. The sentiment was well captured by William Stewart (then assistant secretary for health and medical affairs at HEW), who wrote in 1963: "From the 1880s onward, the public health movement always included rebels: men and women ready to strike out with new approaches to the roots of evil; crusaders who never lost faith that the movement possessed the breadth of vision, as well as the spirit and competence to meet the health needs of a growing and changing society."[25]

A third allure of the centers was their promised ability to demonstrate the viability of a new means of health care delivery. Reformers who dreamed of a nationalized health care system, or at least state-provided insurance (as existed in Canada), saw in the health centers a battle-front on which to confront the reigning wisdom of health care delivery. Some 20 percent of the American population had no health insurance in 1967, beyond those covered only through government programs such as Medicare, Medicaid, and veterans' benefits. Given the slowing of growth in private sector coverage, many planners believed that this 20 percent represented a hard-core group of uninsurables—self-employed people, above the poverty line, whose incomes were inadequate to purchase private policies. Their ranks might decrease a bit over the next decade through growth in the private insurance industry, but there must come a time when all who could qualify for private insurance and afford to buy it would have done so. The remaining population would be vulnerable to catastrophic medical events—accidents, cancer, surgery—which could quickly produce billings high enough to bankrupt a family.

Community health centers represented a non-market-based response to the challenge of the uninsured. In the community health center model, clinicians, planners, and social workers could all work to promote the health of the entire community, rather than of only those patients who could afford their services. Some advocates of the centers, the historian Alice Sardell notes, hoped that they would "stimulate the reorganization of the entire health care system."[26]

Community health centers received their first large infusion of funds from the Community Action Program established by the Economic Opportunity Act of 1964. The program made grant money available to community groups willing to establish centers based on certain service criteria, including basic primary medical care, diagnostic and laboratory services, referrals, and case management. The first program grant was awarded to the Columbia Point Health Center in Boston, established by Jack Geiger of Tufts Medical School. A half-dozen more followed within the year, and by 1966 the program was expanded at the behest of Senator Edward Kennedy (D., Mass.), with a new Office of Health Affairs established within the OEO. In 1968 the Public Health Service initiated its own grants program for health centers (tied to the health planning act of 1966), which evolved into the Community Health Service within HEW by 1970. Centers could tap into money from either of these programs, or by qualifying for Medicaid and Medicare reimbursement, as well as by attracting private grants and funding from local government. In theory, privately insured patients (as well as self-pays) could use the resources of the centers too, but this rarely happened. By 1968 fifty centers were in existence, and by 1971 the number topped a hundred, with funding streams guaranteed through 1975.[27]

Not surprisingly, organized medicine opposed the centers as one more incursion into their own professional control of the health system. Grappling with the substantial shift in the government's role in health care brought on by the passage of Medicare and Medicaid, physicians were intolerant of yet more experiments in government delivery of, or payment for, medical care. Medicaid and Medicare had been carefully negotiated so as to allow the profession to retain maximum control over clinical decision making as well as the central institutions of medical care delivery—hospitals, clinics, and medical schools. By contrast, the community health centers seemed designed to achieve just the opposite effect. The program was small at first, and it brought care to patients living in neighborhoods and areas where few private physicians practiced, and thus attracted little attention within the American Medical Association (AMA) and its state affiliates. But those doctors who were aware of the nascent program would attack it. One doctor in Denver dismissed the local community health center as "just another step toward socialism," and the AMA's president stated his opposition to the "doling out of tax funds to the wealthy and the well-to-do," which he saw as a danger because the community health centers typically lacked formal guidelines for means testing.[28] Medicaid, after all, was already providing the neediest with adequate care.

The community health centers which dotted the nation by 1970 came in a vast array of sizes and shapes. Serving anywhere from a thousand to fifteen thousand patients a year, the centers were located in church basements, converted movie theaters, storefronts, superfluous hospital wards, free-standing clinic buildings, deserted YWCAS, and old farmhouses. Centers had been founded under the auspices of a great number of institutions, including religious groups, community groups, local hospitals, local governments, progressive physician organizations, and visiting nurse associations. In Newark students at the Medical College of New Jersey founded a center to provide charity care as well as to increase training opportunities for themselves, while Montefiore Hospital in the Bronx chartered a center as part of its commitment to community outreach. The Denver Health Department founded two centers explicitly aimed at increasing access to pediatric care for poor families, while in Chicago half a dozen churches and community organizations founded free clinics targeting specific ethnic groups such as blacks, Mexicans, and Puerto Ricans. Funding for these efforts was drawn from a variety of resources; all drew on the OEO grants and the HEW program, but most benefited as well from local government support, private philanthropy, and existing charitable groups.

Virtually all the centers shared a commitment to social justice beyond the mere delivery of charity health care. To this end, they saw themselves as diverse hybrids that functioned as youth centers, offered jobs and job training, facilitated community action, and advocated for better housing and racial justice. In Lubbock, Texas, the local community health center organized a program among its teenaged patients to build garbage-can racks out of lumber salvaged from condemned houses, then sell the racks for the benefit of the center.[29] Likewise, in Denver the center initiated an intensive training program for local residents to qualify them as health aides, nursing assistants, medical records keepers and neighborhood aides.[30]

Such social activism, laudable as its goals were, created inevitable confrontations between those who strove for professional excellence and those for whom that was subordinate to social inclusion. Ghetto residents generally lacked not only formal education but also the basic habits of living that correlated with success. Administrators of training programs were torn between a natural inclination to recruit the most qualified applicants to their programs and a more altruistic inclination to recruit those who most needed the job, and often they opted for those with better qualifications. At the same time, community activists and leaders, who sometimes valued the community-building goals of the centers more highly than they did the clinical goals, tended toward inclusiveness. The tension erupted into confrontation in at least one community center, when black and Puerto Rican leaders demanded that the Montefiore center hold minority applicants to a lower, "compensatory" standard of achievement—to rectify past discrimination and prejudice—and organized a strike. Montefiore officials held firm, and the strike was concluded peacefully.[31]

Community health centers enjoyed mixed success in their early years. On the one hand, patients who used them saw physicians more frequently than they had done before the centers were established, and as a result they received better preventive care.[32] On the other hand, staff turnover was high (as much as 30 percent a year at some centers), and qualified administrators scarce. But the greatest barrier to the centers' success was the sheer magnitude of the challenges, and the dearth of adequate funding for the project. By 1970 there were about a hundred centers funded by OEO, with a median patient population of eight thousand. HEW estimated, however, that the nation would need eight hundred such centers, each serving thirty thousand patients, for the program to meet the needs of the population. This was unrealistic given the level of federal commitment to the program: annual funding for OEO had been increased in 1968 to $57 million (which was matched by approximately $150 million from local government and outside sources), but the required funding for eight hundred centers would top $800 million. A White House task force recommended in 1968 that a federal commitment of $200 million be made to the program by 1975 (to be matched by $600 million in outside funds), but the funding was ultimately held near the 1968 level. In many ways the program never grew beyond the demonstration stage.[33]

Community Mental Health Centers

Mental health centers grew up in parallel with the community health centers after passage of the Community Mental Health Centers (CMHC)

Act of 1963. Similarly modeled on a more politically progressive conception of health care delivery, the centers were designed to offer a full range of therapies, from outpatient to inpatient to education and outreach, all within the home community of the afflicted. Staffing funds were continued by legislation in 1965, and then twice again over the next half-dozen years. By 1969 there were 330 centers throughout the nation, and by 1980 more than 600.[34]

Optimism for the CMHCs ran high in the early years, as hopeful psychiatrists looked to the new institutions to facilitate re-entry into normal living for long-term psychiatric patients. While the movement never inspired the same degree of idealistic rhetoric that the community health centers did, it attracted its own brand of loyalists. "Young Turks" in the American Psychiatric Association looked to the centers to reorient the power dynamic in the psychiatric relationship, and social workers saw in the centers a renewed endorsement of their own role in mental health care.[35] One rural physician from Harlan, Kentucky, wrote of the suicide of an elderly patient the previous year—a man whom the physician had recently given a clean bill of health and sent home—and the hope which a CMHC could now offer to such patients: "On Christmas day in a tar-paper shack in an abandoned coal camp he blew out his brains with a shotgun," the doctor wrote. "Now we have a new comprehensive mental health center. They have tax money, trained psychologists, and an ongoing suicide prevention program. I am appreciative."[36]

The CMHCs, like the community health centers, had mixed success. Psychiatrists soon realized that the patients seeking treatment in the centers were not the same ones recently discharged from the state hospitals. Those patients had often been assigned Medicaid funds and been placed in long-term care facilities, essentially displacing the old state hospitals not with CMHCs but with nursing homes. Patients seeking care in the centers were more likely to be outpatients—the "worried well" in the parlance of the day—rather than the seriously ill psychotics whom the centers were designed to serve. The most severely ill patients often lacked the strong community ties which the centers' designers assumed existed—either the patients' families had long ago broken off relations with them, or they had never had those ties in the first place. Discharged from what were often the only homes they had ever known as adults, these former inpatients began a cycle of admission and discharge, often living on streets or in shelters, infrequently medicated properly, and sometimes becoming part of a growing homeless population. States pursued community mental health care in the hope that it could offer more promising results than long-term custodial care, but also because of the lure of federal financing though Medicaid. One cynical journalist in Denver wrote of the program: "The best psychiatric therapy we know is watching full-grown, degree-laden doctors fight like children over who gets to splash in the river of tax money Washington sluices this way for the greater glory of mental health."[37]

Besides the naïveté underlying CMHCs, the program fell short of its goals for two familiar reasons: inadequate political commitment and a failure to adequately coordinate the centers with private mental health care. In theory each CMHC was supposed to draw from a catchment area of approximately 100,000 people, thus requiring a total of some 2,000 centers to adequately serve the country. As late as 1969 this number was still being projected as a reasonable goal for the program, and planners continued to push for funding to maintain a large-scale building program. But by that year, when only 330 centers had been built, support for continued construction was waning in both the state legislatures and Congress. The states, which were required to fund half the cost of the centers, were unwilling to devote such substantial funds to a project which many legislators and mental health professionals continued to regard as experimental, while Congress, particularly under the leadership of the Nixon administration after 1969, saw its role as that of start-up rather than long-term benefactor. Nixon's secretary of HEW, Caspar Weinberger, suggested that the initial intent of the federal program had been to provide "demonstration grants," and that these had now effectively concluded. Nixon reduced funding for the centers in 1973, and their number remained at just over six hundred.[38]

The relationship of the centers with private psychiatry was also problematic. Since no means test limited use of the centers, middle-class patients, hitherto unable to afford private psychiatric care, suddenly found it within reach and flocked to them to receive subsidized care. Yet the neediest (and poorest) patients frequently lacked the fortitude, or mental health, required to obtain services, and often wound up undertreated and undermedicated. Private psychiatrists thus viewed the centers with mixed emotions. In theory, the centers supplemented their own private services, but in reality they acted as stealth competitors. Lacking commitment from the most powerful mental health professional group, the centers lost a potentially powerful ally in lobbying for legislation.

Community health, for both mental and physical ailments, never quite surpassed the political rhetoric and idealism which surrounded its conception. The community health centers movement remained a child of social activists, anti-authoritarians, and national health aspirants, while community mental health centers lost the natural advocacy of state mental health bureaucrats (who remained loyal to the large state psychiatric hospitals), private psychiatrists, and other mental health professionals. The true natural constituency of both types of centers, beyond the patients they served and a few community leaders, was social workers, who saw their own currency rise with the new demands for case management, counseling, and assisted living which both types of centers created. Social workers had never held particularly strong or influential positions within the health or mental health systems, however, and their professional commitment and advocacy for the centers was only a middling asset. Only the federal government had the money and power to fundamentally change delivery of poor care, and the government was showing itself a fickle partner in both enterprises.

6

Charity Care and Comprehensive
Reform under Nixon

Charity Care in 1969: A Snapshot

By 1969 the Medicaid program was posting a mixed record of success and failure. Vital health statistics in general were improving. Maternal mortality had fallen from 68 deaths per 100,000 in 1953 to only 28 per 100,000, and life expectancy had increased from 67 years to 73.5 years during this same period. These improvements were in part due to the increased accessibility of medicine to the poor. The improvements were not to be celebrated, however, as according to both measures the United States only ranked about tenth worldwide, with lack of adequate maternal and prenatal care the chief culprit. Infant mortality, for example, the single best indicator of the availability of preventive care (particularly prenatal care) to the widest spectrum of people, was 22 deaths per 100,000 births in the United States, almost double the rates of top-ranked Norway and Sweden.[1]

Medicaid was helping poor people to gain access to medical care, but the quality of the care was hardly comparable to the care purchased by non-Medicaid patients. The most basic criterion for competent medical care—access to a private physician—showed markedly different rates between the two populations, with only 23 percent of Medicaid patients using a private physician in 1969, as opposed to 85 percent of non-Medicaid patients. At the same time, 19 percent of Medicaid patients recorded using a hospital outpatient clinic or emergency room for basic medical care that year, as opposed to 1 percent of non-Medicaid patients.

And oddly, these numbers were actually getting worse. While the drop in use of private physicians probably reflected a growing use of community clinics and community health centers, it nonetheless demonstrated the persistent gap between how poor people and the rest of the population obtained their medical care.[2] More encouraging were the rising rates of childhood immunization under Medicaid. In 1967, for example, 81 percent of pediatric Medicaid patients reported having received a DTP (diphtheria-tetanus-pertussis) shot, while in 1969 the number had risen to 93 percent. Immunization rates for smallpox, polio, and measles for Medicaid patients had all risen as well.[3] Rising rates of immunizations were good for the public's health, and the fact that the non-Medicaid population showed only nominal increases in immunization rates during these years, or actual declines, suggested that the various Medicaid programs could claim credit for this public health advance.

Not all clinical advances were necessarily good. Medi-Cal, the giant California Medicaid program, was helping poor people to afford hospital stays, and they were staying in the hospitals more frequently, and for longer periods. Between 1968 and 1970 the annual rate of admissions per 1,000 Medi-Cal patients rose from 217 to 246, while the rate for non-Medi-Cal patients remained static. By contrast, Medicare patients, also newly benefiting from a hospital payment program, increased their hospital admission rate by only 10 per 1,000.[4] In part this was because Medicaid patients, being poorer, often arrived at physicians' offices when their illness was at a more advanced state, and thus required hospitalization more frequently. But most health researchers concluded that poor people were simply displaying signs of the "tragedy of the commons"— overusing a free resource. If this was so, even greater government control and regulation of health resources would be needed in administering the Medicaid program. This scenario had not been foreseen when the program was designed.

Cost Overruns and Bureaucratic Inefficiencies

Beyond the clinical shortcomings of the new Medicaid programs, the most serious threats to their survival were the cost overruns which began almost immediately after states implemented them. Cost overruns were partly due to general medical inflation, which had tripled hospital fees and doubled physician fees since 1957, as well as doubling the share of the nation's GDP committed to health care (from 3.5 percent to 7 percent).[5] Most of the rise in medical spending could be attributed to growth in private insurance coverage and to the inflationary pressures of Medicare. Improved technology, more highly specialized clinical training, and greater budget allocations for basic research also added to the growing burden. In a sense, the growth in Medicaid spending was simply consistent with the growth in all health spending during these years.

But Medicaid faced the problem of public accountability which private insurers did not. If Blue Cross or Aetna needed to increase its premiums, it simply did so and passed the cost onto its policyholders— generally large corporations. By contrast, if a state's Medicaid budget exceeded expected allocations, the only recourse was to cut reimbursement rates (sharply limiting the number of providers willing to treat the patients), tighten eligibility restrictions, or increase taxes. More troubling was that the rate of growth in the programs appeared to be increasing by 1970. The cost of Medi-Cal, for example, doubled from $600 million in 1966 to $1.2 billion in 1971, provoking Governor Ronald Reagan to call the program "an alimentary canal: an appetite at one end and no sense of responsibility at the other."[6]

Whether by increasing eligibility requirements, decreasing reimbursement, requiring second medical opinions, or forcing physicians into a capitated arrangement, state governors began to tame the most threatening item on their budget in the early 1970s while at the same time demanding more generous matching funds from the federal government. As states had different levels of eligibility to start with, and different reimbursement schedules, each state attacked the problem differently, with varying degrees of success. In New York, for example, a commitment to generous social welfare spending precluded Albany from overly constricting the program, and the legislature voted instead to shunt some of the extra cost back to the localities and municipalities, particularly New York City. The strapped city in turn developed a new "ghetto medicine" program to help fund its part of the local Medicaid disbursements, while deferring maintenance on infrastructure projects and nearly defaulting on its debt load. By contrast, Governor Reagan responded in

California by forcing Medicaid providers into a strict rate schedule (a sort of precursor of the diagnosis-related group, or DRG, system), thus reducing their incentive to overprovide and overbill, and holding the program's budget nearly flat for 1972.[7]

The federal government too bore the cost of the increases. Less hampered by tax limitations than state governments (Medicaid expenditures constituted less than 3 percent of federal expenditures in the 1969 budget), the program's growth nonetheless attracted the attention and concern of the Nixon White House. Because eligibility standards had been defined by Congress as a floor but not as a ceiling, any state had the prerogative to provide more generously for its residents than the program mandated, and to pass at least half the cost on to Washington. Additionally, the "prevailing charge" standard of reimbursement made the federal government financially beholden to a large sector of the economy which was exhibiting double-digit growth. As early as 1969 President Nixon's economic advisor Arthur Burns informed him that various state actions could result in "uncertain but potentially great increases" in the program's costs, and that such increases needed to be addressed with greater federal regulation of the program over the long term.[8] Ultimately, however, it would be the much larger increases in the Medicare program which would prompt focused attention from the federal government on the issue of health care inflation.

Compounding the cost overruns was general bureaucratic inefficiency associated with the various Medicaid programs. While some glitches were to be expected in starting up such a diverse and extensive series of payment schemes, physicians and hospitals had been spoiled by the efficiency with which the Medicare program had been implemented. Medicare payments came relatively promptly, for billed amounts, with few questions or challenges. By contrast, delays in Medicaid reimbursement were legendary, with some providers waiting months to receive reimbursement for standard billings. A major culprit was the lack of a fiscal intermediary in the Medicaid program. Medicare, from the start, contracted with Blue Cross (and later Blue Shield) plans to reimburse its providers. With their decades of private sector experience, the Blues had a relatively easy time building Medicare reimbursement systems into their existing functions. Medicaid, by contrast, was reimbursed directly from the state agency to the provider, and as a result was saddled with all the usual inefficiency and bureaucracy of a government office.[9] While one pollyannaish welfare commissioner, Ellen Winston, wrote of the advantages of a decentralized, state-administered charity medicine program (more discretion at the local level for setting eligibility standards and reimbursement rates),[10] most providers vehemently disagreed. One dentist on Long Island, for example, questioned the decision not to use a private sector intermediary for Medicaid, despite his profession's endorsement of the program: "Instead, huge and unwieldy welfare staffs were hastily created," he wrote in an editorial in 1968. "They were unable to function efficiently and created serious problems for those dependent on prompt payment for services rendered."[11]

There was no easy solution to the bureaucratic barriers. Medicaid had never been envisioned as a federal program, but rather as a federally coordinated series of state programs, and thus could not be made consistent and coherent at the federal level without fundamentally violating its intent. Moreover, it was essentially a welfare program, not an insurance program, and thus needed to be tightly wedded to existing welfare programs (AFDC, Food Stamps, SSI) within the state bureaucracies, lest eligibility standards diverge. Medicare, by contrast, was really national health insurance (albeit for only the senior portion of the population), with a nationally unified product that could be easily delivered, under contract, by a third-party payer. A task force report on problems with Medicaid in 1970 did suggest a certain amount of reorganization with HEW—perhaps a new undersecretary for health and scientific affairs could help, along with a national council of health advisors—but these measures could only improve matters to a limited extent. The task force endorsed decentralizing the program through existing public agencies (that is, state-level bureaucracies) with only nominal guidance from the federal government.[12] At best, the federal government was willing only to reemphasize the need for primary care over specialty care, and express hope for regional cooperation in setting standards.

A more subtle barrier to programmatic efficiency was a changing attitude among physicians toward charity care—a change which Medicaid itself had facilitated. Historically, doctors had maintained a commitment to pro bono care; the Hippocratic Oath itself enshrined and mandated allegiance to the principle. While individual doctors' level of commitment to the principle had varied, most had been willing to alter their fee scales, write off bad debts, serve gratis on hospital rounds, and lend their time and expertise to training residents. No other profession had recorded such a long and noble catalogue of public service. But Medicaid, in the minds of many doctors, had changed the equation. With the backing of the federal government, millions of former charity patients had become potential private wards, and thus no longer merited free care. Thus when states delayed payments on bills, or reimbursed at rates substantially below the market, physicians responded with a marked lack of charity. While patients might be poor, resentful doctors argued, state governments were decidedly not, and bureaucratic inefficiency and political bickering did not make a persuasive case for dispensing uncompensated care. As a result, certain poor patients actually saw their access to medical care decline under Medicaid, as they lost the elevated charity standing which had previously entitled them to free care while failing to receive adequate compensation from impecunious state programs. Recategorized as beneficiaries of federal or state charity programs, these poor patients could not reasonably be recognized as medical charity cases. "The concept of the federal government as a charity case is ridiculous," wrote the editors of the *New England Journal of Medicine* in 1967.

Changes under Nixon

The ascendance of Richard Nixon to the presidency brought change to welfare programs, to charity health care, and to government generally. Nixon looked askance at many of the Great Society programs initiated by his predecessor, questioning not so much the cost of the programs as the theoretical foundations on which they rested. For Nixon, want was a relative condition whose most effective remedy was work. "You can see why I believe so deeply in the American dream," he declared in accepting the Republican nomination in 1968. "The American dream has come true [for me]."[13] For impoverished minorities, multigenerational welfare recipients, and those who lived within a culture of poverty, Nixon felt contempt. "Work, work—throw 'em off the rolls. That's the key," he told his aide John Ehrlichman in 1971.[14] Welfare, in his opinion, as construed and delivered in 1970, served little purpose but to morally enslave its recipients and deny them dignity and self-respect.

Medicaid and other Great Society programs offended Nixon for two reasons: unnecessary federal control and a tendency toward dependency on government. Nixon was the first national political leader since the 1930s to question the efficacy of the New Deal not on ideological grounds but on administrative ones. A states-rights activist before the term was widely used, the president held suspect all programs administered at the federal level that lacked an obvious need to be so administered. Programs such as Head Start, neighborhood health centers, and Aid to Families with Dependent Children (AFDC) drew his skepticism, not so much because they represented a more expansive welfare state than he might have otherwise designed but because they carried with them the taint of unnecessary federal intrusion into affairs of the states. His overarching approach to domestic policy, later dubbed the "New Federalism," was to return as much discretion to state and local policymakers as possible, without compromising necessary federal controls.

But Nixon's more fervent critique of welfare was grounded in a profound personal belief in self-sufficiency. As one who understood the vagaries and insults which life held for many people, he also believed that the path to transcending these challenges lay in work, self-reliance, and personal motivation. Any program which encouraged dependence upon an outside agent, be it private or federal, ultimately undermined the ability of people to achieve personal dignity. New Deal welfare programs were pernicious for the multigenerational dependency that they encouraged on government, social welfare agencies, and social workers, robbing people of the incentive to take responsibility for their fortunes and misfortunes. Drawing a distinction between "welfare" and "general welfare," he described his objection thus: "In a welfare state, the government absorbs the citizens and private groups. It may smother them with honey, but nonetheless it smothers them. They are regulated from cradle to grave. In the general-welfare state, the government is the servant of the citizen. It seeks to help, not to control."[15] For Nixon, welfare programs must aid without "smothering" to be worthy of support. Tax credits (or a negative income tax) would be preferable to chits, vouchers preferable to government-owned housing, and publicly financed insurance preferable to publicly financed doctors. Vividly remembering families who weathered the 1930s on "black-eyed peas, turnip greens," he understood the need for government to help those in need, while at the same time emphasizing the dangers of providing help where none was required.[16]

Medicaid violated a number of precepts which the Nixon administration set for acceptable domestic policy. For all of its growing size, Medicaid had left large gaps in the nation's health insurance net. Although designed primarily to aid the nation's poor in purchasing health care, the disabled and long-term elderly care built into the program were absorbing a disproportionate share of the program's expenditures, leaving only 19 percent of the program's resources for pediatric care by 1971. And because of its reliance on AFDC eligibility standards (which effectively excluded married couples and unmarried men, no matter how poor), it failed to cover a large number of the nation's needy. As a result, by 1971 nearly 60 percent of the nation's families with incomes of under $3,000 had no health insurance (including Medicaid), while 40 percent of families with incomes between $3,000 and $5,000 lacked health insurance.[17] A strange amalgam of eligibility standards, poverty thresholds, and marriage penalties created disincentives to marry, to work, to acknowledge child support benefits, and to report taxes honestly, and created an odd notch among working Americans. Those in the notch failed to receive benefits from their employers and could not afford private health insurance, yet earned too much money to qualify for Medicaid.

Nixon's response was a more general national health insurance program for families of limited means, ranging from true destitution to approximately the median family income. Entitled the Family Health Insurance Plan (FHIP) and formulated in the White House Domestic Council's Health Policy Review Group in 1970, the program was presented to the president as a sort of Medicare program with graduated subsidies that families and individuals with incomes below $8,000 a year could buy into. True to Nixon's parsimonious tendencies, the program included cost control measures such as co-payments, deductibles, and partial reimbursements—all in an effort to make both patient and physicians more conscious of underlying costs.[18] The program would subsume Medicaid and add about $3 billion a year to the government's health bill, but in return it would vastly diminish the rolls of the uninsured, draw patients away from public emergency rooms and hospitals, and ultimately reduce the nation's health bill by encouraging preventive treatment.[19]

But many politicians failed to view the problems in the American health system as particularly pressing. True, a sizable portion of Americans lacked private health insurance, but this was not tantamount to being denied all medical care. Patients could pay cash for services, or turn to the web of public and charity services and facilities throughout the nation such as community clinics, municipal hospitals, and private emergency rooms. American life expectancy and infant mortality rates were not the best in the world, but neither were they reprehensibly high. Infectious disease was a diminishing threat, smoking and drinking were in decline, a growing number of Americans were receiving private health coverage through employment (although the proportion had reached a plateau), and childhood inoculations were nearly ubiquitous. Gaps in Medicaid for the working poor and working classes were unfortunate, in this view, but they hardly constituted a crisis.

Inflation in the Health System at Large

The more threatening problem was health care inflation. The cost of medical expenditures had risen markedly in the final years of the 1960s, owing largely to the inflationary pressures of Medicare (and to a lesser extent Medicaid). While before 1965 health care cost increases had averaged 3 to 4 percent annually, since the advent of Medicare the figure had jumped to 10 percent. Even with the high inflation of the early 1970s, health costs regularly rose faster than other costs, and health planners warned that this trend was getting worse. Numerous hospital expansion programs nationwide promised to exacerbate the inflation, and growing pools of physicians seeking specialty and subspecialty training suggested increases in physician reimbursement rates as well. And while private insurers could pass along the rising costs to their policy holders, governments—both federal and state—had no choice but to go back to the taxpayers or increase their outstanding debt. "The health care crisis is upon us," the journalist Godfrey Hodgson wrote in 1973.[20]

While taxpayers and consumers bore the cost increases through higher taxes or higher-priced consumer products and services, certain people and institutions benefited. Patients to some degree benefited from new facilities, although one White House analyst estimated that only 30 percent of all new costs could be explained by improved medical care and services. Medical care professionals, particularly specialists, experienced an extraordinary rise in their incomes, with nurses' incomes rising by 100 percent between 1959 and 1969 and physicians' incomes rising by even more during the same period. But it was the private hospitals which experienced the most notable increase in revenues. Bill Fullerton, a member of Wilbur Mills's staff, noted that after Medicare, hospitals were for the first time "really making money." As noted in chapter 4, hospital adminstrators saw Medicare as affording them the opportunity to "start checking . . . off" expenditures and improvements that they had been deferring.[21]

Both Congress and the White House recognized the looming problem, and responded with quick fixes to stem inflation in the industry. Congress established Professional Standards Review Organizations in 1973 throughout the nation in an effort to better control health care use and capital expenditures. The White House adopted a variety of strategies to train more physicians' assistants and other nonphysician medical personnel.[22] But by the early 1970s officials in the Nixon administration recognized that health care inflation was probably symptomatic of deeper flaws in the production and delivery of health care. One prescient White House analyst, noting in 1970 that inflation in the health care sector would probably exceed 13 percent a year over the next five years, pinned the blame firmly on one of America's most beloved community institutions—the private hospital: "We have a medical system based on the highest cost facility—the hospital," the analyst wrote. "We need preventive and outpatient services that cut down the need for hospital care."[23]

Nixon rightly perceived increases in health care costs to be the true impending "crisis" of the nation's medical care system. Although the number of uninsured was troublesome, it didn't require a structural change as much as a simple expansion in one of the many programs then being offered by the government to deliver health care—Medicare, Medicaid, neighborhood health centers, or veterans' benefits. Most every proposal introduced in Congress in the early 1970s would alleviate, if not totally rectify, the problem. But rising health costs suggested a far more pernicious problem requiring a more profound (and more difficult) solution. It called into question the efficacy of third-party payment, the bulwark on which the nation's medical delivery system was based. Third-party payment induced doctors to overprovide, patients to overconsume, hospitals to overbuild, and medical schools to overtrain, yet discontinuing the system of private insurers was politically unfeasible. A payment mechanism which had made perfect sense in the depressed economy of the 1930s, when hospital care was cheap and physicians largely rural and oriented toward general care, had given birth to a giant hydra which consumed a growing share of the nation's GDP to enrich a medical system which was improving America's health status at an ever-slower rate.

Comprehensive Health Reform

By 1972 several flaws in the charity health system and the health system at large combined to create momentum for comprehensive reform. Medicaid had failed to cover a large number of needy individuals, and health costs were ballooning. In addition, medical manpower was inadequate and getting more so, vital statistics were growing (comparatively) dire, and lack of coordination between private insurers, public payment programs, and nonprofit community clinics was creating inefficiencies in the delivery of care. In manpower alone, the United States was producing little over half of the necessary fourteen thousand medical graduates needed each year to staff intern and residency positions in the nation's hospitals, forcing it to import graduates of foreign medical schools to make up the balance. "It seems strange, doesn't it," wrote a columnist in the *New Republic*, "to send U.S. foreign aid abroad and drain away its physicians."[24]

One indication of growing dissatisfaction with the health care system on the whole (as opposed to isolated components of the system) was the consistency of calls for reform across the political spectrum. While social progressives, policy scholars, and academic economists had repeatedly called for comprehensive reform, since at least the 1920s, even conservative business and community leaders began to do so by the early 1970s. In California, Governor Ronald Reagan proposed a statewide catastrophic care bill to cover the state's middle class, who were excluded from Medicaid but too poor to cover their own catastrophic needs or afford private coverage. Breaking with his business colleagues, the chairman of IBM, Thomas Watson Jr., a self-described "dyed-in-the-wool free trader and free enterpriser" who had long rejected calls for a national health plan, changed his mind. "I accepted that argument in 1949," he told an audience, "and I bet nearly everyone else in this room did, too. But on the evidence—particularly the international evidence—I cannot accept it in 1970."[25]

For progressives the idea had long been attractive. Stymied in their efforts to pass national health insurance legislation in the late 1940s, when Truman had given top priority to the measure, they had waited two decades for the return of a political and economic climate favorable for reform. The Vietnam War had forestalled a great deal of domestic legislation in the late 1960s and early 1970s, but with the war winding down and the economy floundering, the moment seemed propitious for introducing new legislation. Moreover, the movement had been given added force by the clear inequities between what the poor obtained through Medicaid and what the well-to-do obtained through private insurance. Despite its initial promise, Medicaid was providing the poor with lower-grade health care in lower-grade facilities, and planners found the growing discrepancy unacceptable.[26] "I take it that our goal is to achieve a situation where the amount and quality of medical care that an individual receives is not a function of his income," wrote Rashi Fein, a health care economist at Harvard, in 1972.[27] A growing number of planners were agreeing that such a goal could not be achieved by creating a separate system of poor care for the nation's least well-off.

Paradoxically, a strong impetus to comprehensive health reform—notably in the form of compulsory health insurance—was the growth of private health insurance over the previous two decades. From 1950 to 1970 the percentage of all hospital costs covered by private insurance had risen from 34 to 71, the percentage of physician costs covered from 12 to 43, and the percentage of health care costs as a whole which were covered from 12 to 37.[28] Coupled with Medicare and Medicaid reimbursement, health insurers now dominated the market for purchasing health care, making the noninsured worse off than they had been thirty years before.

Effectively, the standard had shifted. Physician training, capital investment in hospitals, and pharmaceutical research were now conducted with the expectation that new procedures, drugs, and equipment would be reimbursed through an insured populace with far greater medical purchasing power than a noninsured population could have. Specialty and subspecialty training assumed this trend, as did investments in more sophisticated surgical suites, diagnostic equipment, and medical devices. Prices had not risen for long-existing products and procedures; but new, more expensive products and procedures, necessitating third-party payment if they were to become affordable to most middle-income Americans, had displaced the old. Uninsured patients were not worse off medically in 1969 than they had been in 1939, but the discrepancy between the quality of care that they could afford and what was available to the insured population had grown substantially.

With third-party payment now the norm, a grand leveling effect was evident throughout much of America's medical care landscape. For the privately insured (as well as for Medicare recipients), wealth had ceased to be a significant factor in the purchase of health care. Blue-collar workers were treated in the same hospitals as corporate executives; middle-class wage earners could seek care in the same private psychiatric clinics as the moneyed few. For much of the population, health care had ceased to be a discretionary purchase and become part of the basic fabric of residency. To be born in the United States with private health insurance in 1970 was to be born with access to unlimited hospitalization in accredited hospitals, unlimited care from a corps of physicians with medical training unparalleled in the world, and access to all the benefits accrued through the largest program of biomedical research ever, anywhere. True, the very wealthy could spend themselves into private rooms during hospital stays, with private nursing, but beyond that their care differed little from that of the middle class. Health outcomes and expectations leveled accordingly.

This social leveling effect spurred a number of health reformers to suggest that Medicaid, or any program specifically targeting the poor (such as neighborhood health centers), was fundamentally at odds with the long-term goals of American medicine. Segregation by income would inevitably result in an inequitable system of care: the "two-tiered" system which poverty advocates had long warned against. While incremental improvements could be made to the poor care system, the better goal was to do away entirely with poverty care, and Medicaid, and work instead for a true national health system. In 1974 Nixon's commissioner of the Medical Services Administration, Howard Newman, spoke for many moderate political leaders when he wrote that "no health program designed specifically for the poor can be successful," but rather that poor care must be accomplished by a "broader, probably universal solution."[29] Kerr White, public health professor at Johns Hopkins, had made a similar prediction a few years earlier: "it seems almost inevitable that this country will have a National Health Insurance plan, financed through statutory employee-employer contributions and general taxes."[30] Flaws in Medicaid spurred such thinking, but so too did a large-scale shift in the nation's perception of medical care insurance as a basic right.

Nixon responded with a Comprehensive Health Insurance Plan (CHIP), which included a Family Health Insurance Plan (FHIP), an Employee Health Care Insurance Plan (EHIP), and an Associated Health Care Insurance Plan (AHIP). The three plans together constituted what would today be known as a pay-or-play approach: employers above a certain size would be required to enroll their full-time workers, or pay a tax to help fund the AHIP program, which would provide private insurance to all families with income below $5,000 at no cost to the insured (except for a sliding-scale deductible based on income). At incomes between $5,000 and $8,000, families could buy into the federal program at annual premiums of $300 per person, until their income rose enough to qualify them for the EHIP program. The program was attractive in that it would supersede the existing Medicaid program, with all of its state-to-state inequities and bureaucratic barriers, while at the same time preserving the private insurance market, which would be a formidable political opponent in any legislative fight over comprehensive reform. It would also delegate managerial authority to the private sector, where cost containment could be allied with profit-making motives.

The problem with CHIP was that it was not the single-payer system desired by the most avid proponents of health reform. These individuals looked to Canada particularly but also to England, New Zealand, and

Japan for inspiration, and found the state-based (or province-based) single-payer model highly attractive. Under that model one nationwide universal payer, funded entirely out of general taxes, paid for all physicians, hospitals, and pharmaceutical care, all of which continued to be provided by private professionals and firms. Gone was the administrative redundancy found in a competitive, market-driven system such as America's, and gone too was the association of health coverage with employment. In Canada to be alive was to be insured, with no requirements beyond citizenship. Such a system severed health insurance from jobs and thus facilitated movement in the labor market, while allowing provincial health authorities, through universal budgeting and bargaining, to hold down costs. And indeed Canada was holding down costs better than the United States was, while insuring all residents and providing medical care of high quality. The question of whether the quality of care was comparable to that produced in the United States was the one great challenge to the idea.

Astute political observers recognized that a more likely avenue for health reform was increasing the number of primary-care physicians and nurses in the country, whose thinning ranks (relative to the population) were preventing so many Medicaid beneficiaries from getting reasonable care. Despite the huge investments made in medical care since the Second World War, the number of primary-care physicians per capita had fallen drastically since the pre-war years. In 1931, for example, there were 94 pediatricians and internists per 100,000 people in the United States; by 1967 this number had fallen to 53.[31] A near-reversal in the ratio of generalists to specialists was partly responsible (by 1967 nearly 70 percent of all medical school graduates applied for specialty residency training upon graduation; in 1931 the figure had been less than 20 percent), as was a failure to establish new medical schools despite substantial population growth. In addition, American medical schools' almost obsessive focus on research to the exclusion of teaching meant that virtually all the growth in faculty had served to expand research output but not class size. "Some of our best and most lavishly funded medical schools are training a ridiculously small number of physicians," said James Cain, a physician at the Mayo Clinic, to the Association of Military Surgeons in Washington. "It seems absurd that our great country is an importer rather than an exporter of medical talent."[32]

By the time Nixon left the White House in 1974, charity care was being pulled in two directions. For some reformers, charity care was part of a larger array of services to be offered through welfare agencies in an effort to empower local communities, increase professional opportunities, and not incidentally serve medical care to the sick. For those who felt this way, Medicaid rightly remained at the state and local level, delivered though a welfare agency, and further filtered through the institution of a community or neighborhood health center.

Others, however, questioned the very existence of charity care, and viewed the existence of programs such as Medicaid and uncompensated care funds as an indictment of a system which failed to care for everyone equally. For reformers who held this view, flaws in charity care were less a problem in themselves than a symptom of a system fundamentally misconstrued. Members of this group saw private health insurance as an inadequate mechanism by which to finance a nation's health services. Remedies ranged from a single-payer system along Canadian lines, to a pay-or-play system, to a nationally mandated catastrophic plan to cover the worst problems for everyone, but in each case the remedy reflected a lack of faith in the ability of market forces to equitably deliver medical care.

Those who looked to comprehensive reform also feared the medical inflation which was threatening the stability of state budgets, and ultimately the ability of the federal government to meet its commitment to Medicare recipients. Health scholars with a variety of views all saw that the third-party system created disincentives to deliver care economically, and in fact encouraged abuse of the medical system on the part of both provider and patient. Such a threat drew bipartisan attention, and political leaders from diverse camps argued that any meaningful reform must begin to eliminate the forces driving inflation in the sector. The system as it stood in 1974 delivered too much care to those with private insurance, and not enough to those without.

7

Health Planning and Community Medicine in the 1970s

Gaps in Coverage in 1975

In its tenth year Medicaid could boast of multiple accomplishments. The long-running disparity in the use of private physicians between the poor and the nonpoor had been eradicated, and sometimes reversed. Before 1965 the nonpoor visited physicians 20 percent more often in a given year than the poor did; by 1975 the poor were visiting physicians 13 percent more often than the nonpoor. Poor children had increased their average annual physician visits from 3.3 in 1964 to 3.7 in 1974. The portion of the poor who had not visited a physician for at least two years had fallen from 28 percent in 1964 to 17 percent in 1974, while the portion of impoverished pregnant women visiting a physician during the first trimester of pregnancy had risen from 58 percent to 71 percent during the same period. By any measure, the primary mission of Medicaid—to increase access to the private medical system for the nation's poor—had been accomplished. The health policy expert Karen Davis wrote in 1976 that the program had had a "major impact" on the health of the poor, whatever its shortcomings might be.[1]

Not all was well and good. Although the poor were using more health care resources than the nonpoor by 1975, they also required more health care given their generally worse state of health, and many health analysts suspected that they were still not getting enough. Of greater concern was the substantial number of poor people who were not benefiting from expanding programs or alternative charity care services, such as neighborhood health centers and municipal clinics. As eligibility for Medicaid was linked to state-determined eligibility for other welfare programs (AFDC and SSI), those poor who failed to qualify for the cash assistance programs generally failed to qualify for Medicaid as well. Half of the states limited AFDC to families in which the father was not present, meaning that two-parent families with unemployed fathers failed to qualify, regardless of their level of destitution. Moreover, the income eligibility limit for AFDC and Medicaid ranged widely, from $2,208 for a family of four in North Carolina to $5,472 for that same family in Wisconsin. Families qualifying under special "medically needy" provisions also faced divergent standards: Tennessee defined the limit at $2,200 while Wisconsin, again, granted benefits to families with income up to $5,600. As a result, nonqualifying needy persons included such assorted groups as widows under sixty-five, two-parent families (which constituted more than 70 percent of the rural poor), families with fathers earning marginal wages, pregnant women with no previous children, and children of non-AFDC families in the thirty-six states with no "all needy children" provisions.

The result of these many coverage gaps was that by 1975 a third of the nation's poor—over eight million people—failed to qualify for Medicaid. In some states the situation was far worse. In Alabama, Arkansas, Louisiana, Mississippi, South Carolina, and Texas, fewer than one poor child in ten was included in the program in the early 1970s. HEW estimated that in seventeen states fewer than one third of the poor residents were enrolled in Medicaid. And of those who did qualify, tens of thousands failed to seek care for want of transportation, ignorance of the system, aversion to medical authority, or fear of abusive interactions with doctors. In one notorious case, a gynecologist in rural South Carolina demanded that all of his pregnant welfare patients with three or more children submit to "voluntary" sterilization or forgo further prenatal care. With the closest physicians more than twenty-five miles away and public transportation nonexistent, sixty-seven women, mostly black, submitted to the procedure over a two-year period.[2] Poor southern states, such as Mississippi, Alabama, and Arkansas, funded the program at as little as $50 per child per year (versus almost $500 in New York) and at just under $500 per AFDC family per year. The social scientist Beverly Myers described Medicaid at the time as a "poor program for poor people."[3]

Another flaw in the programs, as they evolved, was the inequitable way in which they skewed payments to whites, urbanites, and Northeasterners. Nationally, whites who enrolled in the program received nearly 75 percent greater annual benefits than blacks, and rural white enrollees' benefits exceeded rural black enrollees' benefits by over 100 percent. While part of the discrepancy could be explained by racially skewed settlement patterns of state residence, whites did better even within the same region, or the same state. In the Northeast, for example, whites received $362 while blacks received only $205. For Medicaid recipients in nursing homes, whites received $2,375 compared to $1,857 for blacks, and physicians seeing white Medicaid patients were paid at rates 40 percent higher than those seeing black patients. At least some of these discrepancies were mitigated by the tendency of blacks to qualify for Medicaid at higher rates than whites, because of their higher rates of divorce and out-of-wedlock births. Even so, racial discrimination prevented many enrolled blacks from seeing the most proximate or best-qualified physicians and nurses. Despite Medicaid's many accomplishments, there was "little doubt" that it had fallen short of the "original high expectations" for it, Davis noted in 1976.[4]

As the Medicaid program grew, it began to fundamentally change the manner in which medical care was purchased and delivered, first for the poor but ultimately for everyone. Public hospitals lost many patients to private institutions, as newly qualified Medicaid beneficiaries seized the opportunity to purchase care in the private sector, and municipal governments became purchasers rather than providers of care in urban areas. Government in New York City, for example, accounted for 60 percent of all medical care purchasing in the city in 1975, as opposed to only 30 percent in 1965, and government purchasing in Detroit, Washington, and Baltimore exceeded even this. At the same time, over half of all government medical care funds were flowing into private hospitals by 1975, as opposed to only a fifth in 1965. The patients continuing to seek care in public hospitals were disproportionately poor, uninsured, often illegal, and incapable of qualifying for state and federal charity programs. Medicaid had effectively taken federal aid from the public hospitals and given it to the private ones.[5]

This diversion of funds from public to private hospitals created one of the great paradoxes of Medicaid, for in improving access to private-sector institutions for the poor, the program concomitantly impoverished public institutions, the traditional purveyors of charity care and community services. While the framers of Medicaid had always envisioned the program as a conduit to move the poor into mainstream medicine, they had failed to realize that it would inevitably weaken the existing charity care system. Were Medicaid a comprehensive system of poor care, then the effects on public hospitals would have been inconsequential to charity patients—the hospitals would have slowly closed down as poor patients found care elsewhere. In fact, the one third of the nation's poor who failed to qualify for Medicaid programs now disproportionately filled the wards of city hospitals, making it even more difficult to collect revenue. City hospitals and hospital systems were now caught in a trap—unable to close their doors to the remaining needy, they found that traditional funding streams were being redirected to institutions which they had never had to compete with in the past.[6]

Foreign Medical Graduates, Long-Term Care, and EPSDT

Although the poor were getting substantially more care in the private sector in 1975 than they had in previous decades, the care was still not at the same level as that received by the nonpoor. Medicaid payment rates had not maintained parity with private insurance reimbursement, and this, along with the bureaucratic complications of applying for Medicaid reimbursement, kept many of the nation's most highly qualified doctors from providing care for Medicaid patients. Rebuffed by the most exclusive private physicians, Medicaid recipients turned to graduates of foreign medical schools (FMGs), who began to establish offices and clinics in inner-city and immigrant neighborhoods in large numbers in the 1970s.

The presence of FMGs in the United States was an unforeseen consequence of federal legislation in the 1960s designed to ward off predicted physician shortages. While the long-term solution had always been to fund new American medical schools (of which over twenty-five were established in the decades after the Second World War), a parallel program to thwart physician shortages was the opening of residencies in the United States to graduates of foreign medical schools in the 1960s and 1970s. The FMGS took the nearly one quarter of all residency spots which hospitals had been unable to fill with graduates of domestic schools (disproportionately in urban public hospitals), with the understanding that upon completion of training many would return to their native countries. Many of the FMGS elected to stay in the United States, however, to help meet the growing medical needs of Medicaid recipients and other underserved portions of the population.

By 1976 a disproportionate number of all Medicaid physician visits were taking place at offices of FMGS, with over 60 percent of all Medicaid patients seeking care in practices which were over one-third Medicaid. One rigorous study of the trend in Maryland found that over a third of all Maryland doctors willing to treat Medicaid patients (known as Medicaid "vendors") were FMGS, although such doctors constituted only a fifth of the state's medical personnel pool. Moreover, many FMG practices catered predominantly or exclusively to Medicaid patients, leading to the pejorative sobriquet "Medicaid mill." Graduates of domestic schools derided these practices as substandard, impersonal, and sloppy, while failing to acknowledge that their own unwillingness to treat Medicaid patients had effectively created the phenomenon. Charity care advocates expressed concern that the "two-tier" system of medical care, which Medicaid had been explicitly designed to end, was being recreated in a new form.[7]

Despite the grimy locales of the practices, Medicaid mills did not necessarily provide substandard care. A study sponsored by the Health Care Financing Adminstration (HCFA) in 1980 found little evidence that Medicaid patients were receiving incompetent or inadequate care.[8] A study by the Congressional Budget Office similarly found "no link" between the proportion of Medicaid patients in a practice and the quality of care.[9] The impetus to create Medicaid mills run by FMGS had mostly been the preference of private patients for American-born doctors, as well as the disproportionate share of FMGS who had gone into either general surgery or primary care. In addition, a large number of American-born doctors simply did not wish to treat Medicaid patients, regardless of fees. The patients frequently failed to show up for appointments, follow medication regimens, or follow through on referrals and tests.[10] One survey of California doctors found that although three fourths claimed a willingness to treat Medicaid patients, only 40 percent of all doctors actually saw ten or more Medicaid patients in a given month.[11]

A second major shift in the provision of medical services had resulted from Medicaid by 1975: the large-scale movement of the nation's elderly into nursing homes. Medicaid expenditures on nursing home care nearly tripled from 1970 to 1976, funding over half of all nursing home patients by mid-decade, and over 40 percent of all nursing home costs. The very existence of Medicaid had accelerated the growth in the use of nursing homes by the nation's elderly, which had been under way since the Second World War. By making nursing home care free for all senior citizens without assets (which was nearly half of the elderly by 1975), the program provided a powerful inducement to families to institutionalize parents who might previously have moved in with grown children or sought the part-time care of a home health aide. Along with the elderly, many mentally retarded and long-term mentally ill persons also moved into nursing homes during this period, as states sought to defray their psychiatric hospitalization bills with the federal funds available through the Medicaid programs. Indeed, while the numbers of elderly living in nursing homes increased by 40 percent between 1960 and 1975, the increase for the mentally retarded during this same period was over 600 percent.[12]

The other significant change in medical care wrought by Medicaid was the increased attention paid to children. Pediatric health had long been the ignored backwater of poor care. Lacking the compelling immediacy of prenatal care, or the political attractiveness of elder care, pediatric care beyond routine immunizations and appointments with the school nurse had often been dismissed as superfluous, given the generally rosy appearance of most preadolescents. To remedy the failing, HEW created the Early and Periodic Screening, Diagnosis and Treatment Program (EPSDT) in 1971 to fund preventive care for poor children through Medicaid, even for those children whose parents otherwise failed to qualify for the Medicaid program. While some states had funded pediatric preventive care all along, the new program worked to expand the number of states so doing, and resulted in lowering the incidence of childhood afflictions such as rubella, otitis, anemia, uncorrected vision and speech disorders, and congenital heart defects.[13]

It should be noted that health gains produced by Medicaid during the program's first ten years were not made in isolation. The varied programs of the war on poverty had produced marked gains for the poor during this period, resulting in a one-third reduction in their ranks between 1960 and 1975, most dramatically in 1965, when the poverty rolls declined by five million in just one year.[14] Aided by the Supplementary Security Income (SSI) program of 1971, the nation's poor enjoyed improved access to adequate nutrition and safe housing, which along with Medicaid helped to ease their condition. While the poor still lived lives of deprivation (the poverty threshold for a two-parent family with six children was only $9,588 in 1975), more and more they were free from want for their most basic needs.[15]

And yet, as the base rates of poverty (as measured by income) declined during these years, the rates of social pathology and family breakdown increased.[16] Deaths from suicide and homicide among the poor increased after 1965, as did rates of adolescent drug use, out-of-wedlock births, adolescent pregnancy, and school truancy. These developments detracted from the gains made by Medicaid and other antipoverty programs, and threatened to undermine public support for the vestiges of Johnson's antipoverty agenda.

The end of the Republican administrations of Nixon and Ford began a time of uncertainty for poverty programs in general, and poverty medical care in particular. The high inflation and unemployment of the mid-1970s threatened to more than undo the gains made in social equity over the previous decade, and a nation ill at ease with its own government looked skeptically to any overly activist agenda of a new administration. State governments sought areas in which to cut budgets as they faced tax revolts, growing unemployment, and a diminished national sense of self-confidence. Rising health costs in all sectors compelled a national re-examination of how medical care was produced and purchased, and a growing pool of radicalized social welfare advocates pressed for a significant restructuring of the entire health system. The future for poor care was uncertain, and unpredictable.

Health Planning and the "Right" to Health

As Medicaid grew, and as neighborhood health centers, community mental health centers, and mobile health clinics proliferated, so too did the general use of medical care. Since 1965 health care had grown at a prodigious rate, doubling its share of the American economy to nearly 9 percent by 1976. Every aspect of medical care, including research, capital investment in technology, training, and nursing care, had grown substantially in cost since the inauguration of Medicare, and the system's expansion showed no sign of slowing. Through the early 1970s the national cost of hospital care grew as much as 18 percent in a single year, while health insurance premiums for employers and individuals rose concomitantly. The cost increases in charity care reflected, to some degree, growth in the system as a whole.[17]

Accompanying the increases in costs for capital expenditures, personnel, research, and training was an expansion in the general mission of medicine. As has already been discussed, public health had been moving during the postwar decades from an infectious-disease model of the profession to one more concerned with social pathology. As part of the same trend, certain physicians and medical institutions in the 1970s began to perceive the whole of society, and not merely the individual, as their patient. Within these enlarged parameters of professional concern, environmental degradation, crime, filth, human misery, and natural hazards all came to be seen as within the purview of the medical doctor, or of the neighborhood health center. In 1967 the National Commission on Community Health had declared that reasonable health care could not be provided in a "contaminated environment," be it degraded by nuclear radiation or everyday dirt.[18] And in 1974 a team investigating health hazards in poor neighborhoods of New York City reported on the dangers inherent in peeling paint, broken stairs, rotting window sills, defective plumbing systems, inadequate heating, and insect infestation. Animal excreta could exacerbate allergies, unsound woodwork could lead to trips and falls, paint could cause lead poisoning, and leaky waste pipes could contaminate local areas with fecal matter and other effluvia.

Public health engineers had been addressing such hazards for decades, and considered these sorts of environmental health risks the central challenge of their profession. What was new in the early 1970s was the change in the perception by the medical community of these artifacts of poverty. Having begun with an almost hyperscientific approach to illness and disease, portions of the medical community were beginning to move to a broader and less literal understanding of their charge to heal the sick, replacing a disease model with a human misery index. Physicians with little or no formal training in public health or epidemiology began to view community medicine as a valid medical specialty, equal to surgery, nephrology, or pediatrics. For physicians with this broader outlook, the Hippocratic Oath compelled them to do more than simply heal the sick: it required healing society as well. "In order to have a measurable impact on improving the health status of a community," members of a community medicine research team wrote in 1974, "the health professionals must assume a vigorous leadership role in correcting those environmental defects—particularly in housing—which produce identifiable health problems."[19]

Underlying the case for an expanding medical purview was a growing "right-to-health" movement, which had emerged out of the war on poverty in the late 1960s. As has previously been discussed, the existence of an enshrined right to medical care had been postulated as early as the 1930s, when the Committee on the Costs of Medical Care (CCMC) offered its sweeping vision of a rationalized and centrally controlled American medical care system (although in Europe the perception went back farther still), but the country's receptiveness to this notion waxed and waned over the subsequent fifty years. With Medicaid firmly in place, and an ensconced bureaucracy of civil servants, nonprofit administrators, and professional poverty advocates all lobbying for due care for the poor, the idea of health as a basic right was finding greater social acceptance by the mid-1970s. Arthur Okun, an economist at the Brookings Institution, wrote in 1975 that all people required a "right to a decent existence—to some minimum standards of nutrition, health care, and other essentials of life," and that "starvation and dignity do not mix well," while the health policy analysts Karen Davis and Catherine Schoen wrote that "some minimum standard of health care for all seems essential to the preservation of social order and justice."[20]

Opponents of this view argued that the supposed right was a sham—a shrouded call for expanded welfare benefits. While such a right might be granted by legislative fiat—as similar rights effectively had been by the AFDC, SSI, Food Stamps, Medicaid, and public housing laws—an action of Congress was different from an inalienable right. Various physicians, many of whom took seriously their obligation to provide care pro bono for the poor, argued against the rights-based terminology, even as they acknowledged their own moral compulsion to serve those in need. Rights-based medicine was "adversarial," the physician-philosopher Mark Siegler suggested, and presupposed a "radical individualism" which laid claim to the physicians' skills. By contrast, medicine had traditionally been based on a covenant of reciprocity, intended to maximize universal health, in which patient and doctor each had obligations to the other.[21] Similarly, the public health physician George Pickett warned against furthering a rights-based rhetoric when speaking of medicine: "Rights are hard to live with because we must all yield a degree of freedom to protect them," he told an audience in Washington in October 1977. "The right of access to medical care will cost us more than money."[22]

The call to rights was effectively a call for planning. The holy grail of health policy visionaries since the 1930s, effective health planning had long promised cheaper, better, and more broadly accessible medicine. From the dispensary movement of the 1920s, to the CCMC recommendations of 1932, to the comprehensive reform bills of the 1940s, health care advocates had maligned the slipshod market response of the medical care anti-system, in which hospitals and high-cost specialists proliferated in wealthy suburbs, leaving vast swaths of the rural midland and most urban ghettos underserved. To rectify these imbalances required a national planning model, in which government—federal, state, and local—would designate regional health centers and establish lines of referrals from general community hospitals, rural clinics, private physicians' practices, and public health nursing units. This utopian system would blanket the country with perfectly allocated health care personnel, taking from those communities blessed with abundant physicians and hospitals and giving to those which had few or none.

The vision never came to pass, but certain of the most acute needs had been alleviated. Many rural areas, for example, had received subsidized hospitals built courtesy of the Hill-Burton program during the 1950s and

1960s, and Medicare subsidies to teaching hospitals had provided substantial funds for urban academic health centers which catered primarily to the poor after 1965. A concomitant reduction in facilities and personnel in those areas which had long had an overabundance of health care resources never happened, however, and by 1975 the more pressing challenge for health planners was not distributing hospitals, doctors, and nurses to impoverished areas but rather controlling their growth in areas which already harbored more than their needed share.

The legislative response to this runaway growth was the National Health Planning and Resources Development Act of 1974 (P.L. 93-641), which attempted to limit new investment in health care infrastructure and equipment through a newly created certificate-of-need (CON) process. A CON granted by a local Health Systems Agency (HSA) was now required for most new construction, purchasing of major medical equipment, or institutional realignment. The HSAS, consisting of local clinicians, providers, purchasers, concerned citizens, academics, and community leaders, evaluated the need for proposed expansions by using a complex algorithm incorporating population density and the demographic characteristics of patients, the existing number of beds, the presence of proximate and competing institutions and of a regional tertiary care center, and other variables to arrive at a fair decision for granting the CON. In theory the process limited the number of new hospital beds, imaging clinics, and other expensive revenue generators, and in doing so capped the growth of the health care system. While P.L. 93-641 was hardly the comprehensive planning act envisioned by the most radical advocates of health planning, it was at least a step in the right direction.

The CON program was criticized by nearly all interested parties. The HSAS in particular were attacked by public health professionals for their citizen makeup, ostensibly because the job was best left to professionals trained in public health and health planning; by patients' advocates for being instruments of government control over access to health resources; and by physicians for their potential to usurp the preeminence of the medical staff in dictating hospital policy.[23] Daniel Rubenstein, for example, a physician in Boston, expressed concern over the "inflexible regulatory processes" implicit in the program.[24] And political scientists, cognizant of the micropolitical tussles present in all community boards and institutions, viewed skeptically the dominance of the HSAS by clinicians, providers, and hospital representatives. "In government, anatomy is destiny," wrote the public health analyst and future HCFA administrator Bruce Vladeck. "Congress has provided for the institutionalization of existing structures of power."[25]

Accompanying the National Health Planning Act was the Emergency Medical Service Systems Act of 1973 (P.L. 93-154), which mandated local planning efforts in constructing comprehensive emergency medical systems for localities, and provided funding to assist in the task. Incorporating citizens' representatives as well as local clinicians and patients, the program was charged with an open mandate to plan emergency medical services. While progressive "good government" types applauded the initiative, free-market critics withheld their endorsement or openly criticized it. "It is likely that the act will bring about profound changes in the emergency medical system," wrote Michael Eliastam, a professor at Stanford University School of Medicine. "But whether all or even half of these changes will be of benefit to patients is not at all assured."[26]

Underlying the squabble over the constitution of HSAS and other planning bodies was the public's discomfort with planning in general, and health planning in particular. Anti-planning sentiment tended to dominate municipal and county government, particularly in the South and West, with regard to land development, water usage, zoning, business, and commerce. Medical and hospital care had traditionally fallen within the category of demand-driven goods and services best left to the private sector to produce and deliver, and many Americans were reluctant to elevate medical care to the status of public good. Health planners, accountable to no one once appointed, would be free to impose their visions and designs on the health system—still the world's best, in the view of many. "Planners could easily become very dictatorial and bureaucratic if given too much latitude in this matter of authority," wrote Robert Corbett, counselor to the Kansas Health Board.[27] Other critics suspected the opposite outcome, in which emasculated boards would accomplish little beyond validating the desires of influential players and institutions within the health system, making the prospect of true reform even more distant. Vladeck, of this latter camp, dismissed the whole HSA design as an "institutional forum" for legitimizing "existing patterns of power distribution."[28]

Without planning, however, government effectively ceded its role in poor care to well-meaning individuals and philanthropic groups, many of which were incapable of shouldering the increasingly complex task. The nation had been convinced by the Social Security program, which had extraordinarily high approval ratings, that retirement security could no longer be left to individual investors, and by the G.I. Bill that the government could play a constructive role in providing higher education. So must health care follow, regardless of personal ideology. "The government, in its cumbersome way, is attempting to address itself to the attainment of mental and social well-being, rather than treatment of disease," wrote Albert Anderson, a professor of medicine at Columbia University. "Let us not shrink from the recognition that health care is a political issue."

Changes in Medical Delivery: NHCs, HMOs, and the Rise of Community Medicine

Although charity care was being delivered predominantly on a fee-for-service basis by private-sector clinicians by 1975, it continued to be delivered by other means as well. The community health center (CHC) program, transferred from the Office of Economic Opportunity to the Department of Health, Education and Welfare in 1968, had peaked in 1971 with 112 centers nationwide and then declined.[29] By 1975 there were just over 100 of the centers, and although clinical quality (and satisfaction over outcomes) was high, other goals of the program remained elusive. The vision of the centers as akin to social service agencies, replete with employment-training and community-building functions, had fallen into disfavor, and the centers were beginning to resemble public clinics more than anything else. And although some centers continued to take their role as patient-educators and community advocates seriously, for the most part they invested their resources in raising standards of clinical care.[30]

At their best, the centers brought comprehensive care to impoverished communities and dropped it at residents' front doors. Reaching out through school-based clinics, door-to-door solicitation of patients, and the offering of free meals and transportation, the centers were able to bring decent primary care to large portions of the communities in which they were situated. In certain ghetto areas in which CHCs were established, the centers accounted for up to a third of all physician visits by residents of the catchment areas (the remainder being divided roughly evenly between hospital emergency rooms, outpatient clinics, and private physician care), and generally improved the health of the targeted population.[31] In the most impoverished rural areas of the South, for example, care offered through local CHCs was responsible for a decline in infant mortality rates of 40 percent between 1966 and 1970, and in rates of influenza and pneumonia of almost half. "Town doctors here in Gunnison (MS), well they don't take up with us poor folks," remarked one resident, Pearlie Johnson, of her efforts to seek treatment for cataracts in the early 1960s. The local Mount Bayou Comprehensive Health Center had saved her sight by providing free eye surgery and medication in 1965.[32]

The downside of CHCs was twofold: their tendency to increase the use of hospitals by poor patients (contributing to health care inflation), and their expropriation of local private medical practices. With regard to the overuse of hospitals in the early 1970s I will speak more later; for now suffice it to say that the erection of a CHC could double the rate of hospital use for the residents of a catchment area, despite the community health emphasis on prevention and primary care.[33] Local health advocates predicted that the increase would be temporary as previously undertreated residents were hospitalized for existing illnesses, but critics were skeptical.[34]

The migration of physicians and the need to retain them proved more problematic. Poor communities had always been medically understaffed, and CHCs did not appreciably alleviate the shortage. Studies in the mid-1970s showed that the presence of local non-CHC physicians declined at almost exactly the same rate that physicians signed on to work for the centers, suggesting that CHCs merely shifted the already meager supply of poor-care doctors from one venue to another. Moreover, the CHCs had difficulty retaining hired doctors for longer than two years, and many administrators found that the high rate of turnover precluded effective planning and coordination of services.[35] At least one researcher regarded the need to attract and retain young doctors to poor areas as the "principal problem" facing the entire movement, and indeed poor care in general.[36] CHCs might have alleviated the financing challenges for poor care, but they had done little to bring enough qualified personnel to the afflicted areas.

Overall, CHCs were a clear asset to poor communities. Local residents flocked to them once they opened, and found them less intimidating and less culturally alienating than private practice doctors. The social work component of the CHCs, along with their ability to coordinate primary and specialty care, laboratory work, and pharmaceutical services, all made for a more highly regulated poor care environment, which seemed to work to the greater salubrity of the affected patients. The centers represented a "truly remarkable initiative" in the effort to "improve the human condition," a group of social scientists at UCLA wrote in 1982.[37]

The success of CHCs and mobile clinics in providing care to hard-to-reach poor populations led some states to begin experimenting with enrolling Medicaid recipients in private health maintenance organizations (HMOs). From a charity care standpoint, the plans were attractive insofar as they promised to reduce the cost of providing Medicaid coverage while at the same time increasing the providers' abilities to coordinate care in ways similar to the CHCs. California, where HMOs had the greatest market share in the early 1970s, announced a plan to move half of its Medicaid population into HMOs by 1975, although it never managed to move more than 10 percent of all patients. At least thirteen other states followed California's lead in the next few years, such that by 1976 approximately 6 percent of all Medicaid care was being provided through prepaid HMOs.[38]

Outcomes for HMO-provided Medicaid care were mixed. One study of California's program deemed it "scandalous," but many states found that the programs reduced costs and improved health outcomes for the target population.[39] An experiment with enrolling Medicaid recipients in the Group Health Association (GHA) in Washington, D.C., for example, reduced hospitalizations and improved health outcomes for the enrolled group, while reducing costs as well. The GHA enrollees used fewer prescription medications with no obvious loss in treatment outcomes. One group of scholars studying the program wrote, "the decrease in medicine use rates and in other services with no decrease in patient satisfaction may justify enrolling welfare groups in prepaid group plans."[40]

Charity Care as Template?

The expansion of poverty programs, private insurance coverage, and biomedical research funding all contributed to robust national health by mid-decade. Declining rates of infectious disease and infant and maternal mortality, combined with advances in treatment for cancer, stroke, heart disease, and endocrine disorders, meant that people were living longer, dying more slowly, and recovering more frequently from practically everything. "In the year 1974, out of a population of around 220 million, only 1.9 million died, or just under 1 percent—not at all a discouraging record once you accept the fact of mortality itself," Lewis Thomas wrote.[41] This sanguine state presented the possibility of shifting medicine from crisis intervention, disease engagement, and preventing death to life improvement. With medical coverage available to all but the odd few not covered by Medicaid, Medicare, or private insurance, medicine stood poised to convert itself to a mechanism for social renewal.

The success of CHCs, rural clinics, and Medicaid HMOs suggested to some health planners that provider-driven medical care delivery ought to be the goal for the whole of the medical system. Proponents of this view advocated expanding community medicine both as an academic discipline and as a medical specialty. Foundations which funded research into health services delivery began to explore this possibility, with the Robert Wood Johnson Foundation funding the creation of fifty-three hospital-based community medicine groups nationwide in 1975. The project, which created prototypes for physician hospital organizations (PHOs), was granted $27 million over eight years, and ultimately funded seventy-seven community medical clinics.[42]

Physicians divided into two camps: those who decried the growth of community medicine departments, and those who feared that the current path of medicine was creating a profession overconcerned with disease and underconcerned with health. "What we don't need, and I fear we produce, are physicians blinded by the dazzling technology of medicine, which often does not affect, rarely cures, and sometimes causes the disease of our population," wrote David Rabin, a professor at Georgetown Medical School.[43] By contrast, one academic physician decried the growth of "splinter departments" of community medicine, and refused to accord them "the dignity of an academic title."[44] Those who advocated for community medicine saw the battle for poor care as central, not peripheral, to the entire medical enterprise, and cautioned against claiming victories in the war against pathogens at the same time that social pathology threatened to undermine the integrity of community bonds. "A health service system should focus not only on the state of the people's health, but also on the environment and the behavior of the community," wrote Sidney Klark, an Israeli professor of community medicine, in 1974,[45] while a cadre of professors of community medicine urged the profession to support them in their "prodigious task" of freeing those "trapped in our urban and rural ghettos."[46] Whether medicine should arrogate to itself the task of ameliorating the great divide between rich and poor, or rather focus on the limited task of repairing ailing and deficient tissues and biological systems, was one which would divide the profession for some time to come.

Rural Charity Care

Rural health conditions improved in the decade after 1965, with infant mortality often declining by 50 percent or more during this time. The rural poor continued to be sicker than the urban poor, however, for even as rural health had improved under Medicaid and other programs, urban health had improved more. By 1978 rates of chronic mental, musculoskeletal, and spinal disorders were all 10 percent higher in rural populations than in urban ones, and the gap in digestive and genitourinary disorders was almost as severe. And although nearly a hundred new "rural health initiative" projects (sponsored by the PHS) had been funded since 1975, large swaths of the countryside continued to be isolated from physicians' offices and community health centers.[47]

Various factors explained the rural-urban divide, although none did so wholly satisfactorily. Poor, rural households disproportionately had two resident parents rather than one, making them less eligible for Medicaid and welfare programs, and those families which did qualify for Medicaid found that the reimbursement rates were heavily skewed toward urban medical practices. (Annual Medicaid payments per child in the early 1970s averaged only $5 in rural areas, versus $76 in urban ones.)[48] An inadequate number of physician practices and hospital beds did not appear to be a factor in the discrepancy. One study in 1976 found that the Hill-Burton program had spurred sufficient hospital construction over the previous thirty years to supply rural counties with an adequate or slightly excess number of beds, while another study showed that inadequate incomes and excessive travel times were not preventing most rural residents from seeking appropriate health care.[49] Rather, the most likely explanation for the continuing discrepancy between the health status of poor urban and poor rural residents was differing knowledge of hygiene, and the residual effects of malnutrition and lack of prenatal care from thirty years previously.

A paucity in the countryside of state and municipally funded relief programs, as well as charitable institutions, made rural populations all the more dependent on a continued federal commitment to Medicaid, CHCs, and other subsidized charity care programs. Beaufort and Jasper counties in South Carolina, for example, each with a per capita income of just over $1,500 in 1976, faced medical catastrophe when the state threatened to cut Medicaid allocations by nearly a quarter. While the county health departments had cut infant mortality from 62 to 16 per 1,000 live births during the period from 1965 to 1975, their inability to continue these programs after 1976 threatened to return the areas "to the 19th century," in the words of the local attorney Scott Graber. Although the programs had brought potable water, insect control, physician care, and rehabilitative services, state politicians were unpersuaded of their urgency and voted repeatedly to cut funds. "You had [the poor] back in the days of Jesus Christ, you have got some now, and you will have some in the future," U.S. Senator Strom Thurmond noted dispassionately.[50] With Medicaid money on the decline, the centers would inevitably be forced to shrink.

More problematic to rural care generally was the diseconomy of operating small, rural hospitals, for Medicaid patients or anyone else. While

Hill-Burton funds had subsidized the construction of thousands of small hospitals in rural parts of the country, the program had provided only scant operating funds for the hospitals once opened, meaning that the finished hospitals needed to seek operating revenue from patients' billings, state charity funds, and elsewhere. But high rates of poverty in rural areas precluded the hospitals from earning a substantial portion of their revenue from privately insured patients, and low rates of Medicaid (and Medicare) reimbursement made it difficult to balance the operating budgets primarily on the strength of charity billings. Moreover, small hospitals, particularly rural ones, were simply economically inefficient as care deliverers. Hospitals with under 113 beds incurred nearly $10 more in costs per bed per day than larger hospitals, controlling for geography and the mix of patients. Although this differential could be partly offset by greater occupancy rates, rural hospitals by definition were almost certain to have lower occupancy rates than their urban counterparts. Medicare reimbursement rates were more generous to urban hospitals, because they took into account the greater costs of labor and real estate, but rural hospital faced unique costs which were mostly uncompensated by private insurance or Medicare. Furthermore, Medicaid programs in rural states were funded at substantially lower levels than programs in more urban states. Thus in addition to historical disparities in access to medical care, education, and adequate nutrition, the rural poor faced unique challenges in maintaining steady access to primary and hospital care, even after the advances wrought by Medicaid after 1965.[51]

Offsetting these disadvantages were several programs unique to rural areas. Some teaching hospitals established satellite clinics in rural areas beginning in the late 1960s, while others, in conjunction with state health departments, funded roving public health "teams" which would go door to door to provide psychological and neurological assessment tests, nutrition counseling, hearing and vision assessment, and general primary care.[52] In Nebraska rural physicians aggressively used physicians' assistants to help with patient loads, while elsewhere states used funds provided by the federal Rural Health Clinics program to establish small, rural clinics that would serve predominantly poor populations.[53] But overall these programs failed to compensate for the differences in Medicaid funding between rich and poor states. So long as Mississippi, Alabama, and Kentucky funded their Medicaid programs at less than one fourth the levels per recipient of New York and California, they would be unable to provide satisfactory care at all levels to their poor residents, regardless of community concern and commitment.

The single greatest weakness in the rural health net was mental health. Before 1965, when most severely mentally ill patients were committed to large state hospitals, a lack of proximate mental health facilities was irrelevant to a patient's ability to gain access to care. But with large-scale deinstitutionalization in the mid-1960s (resulting, ironically, from Medicaid reimbursement for nursing home care, as well as from new drugs), the severely mentally ill were forced to rely on local community mental health centers (CMHCS) or psychiatric clinics within community health centers. Although the federal CMHC Act of 1965 provided construction funds for the centers, few were built in rural areas, leaving psychiatric patients from rural areas without institutional recourse. By 1976 the national inpatient population of psychiatric hospitals had fallen from 550,000 to 200,000, and many states hoped to reduce their inpatient populations to zero. Where CMHCS *were* built, they were often quite successful, attracting many outpatients to their psychotherapy centers and day hospitals.[54] But shortfalls in CMHC construction, particularly in rural areas, led many states to abandon plans for closing out the state hospital systems.[55] By 1978 a White House commission on mental health reported that mental health services in rural areas were "frequently nonexistent" and "almost never comprehensive," and that the mental health system was "unfinished."[56] Although more money would help, the simple facts of demographic dispersal in rural areas made the goal of universal access to comprehensive mental health services unrealistic.[57]

By 1976 Medicaid had accomplished much, albeit at the cost of imbalanced program funding, discontinuous coverage, abrupt service gaps, and general weakness in rural areas. Both the CHC and CMHC programs had reached a plateau or begun to ebb under the onslaught of congressional budget reductions, and foreign medical graduates were providing a substantial (and growing) amount of care to the nation's poor. While all major health indicators showed an improved health status nationally, particularly among the poor, a stubborn gap in service quality between poor care and private care remained, thwarting the hopes of Medicaid's designers to eliminate the two-tiered system. Adding to the shortfalls, inconsistencies between Medicaid and other welfare programs meant that the poor were left to navigate a strange amalgam of uncoordinated charity programs, each with different eligibility criteria, benefit structures, and administrative hierarchies, creating a bewildering bureaucratic barrier to gaining access to necessary services, for health care or otherwise.

8

Health and Welfare Reform in
the Carter White House

President Jimmy Carter's attitude toward health care was complex. In part he viewed it as a component of the greater social safety net which needed to be funded, like welfare, at adequate levels to ensure access for all; in part he viewed it as a threat to the nation's economic security, absorbing an increasing portion of the nation's resources without delivering obvious benefit; and last, he viewed health care consumption, to some degree, as a measure of moral failing for those who failed to refrain from insalubrious activities. Breaking with most previous health reformers, he declared, in addition to making the usual calls for cost cutting and greater managerial efficiency, that a reasonable government health policy must encourage "health-enhancing behavior" from all citizens.[1]

Carter's initial response to the twin challenges of gaps in health coverage and runaway medical care inflation was comprehensive reform. He entered office, as Truman had thirty years before, committed to a national health payment plan (left conspicuously undefined during his campaign), which would extend coverage to the twenty million Americans who lacked either private or public coverage. Coupled with this goal was a commitment to better distribution of medical care in those regions which lacked enough doctors and hospitals, and improved control of hospital inflation, which at the time was exceeding 18 percent a year. "The American people will not accept, and I will not propose, any health care plan which is inflationary," Carter wrote in mid-1978.[2] Total national health expenditures, which were $162 billion in 1977, were projected to rise to $320 billion by 1983, and possibly as high as half a trillion dollars by 1990. Whatever plan was ultimately developed by his domestic policy and legislative staffs and relevant agencies would need to contain "aggressive cost containment measures" to be acceptable to the president.[3]

From the beginning, Carter's vision of health reform was a mixture of the prudent and the quixotic. Cognizant of the influence of the private insurance industry, he demanded a proposal which would integrate existing carriers and employer-provided coverage into its final form, following the template of what later came to be known as "pay or play" plans. At the same time, he recognized the potential savings to be wrung out of inefficient administration and superfluous hospital building. But unrealistically, Carter committed himself to unimpeded access to physicians for all consumers, be they Medicaid patients, private insurance beneficiaries, or Medicare recipients, even though in 1977 most health reformers believed that the most promising route to cost containment was to limit access to specialists through capitation, gatekeeping, HMOs, and other managed-care techniques. Carter was not able to accept (and indeed never accepted throughout his administration) that cost containment could only come with concomitant denial of choice, and that steering patients toward cheaper doctors, cheaper hospitals, and less highly specialized doctors was the most potent tool at his disposal to limit medical expenditures. In part this reflected the primitive state of managed care in 1977, and in part it reflected Carter's own ideas regarding social equity and human welfare.

Carter's other great failing in his initial approach to health reform was his insistence on comprehensive, rather than incremental, reform. Along with various legislative leaders of the past, such as Robert Wagner, James Murray, John Dingell, and Claude Pepper, as well as Truman, Carter looked to the nationalized insurance systems of Europe as a basic model for an ideal health system. All who had ever attempted such comprehensive reform over the previous six decades had failed to achieve not only a grandiose vision of reform, but any reform at all. By contrast, the incremental reforms of Franklin Roosevelt in his first administration (including an expansion of public health programs), Calvin Coolidge (who oversaw the enactment of the Sheppard-Towner act for pediatric care), and Lyndon Johnson (Medicare and Medicaid) had all assumed a *limited* governmental role, rather than a comprehensive one. The lesson from history concerning health reform at both the federal and state levels was that political leaders should target specific portions of the population which needed more care, and provide them with as much care as was politically realistic. Politicians who had attempted to wholly remake the system, or mandate the provision of care to those who already had access to care, had accomplished little.

Hospital Cost Containment

Dominating the list of health care concerns for Carter was hospital inflation. Over the previous few years hospital costs had risen at a rate of nearly 15 percent a year, bringing current national expenditures to $75 billion and government spending to $18 billion, expected to rise to $30 billion by 1978. If left unchecked, hospital inflation was predicted to drive annual expenditures in the United States to $100 billion by 1980.[4] Driving the inflation was hospitals' increased investment in technology and equipment, meaning that although patient days were staying constant or actually declining in certain cases, the cost per patient day, and per patient admission overall, was increasing quickly. In 1976 and 1977 expenses per admission rose by 15 and 13 percent, and revenue per patient day rose by nearly 16 percent in each year. Notably, the number of hospital beds stayed nearly the same during these years, and outpatient expenses rose by little more than the overall rate of inflation.[5]

By 1975 the United States was spending a larger portion of its GNP on health care than all but three other nations—West Germany, Sweden, and the Netherlands—and growth trends indicated that it would soon overtake even those. At 8.4 percent of all domestic spending, health care had nearly doubled its claim on the nation's resources from 1960, and was vying for preeminence as the single largest sector in the American economy. Whereas France, Canada, and Australia had once spent nearly 60 percent more of their GNP on health care than the United States, since the inauguration of Medicare the United States had surpassed them. The Social Security Administration estimated that within a year the United

States would rank first in the world in the proportion of GNP going to health care expenditures (nearly 9 percent), and no country stood to match the record anytime soon.[6]

Although the Carter administration brought the issue of hospital cost inflation to the forefront of its domestic agenda, states had been grappling with rising health care expenditures for some time already. As Medicaid allocations drew an increasing share of state funds from competing programs through the late 1960s, governors and state treasurers identified hospital bills as primary targets for cost cutting, and began to take appropriate legislative action. Governor Marvin Mandel of Maryland, for example, drafted legislation in the early 1970s to require more uniform hospital accounting, budget review, and reporting for all hospitals in the state receiving Medicaid payments (which was nearly all of them), and Governor Raul Castro of Arizona made similar efforts in 1972.[7] All states throughout the country had implemented CON processes starting in 1972, with varying degrees of success. Any victories were pyrrhic, however. Those states which were actually managing to contain Medicaid inflation were finding that private health insurance costs were rising at rates above the national average, meaning that at least some of the hospital reimbursement savings produced by Medicaid programs were simply being shifted to the private sector.

Many health planners suspected that the single greatest culprit in hospital inflation was rapidly evolving technology, which produced astronomical bills for hospital capital budgets even while it frequently led to revolutionary developments in patient care and diagnosis. Although the postwar expansion of the nation's basic biomedical research budget had brought laudable advancements in many areas of disease treatment, the advances had come at a high price from which the public had been largely shielded. Much of the equipment necessary to apply the scientific breakthroughs to patient care had been purchased by hospitals, and the hospitals had simply passed the costs along through higher billing rates. The result was a growing burden which threatened to undermine the competitiveness of American industry, overwhelm state budgets, and impoverish private patients. While the bills for the advancements had been delayed because of the usual lag between breakthrough in the lab and technological application, by 1975 they were beginning to come due.[8]

Although Carter's domestic policy staff quickly identified hospital cost inflation as the primary challenge in any health care reform, other individuals and groups studying the problem were not so certain. The AHA and AMA both disclaimed culpability for the impending cost crisis, if indeed there was a crisis, and suggested that adequate results could be achieved through the simple exercise of common sense. Physicians proposed a gradual equalization of reimbursement rates between outpatient and inpatient procedures to discourage doctors from admitting patients unnecessarily, and at least one physician suggested that merely returning graduates of foreign medical schools to their countries upon completion of residencies would further help reduce medical expenditures. Other suggestions included consolidating hospital management into a few larger institutions for the sake of administrative efficiency, eliminating Medicare fraud, encouraging more doctors to seek training in the primary-care specialties, and closing superfluous hospitals. But the paramount concern for most health care professionals and administrators was maintaining control of future policy development, regardless of the direction that such development might eventually take. "We as physicians are in the best position to make the changes that will safeguard the health of our patients and foster the continuation of high-quality health care," wrote Vernon Mark, a physician from Boston, in an editorial in JAMA.[9] But the health policy analyst David Mechanic, drawing on data from the Congressional Budget Office (CBO), was unconvinced: "There is little evidence that physicians who practice under fee-for-service reimbursement are taking positive steps to limit the use of procedures of marginal value," he wrote. "Nor is there strong indication that professional standards review organizations (PSROs) are contributing in any substantial way to cost control."[10]

Inflation in Medicaid

Medicaid expenditures had risen by 231 percent between 1970 and 1976. Carter's aides estimated that current growth, if continued unabated, would bring the program to $33.1 billion by 1982—a sum far in excess of the ability of state and federal governments to fund under prevailing tax formulas. Unlike the health sector as a whole, in which increased costs per patient were the primary contributors to inflation, Medicaid inflation was driven equally by increasing costs per patient and the expansion built into the program's mandate. Program enrollment had nearly tripled since its early years, and even in 1975 states still tried to add patients to their Medicaid plans. Because Medicaid was the single largest source of health expenditures for state government (and increasingly the single largest budget item for the states overall), the Carter administration took particular care in formulating a response to the challenges which inflation posed to the program.

One effort at cost control involved moving the program to block funding rather than entitlement funding. Block funding had been proposed during the waning days of the Ford administration, when White House staffers had proposed eliminating sixteen federal categorical programs, including Medicaid, health planning, maternal and child health, and community mental health centers, and converting them all into one large block grant under a new Financial Assistance for Health Care Act. The main advantage of doing so would be to build incentives at the state level for more effective management. Responsibility for poor care would devolve to the states, and Congress would be exonerated from the cuts in charity provision likely to occur in lean future years. Arguing against such a conversion was the prevailing feeling that the federal government had the obligation to guarantee adequate funding for poverty care as enshrined in the Medicaid program, regardless of states' ability to pay. Already the federal government had adjusted its payment ratio upward to match state expenditures at levels higher than had been required under the initial legislation; future guarantees to poor states would be necessary if minimum standards of poverty care were to be maintained.[11]

More radical was the proposal to move Medicaid from a "reasonable cost" to a prospective purchasing system. Prospective purchasing (sometimes referred to as "prudent buying") would allow state governments to purchase service in bulk from large contracted providers (major hospitals and large medical groups), thereby exerting market leverage on the pricing of the services while shifting the risk of adverse selection to the providers from the payers. The resulting capitation would force physicians and hospitals to cut their own costs and ultimately rethink their investment in the inflationary high technology which was consuming so much of their capital investments. While four states at the time were already experimenting with prospective payment systems (California, Colorado, Massachusetts, and New York), those states were structuring their payment forms to more closely resemble what would ultimately become diagnostic related groups rather than contracted capitation. The suggested program would be experimental.[12]

States viewed the idea unenthusiastically. Even as White House analysts urged caution in attempting a prudent buyer scheme—suggesting perhaps that states be only encouraged, rather than mandated, to work toward such a program—the loss of provider choice which would necessarily result threatened to derail the proposal.[13] The United States was not ready in 1977 to admit that cost containment, whether in Medicaid or in the private sector, could be achieved only by fundamentally limiting access to high-priced specialists and hospitals. Despite the already widespread understanding that hospital admissions were driving the costs of health care, health planners were unwilling to confront the political opposition which would result from offering physicians incentives to keep their patients out of hospitals, nor were they willing to create approved lists of physicians and gatekeeping primary-care providers for patients. Such a world still lay in the future.

The approach finally chosen by the administration was a simple universal cost cap of 9 percent on the average charges per admission for all hospitals accepting Medicaid and Medicare patients. Viewed as a "necessary first step" in getting the system under control, and for ultimately creating a receptive environment for comprehensive payment reform (the usual euphemism for national health insurance), the mechanism would be enforced by a 150 percent tax on all revenue produced by outside billings (thus thwarting a simple shifting of costs from government payers to private ones) and would save the government an estimated $10 billion a year by 1981.[14] The approach, viewed as "interim" by Carter's domestic policy advisor Stuart Eizenstat, would be implemented for eighteen to twenty-four months, and then be superseded by a comprehensive payment reform bill being drafted by Senator Herman Talmadge (D., Ga.).[15] Initial analysis of the proposal's political viability indicated that it was supported by labor, business, and the health insurance industry but vigorously opposed by hospitals and doctors. Insurance companies supported it for fear that if the administration limited only Medicare and Medicaid expenditures, hospitals would simply shift rising costs over to the private payers, while hospitals and doctors, as usual, opposed any outside infringement on their decision-making authority.[16]

Carter broadcast the proposal in 1977 in a speech in which he predicted that the program would save nearly $2 billion in 1978 alone ($650 million in federal expenditures, $300 million in state expenditures, and $900 million in private payments), and that savings would grow to $5.5 billion by 1980. He further emphasized that these savings were necessary if he were to later move toward a program of national health insurance— one of the basic points of his campaign platform. While the caps would limit the ability of hospitals to invest in new equipment and building programs, Carter emphasized that they would leave hospital management free to choose the best response for each institution. There would be no micromanagement of medical care.[17]

But the hospital lobby effectively attacked the proposed program while it was being debated in Congress, and persuaded sympathetic lawmakers to amend the bill into banality.[18] A planned capital investment cap of $2.5 billion was raised to $4 billion, far above the sum the industry would have spent over the subsequent years, while the 9 percent cap on operating increases was deleted. "The bill as altered today . . . is a sham," stated the secretary of health, education, and welfare, Joseph Califano, at a news conference the following July. "It is an affront to the American people and the administration's attempt to combat inflation."[19] Although various compromise amendments were offered, nothing substantial ever reached the floor.[20] Gone was the potential savings of $56 billion over five years, and gone too was the possibility of enacting comprehensive insurance reform, for that was impossible in the present inflationary environment.

Comprehensive Payment Reform

The other great issue concerning health care delivery in 1976 was the nation's conspicuous lack of a national health insurance program, be it simply an expansion of Medicare and Medicaid, a pay-or-play program along the lines of Nixon's CHIP program, a single-payer Canadian model, or some combination of these. The great gap in insurance coverage, leading to alarming statistics for unreimbursed care, pointed to either a failing of domestic policy or a lack of compassion for one's fellow citizens. At least half a dozen legislative teams tried their hand at drafting remedies for the gap in the mid-1970s.

The major challenge facing all legislative efforts, including notable efforts by Senator Edward Kennedy (D., Mass.) and Representative Ronald Dellums (D., Calif.), was Americans' fairly high level of satisfaction with their health coverage in 1977. Not only was insurance reform not a high priority for most American voters, it was actually disfavored by many, lest the product be degraded by government involvement. The hospital inflation which Carter deemed one of the gravest threats to domestic tranquility hardly threatened the average American middle-class wage earner, for once deductibles were met both physician care and hospital care were effectively free. Since most families had experienced only constantly improving medical and hospital care throughout their lives, patients were highly laudatory of their doctors and hospitals. However prescient Carter may have been about the underlying instability in the system, drawing attention to the issue would bring little political benefit, and potentially great harm.

A major problem for the administration in supporting the bills percolating through Congress was that it made the president appear to have been "dragged reluctantly" to the issue (in the words of Carter's health aide Peter Bourne), despite his having made national health insurance a central component of his presidential campaign. In the eyes of the administration it would be preferable to launch a major initiative on the issue that would shore up support from blacks, labor, the elderly, and the poor, while confirming Carter's commitment to his campaign promise. In the ascetic culture of the Carter administration, national health insurance would be an example of the president's "giving something" to the voters rather than asking them to "make sacrifices in the National interest."[21] Although Califano had established an Advisory Committee on National Health Insurance Issues within months of Carter's inauguration, and had emphasized that the issue was a "cornerstone in the structure of the President's domestic policy," the first year had been devoted to hospital cost containment, not national health insurance.[22] Bourne reminded the president that failure to act on the issue during his administration's first year had put him in a "bad posture," with most Americans doubting the president's commitment to reform.[23]

The administration's commitment to the issue was predicated on the assumption that most Americans supported national health insurance (despite their reluctance to say so), and that Carter's victory in 1976 had been based in part on support from middle- and working-class voters for a substantial executive action on the issue. The support for the measure was "shallow and latent," however, and had only diminished over the previous decades as progressively greater portions of the middle class had been granted private health coverage by their employers. Although Carter retained a certain quixotic preference for a truly comprehensive reform bill, even more he favored a bill which could pass. "Political pragmatism should primarily dictate the content of the bill," Bourne wrote in 1978.[24] Only a small range of possible actions could win the support of both Congress and the administration.[25]

Califano supported the pragmatic approach. He warned throughout the first half of Carter's term in office that virtually every other industrialized nation which had implemented national health insurance over the past century had done so while conserving the basic payment structures already in place. This had meant conserving the nineteenth-century sickness funds in Germany, and existing private insurers in Japan and France. Only Britain had fundamentally nationalized an existing private system, and this had been done in two phases, with payment reform long preceding delivery reform. (Not insignificantly, that delivery reform in Great Britain had only become politically feasible during the economic gray days of the postwar years.) For the United States, with an enormous existing system of private payers and providers, independent medical schools and hospitals, and self-policing professions and specialty groups, successful legislation would have to acknowledge and mollify stakeholders in the existing scheme while applying pressure to individuals and institutions to reform their extravagant ways. Caution and sobriety would be necessary precursors to comprehensive reform.[26] Health reformers who argued that health care should follow the example of public education failed to see that public education systems were established at a time when few private alternatives existed, and thus could be created whole with little entrenched opposition.[27]

The resulting administration bill, the National Health Plan of 1979, created a new "HealthCare" program which would federalize Medicaid and combine it administratively with Medicare to create a comprehensive national insurance policy for all families earning under 55 percent of the federal poverty rate.[28] Families earning slightly more than this could qualify for HealthCare by paying a modest deductible, and employers could purchase policies for their employees through the HealthCare program as well. The second component of Carter's plan was mandated employer-provided insurance for all employees who worked more than twenty-five hours per week in ten weeks per quarter, and their families. Employees would be required to pay no more than 25 percent of the premium, and federally recognized qualifying private insurers would be required to cover comprehensive services after a $2,500 deductible per family (per year). With these two measures, the administration hoped to cover the majority of the nation's uninsured. In addition, the programs mandated continued private coverage for all employees for the first ninety days after leaving a job, and sought to restrain inflation by means of certain cost-containment measures (such as incentives to use HMOs and hospital investment caps).[29]

Carter's bill was actually a deft compromise incorporating employer-mandated pay-or-play proposals, Medicaid reform, and hospital cost containment, all of which had been proposed under other guises through the years. By preserving the private insurance sector, the bill could potentially win the support of the insurance industry, the hospitals, and the doctors. By mandating catastrophic coverage rather than first-dollar coverage, it could thwart opposition from small business owners. By melding Medicaid with Medicare, it would assuage Medicaid's critics, who attacked the program for providing second-tier medical care. And by promoting primary care, HMOs, and hospital investment caps, it could restrain inflation and pave the way for a more comprehensive, national single-payer model. The proposal reflected a mastery of political gamesmanship and policy expertise. Opponents would include the elderly, who would resent being grouped with the poor, businesses with many part-time workers who worked just over twenty-five hours a week, and political conservatives who resisted any expansion of government involvement in health care, no matter how deft or sensitive.

But despite the deftness of the legislation, it was doomed. No program rectifying a situation which 85 percent of the population did not view as problematic stood a realistic chance of passing Congress, and Carter's health plan was not an exception. It lost its most potentially influential congressional backer by diverging from Kennedy's plan, as well as the support of the elderly, organized labor, and much of the middle class by tampering with a system which pleased most of these groups' members. Weakened by his ineffectiveness in handling the Iran hostage crisis, by his lack of Washington connections, and by his low approval ratings, Carter lacked the political capital necessary to pass such an ambitious and visible piece of domestic legislation, and in failing to do so he irreparably harmed his chances of enacting comprehensive health reform during the remainder of his term.

Welfare Reform

Carter's drive toward comprehensive health reform, predicated on controlling costs in the system, was part of a larger commitment to reform of the social welfare system. The three main components of the system besides Medicaid—Aid to Families with Dependent Children (AFDC), Supplementary Security Income (SSI), and Food Stamps—were begun in the New Deal (or shortly thereafter) and had since been modified repeatedly. By 1977 the three programs had grown far beyond their original targeted populations and were rife with inequities, paradoxical loopholes, counterincentives to socially and economically responsible behavior, and eligibility gaps. The Food Stamp program, for example, which had begun with the express intention of supplementing the nutritional intake of poor families during the Depression while helping to bolster farm incomes and distribute surplus food stockpiles, had shed most of its purchasing guidelines, creating odd opportunities for poor families to use their stamps to purchase luxury foodstuffs. Such purchases might serve a "psychological, sociological, or economic need," one scholar wrote, "but hardly a physiological or nutritional need."[30] As the Food Stamp program was administered under separate eligibility guidelines in each state, different populations were able to qualify for different components of the welfare program depending on their state of residence. New Hampshire,

Delaware, Oklahoma, Arizona, and Nevada provided no food stamps at all, while Mississippi and Louisiana, two states with relatively modest populations, between them distributed nearly 15 percent of all federal food stamp subsidies. Similarly, annual AFDC benefits for a family ranged from $720 in Mississippi to over $5,954 in Hawaii. While cost-of-living differences explained part of the disparity, differing degrees of government largesse explained most of it.

The AFDC program had grown and expanded in unpredictable directions. It had doubled from 770,000 recipient families to 1.6 million between 1959 and 1969, then again to 3.5 million families by 1977. By that time nearly half of all families in the program were either black or nonwhite Hispanic, over 80 percent lived in urban areas, and nearly half lived within the downtown core of aging cities. As originally planned, the program continued to subsidize primarily those families with absent fathers, but the reasons for the fathers' absences had changed over time. While the program was initially envisioned as a means to guarantee the financial stability of widowed mothers, or mothers whose husbands were permanently incapacitated, it now subsidized those families in which the father simply no longer supported the family, or never had. By 1979 only 2 percent of all AFDC families were those in which the father had died, and only 5 percent were families in which the father was disabled. A further 4 percent qualified because the father was temporarily unemployed, and the rest—nearly 85 percent—qualified because the live, able-bodied father simply refused to support dependent children.[31]

The three welfare programs were derided by reformers for being inequitable, inaccessible, and antifamily. They had substantial weaknesses. The dollar amounts of the benefits were often so low as to preclude the recipients from living with any sort of dignity. Families could be disenrolled for seemingly capricious causes. Eligibility requirements for the three programs were inconsistent with each other (meaning that a family might qualify for Food Stamps but not for Medicaid, or vice versa). And the mixture of federal guidelines and state administration guaranteed certain administrative tensions between the different levels of government. Overshadowing these deficiencies was the problem that the programs (AFDC in particular) actually discouraged employment and marriage (either of which was sufficient to disqualify an applicant), meaning

that the system fundamentally encouraged exactly those types of behavior most closely associated with long-term poverty.[32] While the more
naïve supporters of the status quo suggested that the tenacious American
work ethic would counterbalance the disincentives to seek employment
for those on welfare rolls, that belief defied reality. "Such comments are
usually made by those who, one way or another, are so situated in life that
they earn $30,000 or more a year for attending meetings, reading news-
papers, and writing memorandums," one acerbic columnist wrote.[33] So
glaring was the problem that fixing eligibility requirements so as to encourage work (and marriage) became a paramount administration goal
from the outset. "Provide maximum incentive to work," Califano wrote
to Carter in the administration's early months. "Place as many incentives
as possible for keeping the family together."[34]

Carter's initial attempt at restructuring welfare, the Program for Better
Jobs and Income (PBJI) of 1977, would have abolished the existing programs entirely and replaced them with a single jobs-oriented welfare
program which mandated consistent benefit levels among the states. The
program's two major goals—increasing the number of recipients who
held jobs, and increasing the number of recipients who stayed married
(or married in the first place)—would be accomplished by implementing
incentives to work and marry, and by creating a large federal training and
jobs program to offer nearly 1.5 million positions to people in the welfare
system. These proposals were supplemented with a series of administrative reforms that would consolidate Food Stamps, SSI, and AFDC into a
single cash benefit program, purportedly reduce fraud and error, and
expand federal subsidies to the states. The new program would aim to
produce better benefits at only marginally greater costs.

The jobs program was clearly the weak component of the proposal. No
comparable effort had been made since the early days of the New Deal,
when the creation of jobs programs had been facilitated by uniquely high
unemployment rates. Moreover, even in the Depression political resistance to the New Deal had been fierce, and many of the jobs programs had
been largely disbanded by 1936.[35] The creation of 1.5 million new jobs by a
government facing a decidedly jaded electorate, whose trust in government had been sorely tested by the Vietnam War and Watergate, was a
quixotic undertaking from the start. Even the president admitted that the

jobs program was a "substantial undertaking" that would need to be "imaginative" to succeed.[36] In the end, the magnitude of the proposal, coupled with political resistance to so substantial a makeover in the nation's social safety net, proved beyond the political capacity of the administration. The program was rejected in committee.

Over the following year, while Carter focused his personal attention on hospital cost control, administration aides and select cabinet officials (particularly Califano and the labor secretary, Ray Marshall) worked on producing a series of limited measures designed to produce tangible results in welfare reform without alienating opponents. Planners settled on a series of changes designed to improve the system overall, but these did not alter its systemic weaknesses, grounded in ambiguous federal control and lack of coordination. Their recommendations included reducing benefit inequities between the states, through either increased federal subsidies or more tightly regulated federal spending mandates; expanding the earned income tax credit to aid low-income families currently ineligible for welfare; modulating benefit payments to offer incentives to work; and offering cash in lieu of Food Stamps for the ssi population ("cashing out" the program, in agency jargon). By maintaining state control over the three programs as well as continuing separate administration of them, policymakers hoped to ward off complaints by governors, states' rights advocates, and state government lobbyists, all of whom objected to the usurpation of state control of the programs by federal agencies. The final recommendations, delivered to the president at the end of 1978, discontinued separate application for food stamps from the disabled (by cashing out the program), increased cash aid to two-parent households temporarily unemployed, and provided federally subsidized job training and job creation, along with cash incentives to seek work. (The last was accomplished by reducing benefits by one dollar for each dollar earned.)[37]

The scaled-down program would cost only $5.7 billion once implemented—less than half the cost of the failed reforms from two years previous—and reduce poverty rolls by 800,000 families: a respectable, though hardly revolutionary accomplishment. In a bow to political reality, the president acknowledged that welfare reform was a "difficult undertaking," one surrounded by "hopeful rhetoric" which often as not failed to deliver on its promises.[38] The tempered ambition of the new proposal reduced its potential to disappoint, though it also prevented the administration from accomplishing some of its most cherished goals. After multiple amendments and markups, the programs passed in the following year.

The changes to welfare as embodied in the PBJI proposals represented more than merely a step toward more efficient administration of a cumbersomely bureaucratic program; they symbolized an effort to move welfare beyond merely a "means to ward off starvation" (in the words of the social scientist Leslie Lenkowsky) and toward a program of income redistribution. As conceived in the 1930s, welfare had encompassed a certain recognition of the moral worth of the poor (or lack of moral worth), and had rewarded only the deserving accordingly. Poverty alone had not justified eligibility. Rather, poverty required accompanying children, disability, or widowhood to make it worthy. In moving to include married couples, as well as able-bodied and working people, Carter came close to recognizing a claim that all Americans—not just the morally deserving—deserved a minimum income. "To each according to his needs; that was the new ethic of liberal social policy," Lenkowsky wrote in 1979.[39] Congress's rejection of the initial PBJI bill suggested that it, and perhaps the nation as a whole, was not yet ready to wholly divorce welfare benefits from standards of moral worth.

The Child Health Assessment Program

Medicaid, by contrast, had initially signaled a weakening of the association between charity medicine and moral rectitude. By further removing poor care from the discretion of sectarian hospitals—a movement which had been progressing for several decades by 1965—the federal government was proclaiming its unwillingness to make individual discretion and judgment a precondition for medical care. When medical care had added more comfort than remedy to the lives of the ill, the test had seemed sound: only the worthy would be entitled to spiritual comfort and succor. As medical care became highly decisive in recuperation and even life, however, the moral pronouncement had come to seem too harsh. Still, the virtual exclusion of single men and childless women under early Medicaid eligibility requirements suggested that vestiges of the old standards remained.

Carter's commitment to serving all of the poor, and not just the worthy among them, was exhibited in his Child Health Assessment Program (CHAP), which had been conceived alongside the original Hospital Cost Containment Act of 1977. Over three fourths of the twelve million children eligible for coverage under EPSDT were failing to apply or qualify, and consequently at least ten million children were going without necessary pediatric care. Commenting on the situation, the noted child development scholar Jessie Bierman observed, "The Russians will lick us; they will lick us because they take care of their children and we do not."[40] CHAP made children from families above the poverty threshold with two resident, working parents eligible for Medicaid. It was a pragmatic move which recognized that many families which technically could afford basic pediatric care went without it, partly because of competing spending priorities within the home, and partly because states failed to subsidize the families to the extent allowable by federal law. The program lowered the eligibility level for Medicaid reimbursement, raised federal Medicaid subsidies to the states, covered prenatal care for otherwise nonqualifying women, and guaranteed coverage for children even after their families failed to qualify for general Medicaid.

Discussion over CHAP was postponed for several years as Congress shelved Medicaid and health reform repeatedly while grappling with cost containment, but by 1980 the debate had resumed. The Children's Defense Fund lobbied hard for the bill, pressuring the administration to make it a priority and warning recalcitrant members of Congress that they would face the ire of a growing child welfare constituency. Beyond all else, CHAP made fiscal sense: children treated in state-run programs similar to CHAP cost those states 40 percent less in lifetime medical bills than children initially excluded from primary care. A basic pediatric check-up cost $20 in most states, and the total annual cost of CHAP coverage was estimated to be about $325—"less than it costs your Senator to belong to a country club," in the words of Marian Wright Edelman.[41] The bill, passed in both houses of Congress over the previous year, went to conference committee, where a successful compromise was negotiated.

By 1978 Medicaid was exhibiting the same "gap" shortcoming as welfare. As with welfare, some of the poorest people were being cared for while at the same time many were being excluded. But in a situation unique to charity medical care, the excluded had a panoply of alternative institutions to which they could resort. As Medicaid patients departed public hospitals in large numbers to seek care from private urban hospitals, the public hospitals became the refuge of the working poor who could neither qualify for Medicaid nor afford private health insurance. State charity care funds as well filled the gaps in the Medicaid program, as the uninsured and underinsured appealed to the agencies administering them for help in shouldering premiums, co-payments, deductibles, and uncovered services. A study by HCFA in 1980 found that nearly a quarter of all medical care was being paid for out of pocket, with only the Medicaid population escaping the onus of private billing. Some 4 percent of people were paying medical bills which constituted over 15 percent of their family's income, and of this high-paying group, nearly 90 percent belonged to families with incomes below 200 percent of the poverty level.[42] This "notch" paralleled the gap which had prompted Carter to reform eligibility for the welfare system, and Medicaid watchers similarly questioned whether a system so flawed could remain useful. A system which taxed certain citizens without care to provide others with care was "totally wrong," declared the director of Medicaid for New York City, Martin Paris. The city's health commissioner, Lowell Bellin, agreed: "Fewer and fewer people are being served, and the public is getting angrier. The time bomb has to go off."[43]

Carter's efforts to incrementally advance Medicaid, most noticeably in the form of the CHAP program, were both an effort to recognize Medicaid as subordinate to general welfare programs requiring similar incremental reforms and a pragmatic retort to the defeat of his comprehensive payment legislation. In the best of all worlds Medicaid would cease to exist, having been superseded by a unified national health insurance system. In the world of realpolitik, where entrenched political interests (as well as a leery public) resisted large-scale government reform, Medicaid remained a necessary component of the nation's social safety net, and as such needed to be gradually enlarged to care for as large a portion of the nation's needy as was politically and fiscally possible. In the president's words, CHAP was a "crucial first step," though he slyly refrained from defining the ultimate goal as a more inclusive Medicaid program in an all-encompassing national health system.[44]

The late 1970s were dominated by Carter's ambitious plans to both control hospital costs and initiate some form of national health insurance. Both aspirations met with only partial success, but in facing congressional and popular opposition to his proposals, the president learned the lesson that legions of political leaders and health reformers had learned before him—health reform in America was best conducted in small increments. Recovering from the failure of his comprehensive reform legislation, Carter began the slow process of gradually filling in gaps in health coverage by expanding Medicaid, realigning welfare programs, retuning public health efforts, and generally placing resources where they could do some good without intimidating or alienating politically sensitive constituencies. By taking the gradual approach, Carter was able to improve health care delivery for the poor and working class without greatly threatening the integrity of the major participants in the private system. Yet by maintaining that system, he ultimately failed to rectify the extravagance implicit in its market-driven character. America entered the 1980s healthier than before, with a more equitable health system, but with significant discrepancies in the quality of the care delivered to rich and poor, urban dweller and rural, white and black, and privately insured and self-insured. Moreover, inflation continued to loom over the health care sector in the wake of the ineffective cost control legislation enacted in the late 1970s. Charity care by 1980 was good, though hardly excellent, and for the working poor it was greatly deficient.

9

Block Grants and the New Federalism

Financial Crisis

The compromised amendments to Medicaid produced by the Carter administration failed to rectify many of the program's festering problems. By 1981 nearly half of all Americans living in households below the federal poverty line—some twelve million people—had failed either to apply or to qualify for Medicaid. The group included the usual ranks of the excluded—single individuals and childless couples—as well as those odd few falling into the ineligible income gap, or those living in the handful of states which refused to extend their Medicaid programs to provide optional coverage for the working poor. True to the welfare roots of the program, children tended to be more eligible than adults: 65 percent of all of the eligible poor were minors, though only 36 percent of all poor were minors. In addition, certain states had expanded eligibility limits to individuals and households above the federal poverty limit. California and New York, notably, had a disproportionate share of these, claiming more than a third of all such recipients nationally.

The program had grown throughout the 1970s, with the AFDC sector growing at a rate of 9 percent a year to 11.4 million recipients, although in recent years this had leveled off. More worrisome from a budgetary standpoint was the relatively rapid rise in the number of aged, blind, and disabled recipients, which paralleled expanded SSI eligibility standards. Although this group made up less than one third of the total Medicaid population, it consumed a highly disproportionate share of the program's resources. In 1978, for example, disabled recipients cost the various state programs an average of $1,600, versus $920 for the aged poor and $580 for adults in AFDC families. Although the federally mandated benefit menu had remained essentially the same, the cost of many of the required services, particularly for the disabled, had increased substantially throughout the 1970s. Adding to this financial load was the ballooning use of Medicaid to pay for nursing home care, which had risen over 150 percent during the 1970s. By 1978 over 40 percent of all Medicaid outlays were for nursing home care, and budget analysts suggested that this figure would continue to rise. As noted earlier, Medicaid itself was partly responsible for the growing use of nursing homes to house the enfeebled elderly: during the few years following the program's inception, the use of nursing homes had increased by more than 50 percent.[1]

The twin bogeymen of service gaps and rising costs prompted congressional interest in Medicaid reform in 1981. Reform could take a number of shapes, including increased eligibility standards, reduced benefits, reduced reimbursement for covered services, and tighter limits on state programs for which the federal government would pay. The National Health Care Reform Act of 1981 proposed to overhaul the program by providing vouchers to poor persons who would spend them on competing private health plans. The plan failed to elicit support, but the idea of using private sector competition as a means to reduce costs was appealing. Private health insurance purchasers, particularly large corporations, were just beginning to investigate the cost-cutting potential of competing managed-care plans, and it seemed to a number of planners that a similar approach could be used by Medicaid. Cost-reducing mechanisms such as co-payments, gatekeepers, and increased deductibles could all be adapted for use by the Medicaid programs, although certain skeptics wondered whether Medicaid contracts could ever be attractive to profit-oriented HMOs and independent practice associations (IPAS).

A more radical approach would be to make the poor, or relatives of the poor, shoulder more of the financial responsibility for the program. Before Medicaid, most poor elderly had been taken care of by grown children and other relatives, and some planners suggested that these natural caretakers be forced to pay at least part of the cost of transferring their wards to the state. Proponents of this approach disagreed over whether to make only biological children liable for caregiving were a new law enacted, or rather to include stepchildren, siblings, spouses, and nieces and nephews as well. Although the idea seemed promising, authors of a CBO report warned that such a step would be "quite controversial."[2]

A less controversial approach would be to scale down benefits. One could eliminate dental benefits, for example, for a national savings of $360 million, or intermediate care facility services for the mentally retarded— with the mentally retarded returned to the state institutions where they had resided until 1966—for a savings of $1.3 billion. Alternatively, Medicaid could stop trying to compete with private insurers, and refuse to pay customary charges to providers. Or conceivably, the federal government could recalculate its reimbursement formula to the states and return the program to the original, cheaper form of 1966. Lowering the federal government's share in the wealthiest states from 50 percent to 40 percent, for example, would save $700 million a year. Alternatively, the federal government could take over the program entirely, "federalize" it in policy parlance, and try to achieve cost savings by streamlining administrative processes and using increased market leverage in purchasing services from physicians, hospitals, and nursing homes. In a similar vein, the government could convert the whole program to a block grant, and allow the states to make necessary cuts where they saw fit.

The problem with most of these approaches was that they threatened to widen rather than narrow the gaps in health status between rich and poor. No empirical evidence suggested that the poor were overconsuming medical care, despite their rising rates of hospitalization, and indeed a number of policy analysts were convinced that the ultimate elimination of the health gap could only come by introducing much broader Medicaid coverage, if not national health insurance. Early and Periodic Screening, Detection, and Treatment programs (EPSDTS), while helpful, had failed to fully halt preventable and treatable pediatric diseases in poor children, and by 1978 fewer than one third of all eligible children were included in the program, despite continuing efforts to enroll them.[3] One particularly sobering investigation revealed that poor children in 1981 died at nearly double the rate of wealthy children. Across all geographical regions and racial groups, children of mothers who had graduated from high school and children who lived in households earning at least $10,000 a year survived childhood more frequently.[4]

One symbol of the gap in medical services between rich and poor was the limited access to abortions that poor women had after Medicaid was precluded from paying for abortions after 1976. Before the program change, Medicaid had paid for nearly 270,000 abortions a year, at a public cost of $61 million. After the change, poor women were forced to pay for their own abortions, at a cost of approximately $280 each—more than the average monthly welfare allowance for an entire family. One study estimated that the loss of Medicaid abortion funds would result in at least forty-four maternal deaths a year.[5]

In the absence of decisive remedial action from the federal government, urban municipal hospitals struggled to compensate for the gaps in the Medicaid programs.[6] The funds to run the municipal hospitals were drawn mostly from state and local governments, which provided nearly $10 billion a year to these institutions by 1982. Public hospitals, which provided just over 20 percent of the nation's hospital care, provided over 40 percent of the nation's free care by that year, and urban public hospitals, which accounted for just 5 percent of the nation's hospital beds, provided over 20 percent of all the nation's free hospital care.[7] The nation's major municipal hospitals, such as Bellevue in New York, Cook County in Chicago, and General Hospital in Washington, struggled to maintain these free services in the face of strong downward budgetary pressures, by doubling and tripling up patient beds, cutting staff, trimming residency programs, and triaging the overwhelming barrage of patients. The situation produced a "self-fulfilling prophecy of disaster," wrote the political scientist Jewel Bellush in 1979, as morale and the confidence of patients eroded. Overcrowded and underfunded public hospitals could not attract qualified medical and nursing staffs, which only added to the sense of chaos and substandard medical conditions.[8]

Reagan and Block Grants

Beyond fundamentally shifting federal spending toward defense and away from domestic service programs, and sharply reducing marginal tax rates, President Ronald Reagan made a major innovation in Medicaid reform, variously known as devolution or federalization. The change reflected Reagan's bias toward gubernatorial control of domestic spending and a minimal role for the federal government. As governor of a large and wealthy state, he had bristled at the control exercised by federal agencies over what he believed were state administrative functions, and he perceived (correctly) that his feelings were mirrored throughout the legislatures of conservative western and southern states. One grateful state legislator, Robert Usdane of the Arizona Senate, expressed his satisfaction in the "new thinking": "[It will] give our country a new foothold on the brake pedal of inflation and return us to greatness in the world marketplace again."[9] While progressive state officials from the East and upper Midwest voiced concern that federal budget cuts would undermine their ability to provide necessary social services to residents, others celebrated the newfound autonomy of state agencies.[10]

The most powerful devolutionary mechanism used by the new administration was the implementation of block grants to replace older categorical funding mechanisms. Previously, many social service and health service programs had been funded by the federal government through a series of matching grants to state and local authorities. The system allowed a great deal of federal oversight of the state agencies which delivered the programs, but at the same time allowed states to spend indiscriminately and apply for federal reimbursement without limit. Under Reagan, some seventy-seven categorical grant programs were lumped together under six "blocks," encompassing cash assistance, social services, state education, local education, preventive health, and health services (excluding Medicaid). That is, the federal government withdrew its matching obligations as well as its administrative oversight of the programs, and instead gave the states a lump sum payment to spend as they might. The two health blocks included funds for preventive health, maternal and child health, public health and immunization, mental and community health, and immigrant health programs, as well as programs to fight black lung and tuberculosis. Notably, under Reagan's initial plan, total federal spending on all these programs would decline from $1.9 billion to $1.4 billion—a drop of over 25 percent.[11] Democrats in Congress, then in the majority, restored some of the categorical programs, but health spending ultimately dropped by more than 10 percent.[12]

Compounding the challenge for state agency officials was a tax revolt spreading nationwide, exemplified in the passage of ballot propositions in California and Massachusetts limiting tax rates as well as future increases. Caught between declining federal grant support, voters' rejection of tax increases, and burgeoning welfare rolls, state officials were forced to cut their support for programs. "It is time for states and local communities to take the initiative in reshaping the design, administration and financing of human service programs," wrote the Massachusetts secretary of human services, Charles Mahoney.[13] Voters had clearly rejected expanding social service programs both in their presidential ballots and in their votes on tax referenda.

Changes to Medicaid under OBRA ('81) and TEFRA ('82)

Medicaid was never a potential block grant target. The program, which by 1980 cost the federal government over $16 billion, dwarfed the programs intended for conversion to block grants and was too large to wholly devolve to the states. Rather, the administration proposed placing a 5 percent cap on increases in the federal portion, regardless of resulting health care inflation. While Congress rejected the proposal, it imposed reductions in matching payments of 3, 4, and 4.5 percent for the years 1982 through 1984 in the Omnibus Budget Reconciliation Act (OBRA) of 1981, while endorsing eligibility cuts which reduced Medicaid coverage to 750,000 children. More significantly, Congress dropped the onerous burden of requiring states to pay hospitals and providers on a reasonable-cost basis, and granted states the option of applying for freedom-of-choice waivers, giving state governments far more latitude in constructing their Medicaid payment formulas but reducing the likelihood that Medicaid recipients would be able to seek care in the private sector.[14] The resulting Medicaid program was more highly decentralized, less generous, and less inclusive. At the same time, the new controls gave governors new leverage in controlling the spiraling costs of the programs, which had threatened to overwhelm state budgets.[15]

The move to give states more latitude in determining Medicaid eligibility, provider choice, and payment formulas, particularly for elderly nursing home residents, was furthered with the Tax Equity and Fiscal Responsibility Act (TEFRA) of 1982, which allowed the placement of liens against the homes of nursing home residents, the restriction of asset transfer "spend-downs," and the provision of home health care for disabled children. The act impelled the states to experiment with different payment mechanisms including day rates and percentage cost bases, while a controversial "family responsibility" clause allowed states to require family participation in nursing home care. Only Idaho adopted this approach, and then later dropped the requirement.

The experience with nursing home payment reform led directly to similar changes for Medicaid hospital reimbursement. Until 1981 Medicaid had paid hospitals on a cost basis, much like Medicare. After Congress decided in that year that the reasonable cost principle for nursing homes could also apply to hospitals, states moved to lower hospital reimbursements with negotiated (discounted) rates, capped budgets, and average patient cost formulas. While in 1981 forty states followed the Medicare payment structure in their Medicaid hospital payments, by 1991 only four states did so.[16]

Central to the Reagan administration's Medicaid reforms was the belief that Americans were consuming too much medical care, particularly in hospitals, and that the solution was to impose some of the costs on the patients themselves.[17] It is important to note that the intention was not to transfer a significant portion of the Medicaid burden to the patients. Rather, the point was to create a psychological barrier to care—accomplished by setting co-payments as low as one dollar—to dissuade patients from seeking care which they knew to be of only marginal benefit or utility. Within a year, sixteen states adopted co-payments, twenty eliminated at least some optional Medicaid services, and fourteen reduced the rolls of eligible recipients.[18]

Critics of the administration were appalled by the policy reversal, even if the amounts in questions were relatively trivial. In the collective opinion of the opposition, the administration's proposals under the Omnibus Reconciliation Act (OBRA) of 1981 undermined some of the original goals of the program. Nixon's appointee Tom Joe decried the change: "They reduce the incomes of people who are already poor, creating difficulty for families trying to secure the necessities of food, shelter, clothing, and medical care; they eliminate the incentives to work for families trying to earn their way off the welfare rolls, and foreclose opportunities for moving into the competitive labor market."[19] Similarly, Richard Nathan, a professor at Princeton (and fellow Nixon appointee), noted sarcastically that Reagan's budget plan for 1981 was a "historic piece of legislation," in that it marked a "reversal of a long period of growth in programs for the poor."[20]

Governors, state legislators, and state agency executives responded to the changes in Washington with mixed approval. For all states, the Medicaid burden had grown frighteningly fast since the program's inception, often tripling in cost over the course of a decade, and by 1981 Medicaid was the single largest item in many states' budgets.[21] The new flexibility in negotiating fees, rates, reimbursement protocols, and eligibility standards was welcome, although most governors had hoped that the president would grant them even more discretion. "Even with additional flexibility, states have only a limited ability to influence hospital costs that currently are rising at 18 percent a year," wrote Governors James Hunt Jr. of North Carolina and Albert Quie of Minnesota to the White House in 1981.[22] Similarly, Governor Edward King of Massachusetts wrote to Reagan's health and human services secretary, Richard Schweiker, that the new benefit elimination measures, reductions in provider rates, and eligibility cutbacks were "band-aid" approaches, inadequate to rooting out the underlying problems.[23] And the National Conference of State Legislatures demanded that Washington give the states "maximum flexibility" by repealing as many restrictions on the Medicaid program as possible. "We cannot accept a mere broadening of the existing waiver authority which would require states seeking to alter their Medicaid programs to seek and obtain prior permission from the federal government," members of the group wrote to the presidential assistant Robert Carleson.[24] Overall, the demand from the states was for the power to limit services and benefits by enrolling Medicaid recipients in HMOs, or restricting them to a few prepaid providers and vendors who would do the states' bidding at discounted rates.

Critics outside of government tended toward the opposite view. "Don't grow old and don't get sick—that's the ominous message that the Reagan administration has sent us in the Medicare-Medicaid provisions of the 1981 budget act," wrote the liberal columnist Sylvia Porter.[25] Not surprisingly, the AMA was "violently opposed" to the call (in the words of the association's executive vice-president James Sammons), and warned of a massive transfer of Medicaid patients from private to public hospitals.[26] While generally supportive of the 5 percent cap initially proposed by the administration, the association feared the type of broad negotiating powers being promulgated by governors and state Medicaid executives, and urged restraint in ceding too much authority to the states.[27]

Physicians too opposed the cuts. Compelled both by a sense of professional duty and by existing obligations to teaching hospitals with which they had affiliations, many physicians had chafed at the less-than-competitive rates at which Medicaid had reimbursed them for their services, yet the inevitable result of OBRA was even less generous reimbursement. Physicians would either have to discontinue treating Medicaid patients entirely or suffer declines in their incomes, even while Medicaid budgets saw only slightly decreased costs. AMA leaders protested the new policy, claiming that cost overruns were not a product of excessive physicians' fees but rather of natural growth in the program. The increased costs resulted from the "success of the program," Sammons testified to a congressional task force in 1984. Aggregated budget cuts in Medicaid had rendered the original program goal of "mainstreaming" patients a "myth" which would only become farther removed from reality if OBRA cuts were implemented.[28]

But these critics failed to understand that the adjustments in Medicaid (and later in Medicare) merely exemplified a larger administration concern with inflation in the system as a whole. Reagan, like Carter, understood that increasing health expenditures threatened to derail the federal budget, and that controlling the excesses must begin with the federal government's own health programs. As a committed proponent of free markets, Reagan envisioned deregulating the health payment system to allow patients (Medicare patients particularly) to be exposed to a greater portion of the financial burden of care, and thus be forced to exercise their own discretion in purchasing medical care. "Clamping regulatory controls on an overheated health care system is just as futile as putting a lid on a pot that is boiling over," according to one White House policy memo.[29] Thus along with changes in Medicaid, in 1982 there was a substantial restructuring of Medicare payments using preset diagnostic related groups (DRGS); increases in premiums for Medicare part B, co-insurance costs, and deductibles; and lower lifetime maximums.[30] While liberal critics might flail at these adjustments, the more fiscally prudent were circumspect. "Despite the uncertainties, Mr. Reagan's prescription deserves a thorough trial," read an editorial in the *New York Times*.[31] Within two years the prospective payment reforms had become ubiquitous in the private insurance sector as well.

Declining Use of HMOs

One of the most promising avenues to reducing Medicaid costs—contracting with Medicaid HMOs—was declining in import during the early 1980s. Closed staff–model HMOs had never provided care for more than about 2 percent of all Medicaid recipients nationwide, but since 1978 the total number of Medicaid recipients enrolled in HMOs had actually fallen by nearly 15 percent. Only five states—California, Maryland, Michigan, Utah, and Oregon—enrolled more than 5 percent of their Medicaid recipients in HMOs by 1981, and most other states enrolled only trivial numbers of their Medicaid recipients. A related option—enrolling Medicaid patients in community health centers on a capitated basis—attracted scant attention as well, despite the positive reports emanating from the nation's several hundred CHCs serving impoverished communities.

The unwillingness of states to push Medicaid recipients into HMOs was mystifying to health budget analysts, who perceived Medicaid inflation as the gravest concern for most state budget committees and budget offices. The lack of private-sector HMO penetration undoubtedly accounted for some of the reluctance, as did ignorance of the mechanisms of managed care on the part of legislators and agency executives.[32] But at the executive level, ambivalence toward HMOs was probably rooted in Reagan's personal disdain for all bureaucratic oversight. He inclined toward self-pay medicine with widely available catastrophic coverage, which he had tried to make universally available in California for as little as $36 a year.[33] Given this outlook, the administration's general approach toward HMOs was a studied indifference. While federal Medicaid regulations did allow, in theory, for states to apply for freedom-of-choice waivers to move patients into HMOs, few states took advantage of the option in the early 1980s.[34]

Federal Medicaid caps impelled little change in most state Medicaid programs in the years following their imposition. States were still responsible for absorbing the actuarial risk of the programs without being granted the regulatory discretion to reduce their exposure, and nearly all states continued to build total risk exposure into the administration of their programs. Only Texas contracted its whole program to a private insurance agency (as did Indiana to a lesser extent), effectively purchasing for itself a reinsurance policy. One outside investigation of the whole system conducted by Deloitte, Haskins and Sells in 1981 questioned the exclusion of Medicaid from the block grants: "Doesn't it necessarily follow that if the states are expected to absorb substantial reductions in the federal funds available to support Medicaid programs, that they also be afforded the discretion to make adjustments in the program to facilitate the most effective delivery of health services within a reduced sum of monies?"[35] Political lobbying from health providers and organized labor explained part of the anomaly, but a tentativeness on the part of governors and state legislative leaders played a role as well. Medicaid was simply too big, and too complicated, for most state officials to feel comfortable assuming total responsibility for its continued success or failure.

Minority Health

The health of black Americans continued to trail that of white Americans by a significant margin. A study by the Children's Defense Fund (CDF) in 1982 found that black children were twice as likely to die in the first year of life as white children, three times as likely to be poor, and five times as likely to be on welfare; 64 percent of all female-headed black families were poor (versus 40 percent of comparable white families), and 85 percent of black children being raised by a single mother under twenty-five were poor (as opposed to 72 percent of comparable white children). Inexplicably, certain discrepancies seemed to be growing. In 1971, for example, black and white high school graduates were about equally likely to go on to college, whereas by 1982 white high school graduates were nearly 50 percent more likely than black graduates to go on.[36]

Even mundane health factors such as dental prophylaxis showed a startling discrepancy between blacks and whites. In one study by the CDF, for example, 54 percent of black subjects had between six and twenty decayed teeth, compared with 21 percent of whites. Likewise, 36 percent of black respondents were unable to identify dental floss, versus 9 percent of whites. Not surprisingly, 85 percent of white subjects had received their first dental appointment before the age of thirteen, while only 45 percent of blacks had.[37] An equally disturbing study showed that the incidence of high blood pressure was correlated not only with race but with skin tone, as high blood pressure was significantly more prevalent among dark-skinned than light-skinned blacks, independent of wealth, age, or weight. The cause of this discrepancy was puzzling, but its presence reinforced the idea that the black community required targeted health education programs.[38]

What these studies failed to show, however, was the remarkable health gains made by blacks in the twenty years since 1960. In a number of categories, blacks had improved more than whites over this period, sometimes significantly so. For example, while the incidence of infant mortality, arteriosclerosis, and heart disease had declined by similar percentages for both groups, blacks led whites in improvements in influenza and pneumonia (a decline of 67 percent versus a decline of 50 percent), and stroke (53 percent to 48 percent). And black use of hospitals, physicians, and other health providers had increased at nearly double the rate of use by whites, bringing blacks up to near-parity. The most significant exception to this trend was in the prevalence of diabetes, in which white improvement had outpaced black improvement more than twofold. A richer and more highly caloric diet which accompanied improved black economic status probably explained this statistic, and the trend worried public health professionals.[39]

The most troubling health phenomenon for blacks, however, beyond the rising incidence of social pathology and family breakdown, was the continued paucity of black doctors. Although affirmative action programs and recruitment efforts had raised black representation among American medical students from 2 percent to 7.5 percent by 1974, the proportion stubbornly remained at that level and then fell. As a result, by 1981 blacks still accounted for fewer than 3 percent of all physicians in the United States, and these physicians were not distributed appropriately for optimal service to the black community. While 20 percent of all blacks continued to live in rural areas (predominantly in the South), only 4 percent of black doctors practiced in these areas. And while a steady core of black physicians practiced in the heavily black inner cities, a disproportionate number of black doctors, like their white counterparts, practiced in middle-class and well-to-do suburbs, where relatively few blacks lived. As was true of physicians the world over, black doctors catered to the wealthiest members of their racial group, regardless of the need for their services elsewhere, and the resulting shortfalls in rural black doctors stymied the efforts of health planners to adequately serve the population.[40]

The health status of black Americans, particularly poor black Americans, was ambiguous by 1982. To be black in America was to be less healthy than the typical white American, but data suggested that this discrepancy was closing rapidly. While professional advocates for the community emphasized the bad news, and called for an increase in subsidies for medical training of black medical students and research to combat diseases which disproportionately affected blacks, the Reagan administration chose to ignore the statistical differential and concentrate instead on devolution, federalization, and state control.[41] If black health was to be a particular focus of domestic policy programming, it would be primarily at the state and local levels (albeit helped along with federal block grants), while Washington concentrated on tax cuts and national defense.

The Ripple Effect

The changes in Medicaid reimbursement under OBRA '81 and TEFRA '82, as well as the agglomeration of categorical social service programs into block grants, produced substantial changes in state health care and social service programs. In the first two years after regulatory and funding changes were implemented, sixteen states adopted co-payments on optional services, and six adopted co-payments on drugs; thirteen states limited hospital stays; twenty-six eliminated certain optional services; sixteen limited emergency room reimbursement through Medicaid; sixteen limited Medicaid eligibility; nine reduced hospital reimbursement schedules; and twelve reduced nursing home reimbursement. Altogether, some 661,000 fewer children nationwide qualified for Medicaid in 1983 than in 1981, and cuts in various community health center programs, local clinics, and community mental health centers excluded thousands more from treatment. Missouri proposed eliminating lead poisoning and adolescent pregnancy programs entirely, while the District of Columbia, Iowa, Kansas, and Mississippi moved to reduce coverage for crippled children's programs. In addition, nearly 150 community health centers across the nation were scheduled to close by 1984 because of funding cuts.[42] Representative Henry Waxman (D., Calif.) called the cuts in Medicaid, CHCs, and maternal and child programs "devastating," and an invitation to "a disastrous rise in infant mortality and infant morbidity."[43]

Hospitals braced themselves for a deluge of uninsured patients seeking basic medical care through associated community health centers, emergency rooms, and satellite clinics. Unfortunately, at the very moment when hospitals might have been expected to shoulder a greater proportion of the burden of charity medical care, their prospects for raising funds through philanthropy had been diminished. Under changes to the federal tax code passed in Reagan's first year in office, marginal tax rates for unearned income and capital gains had been reduced substantially, making gifts to hospitals and other charitable institutions substantially more expensive for the taxpayer. While public hospitals could look to municipal and state budget authorities to raise their annual allocations and thus compensate for loss in Medicaid revenues, private hospitals had no such option. The president of the American Hospital Association called the changed reimbursement and philanthropic environment "a major redefinition of how hospitals operate," and admitted that prognoses for hospitals' financial vitality in the coming decade looked grim.[44]

Further complicating the hospital landscape was the decisive shift in Medicare reimbursement, followed closely by private insurance reimbursement, to a prospective payment system for hospitals (and later physicians). From its onset, Medicare reimbursed physicians through a system of usual, customary, and reasonable (UCR) fees, and hospitals through a system of reasonable cost allocations, meaning that the federal government would try to match the usual fee of the free market. Such a system was inflationary, as physicians needed to do little more than raise their fees en masse to create a newer, higher customary fee, but the system did serve to lure most physicians to Medicare assignment.

States initially paid Medicaid reimbursement on the same UCR system as used by Medicare, but as early as the mid-1970s states began to set rates (or "fee schedules") which were decidedly lower than those prevailing in the private sector. While the effort did limit the growing cost of Medicaid, it produced growing disparities between Medicare and private sector reimbursement on the one hand and Medicaid reimbursement on the other. By 1980 states with fee schedules had Medicaid-to-Medicare payment ratios between .25 and .75, while states which had maintained UCR for Medicaid achieved parity, or near-parity.[45] (The one glaring exception was Nevada, where the state Medicaid program paid more generously than Medicare, despite using a fee schedule.) Such disparities often dissuaded physicians from accepting Medicaid patients.

Although adopting fee schedules appeared on the surface to be a straightforward tradeoff between cost and access, the action was misleadingly destructive. Physician fees in Medicaid tended to account for a relatively small portion of the overall cost of the programs—somewhere between 10 and 12 percent in most. Thus, shaving 20 percent off the cost of physician care achieved little more than a 2 percent overall savings in general program costs. The savings were achieved, however, only by forcing numerous Medicaid patients into hospital emergency rooms (which were often the only available source for primary care once local physicians declined to accept Medicaid), at a considerably greater cost than even full UCR reimbursement of outpatient doctors. One study by the Urban Institute found that raising payments to physicians might save money in the long run.[46]

The adoption by Medicare (and later by private health insurers) of diagnostic related groups (DRGs) in 1982 briefly eased the payment disparity with Medicaid. The use of DRGs, which together made up a highly detailed fee schedule, initially succeeded in slowing Medicare inflation and making the Medicaid payment schedules more competitive. Even with the reduction in Medicare payments, however, state Medicaid payments continued to lag behind federal and private insurance programs, forcing more patients to turn to hospitals for primary care throughout the 1980s.

Reactions to Medicaid Cuts

Reactions to the cuts, both in Medicaid and in the preventive health programs as implemented in the shifts to block grants, were mixed. Public health and social work professionals expressed concern that reducing payments would create greater obstacles for poor people seeking care. Sara Rosenbaum, a researcher for the Children's Defense Fund, excoriated the changes for "turning the clock back a generation," to the time when a child's economic status at birth would determine his life expectancy, while the *New York Times* decried the cuts as "cruel and foolish economies."[47] Physicians and government officials in Florida, Texas, and Massachusetts expressed concern that declining reimbursement was deterring physicians from opening their practices to Medicaid patients, and the National Study Group on State Medicaid Strategies reported in early 1984 that Medicaid programs nationwide were facing financial default and required "drastic overhaul."[48]

Some critics quixotically called for not only restoring the cut funds but expanding or rebuilding the entire program. The Multnomah County (Oregon) human services director called for distributing government-endorsed vouchers throughout the population to enable the purchase of private health insurance, while in a conference report in 1984 the Southern Christian Leadership Conference (SCLC) called for federalizing and expanding the many Medicaid programs.[49] "We 'wince' for the unremitting intrusions and calloused insensitivities that accompany interactions on the part of the poor with the American 'mainstream,'" the authors wrote.[50]

Such critiques lacked credibility, however, not only because of their frank dogmatism but because health statistics available as early as 1983 failed to support their assumptions. By the late 1970s Medicaid recipients were receiving more physician care per capita than privately insured patients, and two to three years after the implementation of Reagan's cuts there was little evidence that this situation had been reversed.[51] Apart from certain elective procedures for musculoskeletal problems, patients from families with lower incomes who had poor educations and dwelled in central cities had more physician visits than middle-class patients did in 1983. In this regard, the black poor seemed to fare as well as the white poor.[52] Reagan's White House responded to criticism from the Children's Defense Fund by pointing out that while it was true that blacks had a lower life expectancy than whites, this was probably because blacks were murdered at four times the rate of whites, and lived with an unmarried mother at twelve times the rate of whites, not because of inadequate Medicaid reimbursement.[53] On a less belligerent note, the White House admitted that while the great disparity in infant mortality between blacks and whites was troubling, it was a long-standing problem, and hardly due to recent modifications in Medicaid.[54]

The sector most adversely affected by the shifts in Medicaid reimbursement consisted of those hospitals for which Medicaid patients made up a substantial portion of the patient load—generally more than a fourth. These hospitals, invariably found either in central cities or in rural areas where many of the elderly qualified for Medicaid in addition to Medicare, found that the cuts and changes in Medicaid reimbursement policy greatly affected their solvency. Although fewer than 9 percent of all hospitals nationwide had such weighty Medicaid patient loads, these "disproportionate share" hospitals collectively provided over 40 percent of all poor care and incurred over 35 percent of all bad debt. Medicaid cuts for these hospitals brought almost immediate financial distress. As early as 1983 the American Hospital Association called for "advantageous" treatment of these hospitals by HCFA, claiming them to be "anchors" of poor communities which were instrumental in assuring broad access to hospitalization.[55] The Urban Institute concluded in that year that this select group of hospitals was experiencing financial "stress" at more than five times the rate of hospitals with lighter Medicaid loads.[56]

Health Care within the Reagan Revolution

Reagan's general antipathy toward Medicaid was consistent with a growing skepticism toward both New Deal and Great Society welfare programs percolating through the national electorate in the 1980s. A large portion of the American middle class had begun to express dismay at the alarming growth in teenage pregnancy, multigenerational welfare dependency, and familial dysfunction which some social welfare programs seemed to have spawned. Certain statistics bore the naysayers out. For example, poverty had declined faster in the years before the Great Society antipoverty programs were enacted than in the years after, and in fact began to rise in the years after 1973 when most of the programs were receiving their maximum funding. Furthermore, studies by HEW in the late 1970s in Trenton, Seattle, and Denver demonstrated that income guarantees suppressed employment rates.[57]

One new development in the 1980s was a strong movement of intellectual conservatism articulated by a small but vocal group of academics in universities and conservative think tanks. One of its leading figures was the former liberal academic Irving Kristol, who postulated that "the difficulty in giving money only to the poor is that it quickly imprisons them in a 'poverty trap.'" Along similar lines, the Washington columnist Allan Brownfeld wrote, "If a society subsidizes indolence and taxes work, it will have more indolence than it does work."[58] A sizable cadre of neoconservative intellectuals coalesced at foundations and nonprofit research groups such as the American Enterprise Institute, the Cato Institute, the Hoover Institution, and the Heritage Foundation, as well as in the law and business school faculties and economics departments of the University of Rochester, the University of Chicago, and Northwestern University.

The most widely read of the "neocon" intellectuals was Charles Murray, who blamed an expanding welfare state for the deterioration of social structures in the ghetto in his study *Losing Ground* (1984). Murray suggested that the misery of poverty was not caused entirely by lack of money but rather by a lack of inner discipline and character on the part of the impoverished. Thus money alone could not be an effective solution to poverty, as it could not reshape the inner character of the targeted population. "We can do all sorts of things with people who have passed a critical threshold of investment," he told an interviewer in 1985. "What we do not seem to be able to do is cajole people into wanting to make those initial investments."[59] In other words, while the government knew how to teach a child who wished to learn, it did not know how to induce the child to want to learn in the first place. Handing money to these children seemed to undermine any previous inclination they might have had to do so.

Murray was intrigued by the question of free choice, for he felt that people who escaped poverty did so because they wished to, and willed themselves to make the choices which would lead them out of the ghetto. Those who were left behind had, on some level, made a series of choices which inevitably resulted in the perpetuation of their own impoverished state. "Large numbers of poor men impregnate women and *choose* not to take responsibility for the resulting child," Murray wrote in an impassioned essay in *Commentary* in 1985, and "large numbers of poor women who cannot afford to take care of a child on their own nonetheless *choose* not to practice birth control, *choose* not to have abortions, and *choose* not to put the child up for adoption."[60] In the light of these choices, Murray wrote, government must admit its limitations in molding individual character and instead concentrate on creating incentives for people to choose differently.

While the neoconservative movement attracted quite a few young scholars and policy makers to its ranks, most social scientists cleaved to a traditional, government-centered approach to alleviating poverty. Reluctant to abandon a social philosophy which had grounded their worldview since the mid-1960s (and for many since the 1930s), these scholars pointed out the setbacks to the poor which had occurred under Reagan, and demonstrated the underlying heartlessness of the neoconservative philosophy. The AFDC budget, for example, was $1.3 billion (13 percent) smaller by 1984 than it would have been without the cuts made by Reagan; the Food Stamps budget was $2 billion smaller (also 13 percent); Medicaid was $1.3 billion smaller (5.9 percent); and public housing was $482 million smaller (4.3 percent). Exacerbating these funding cuts were elevated eligibility thresholds for virtually all poverty programs. "They gutted out the whole hope of the community," pronounced the Reverend William O. Johnson, a community leader in Bridgeport, Connecticut.[61] One public health social worker, Robert Morris, summed up the reactions of social welfare professionals when he declaimed against the regressive cuts in national social obligations: "The most vulnerable are hurt the most."[62]

Proponents of Reagan's cuts, both within and outside the administration, vociferously defended the underlying philosophy. Adopting a "profamily" stance, White House spokesmen contended that the Great Society programs had splintered rather than solidified family life, and that Reagan's approach would strengthen family ties while increasing employment among the poor.[63] The rhetoric was consistent with the facts. Despite evincing criticism from liberals, Reagan's social welfare budget was nearly 12 percent higher (controlling for inflation) than Carter's had been; Food Stamps were available to five million more people than they had been in 1975; and the infant mortality rate was dropping. And while it was true that the wealthiest Americans received a substantial tax break in 1981, many middle-income and upper-middle-income Americans were actually paying slightly higher taxes as a result of OBRA and TEFRA than they would have been had the tax code remained unchanged.[64] In fact, most of the welfare cuts had fallen on those at the top of the eligibility scale (rather than on the "poorest of the poor," as often claimed by administration critics), and thus removed the social safety net from exactly those most capable of supporting themselves. In theory, the administration was reserving government largesse for those, and only those, who could not possibly survive without it, while denying it to those for whom it acted as an unhealthy crutch and a disincentive to work. The conservative scholar Michael Novak noted in 1983, "As Roosevelt is sometimes referred to as the liberal who saved capitalism, Reagan may some day be known as the conservative who saved the welfare state intact for the poor."[65]

Nonetheless, in at least one area the cuts posed a direct threat to the welfare of the poor. Infant mortality, the single starkest measure of the health, social equity, and fundamental fairness of a society, had always been embarrassingly high in the United States. Despite per capita health spending substantially higher than that of all other nations, the United States typically ranked between fifteenth and twentieth in a comparative international measure of national health (depending on the year). By the early 1980s epidemiological studies had demonstrated conclusively that the best predictor of infant mortality was low infant birth weight, and this condition in turn could be directly influenced by various government supplementary food and medical programs.[66] Reductions in Medicaid, Food Stamps, and especially WIC eligibility threatened to undermine public health efforts at reducing infant mortality, and promised ultimately to increase government spending as an increasing number of low-birth-weight infants demanded intensive and chronic care. A computer model generated by researchers in 1987 showed that in 1981 Medicaid had probably averted over 23,000 infant deaths, while WIC had probably averted over 3,000. In 1982, under Reagan's more austere budgets, 2,000 fewer infant lives would be saved.[67] These stark figures threatened to undermine the pro-family successes of Reagan's approach.

Thus the competing forces of cost containment and pro-family welfare reform whittled away at Medicaid and other welfare programs in the early 1980s. Buffeted by a generational backlash to the perceived liberal excesses of the 1960s, and the very real medical excesses of the 1970s, many poor people found themselves the unwitting victims of social forces beyond their control. While Medicaid as a program constituted only a very small portion of the federal budget, when coupled with Medicare it took on the cloak of a medical inflation driver, and thus opened itself to assiduous cost-cutting. At the same time, pleas for greater compassion to the poor fell upon disbelieving ears in an administration which leaned toward self-sufficiency and local responsibility for all but the neediest of America's underclass.

10

Recovering the Cuts, Managed Care,

and Comprehensive Reform

Program Expansions, 1984–1989

The effects of Medicaid cuts enacted during the first Reagan administration were apparent by 1985. The proportion of America's poor covered by the program had dropped from 63 percent in 1976 to just over 50 percent by 1985, and over two thirds of poor people responded in a survey that year that they had needed medical care in the previous year but had not received it.[1] Over 250 community health centers had been closed in the three years after the passage of OBRA '81, and over one million children had been made ineligible for WIC and other government-subsidized meal programs. In a similar trend, 500,000 people had been dropped from AFDC. "The health of poor Americans is getting worse," wrote Mary O'Neil Mundinger, a public health scholar at Columbia University, in 1985.[2] The *Los Angeles Times* admonished in an editorial that spring: "The nation should not be cutting back on immunizing poor children against disease, on helping teenagers learn about birth control, or preventing infant deaths by providing impoverished pregnant women with proper nutrition and health care."[3]

Just as troubling as the reduced eligibility limits for Medicaid was the program's greatly diminished reimbursement to physicians. In California in 1986, for example, Medicaid paid $353 for an appendectomy and $519 for a normal vaginal delivery, while Blue Shield paid $902 and $1,330 for the same procedures. In other states the discrepancies were nearly as large. Extremely low payments discouraged physicians from accepting Medicaid patients, even when they might have been willing to accept a certain amount of pro bono billings, and provoked feelings of resentment among members of the profession that they were being asked to shoulder an unfair responsibility for society's needy. Furthermore, even when doctors were willing to accept low fees, payments were often greatly delayed. "The three biggest complaints are low pay, slow pay, and no pay," stated a spokesman for the American Academy of Pediatrics. Some doctors went as far as dispensing with payment entirely rather than spend valuable hours billing state agencies and appealing to overworked bureaucrats, but this approach was unrealistic for the primary-care providers who treated most Medicaid patients. The more usual response was for the doctors to simply withdraw from the program, creating bottlenecks and waiting lists as Medicaid recipients sought basic primary care. "What good is a generous Medicaid program if you don't have providers who are willing to participate?," queried Jane Perkins, a public health advocate in Los Angeles.[4] All the more galling to advocates for the poor was that the annual tax deduction granted by the federal government for private health insurance amounted to $29 billion—$8.7 billion more than the federal government's entire Medicaid bill.[5]

Concerned members of Congress responded by passing a series of bills between 1984 and 1989 which expanded Medicaid eligibility and partially offset the austerity cuts of the early 1980s. In the Deficit Reduction Act of 1984 (DEFRA), the Consolidated Omnibus Reconciliation Act of 1985 (COBRA), the Sixth Omnibus Reconciliation Act of 1986 (SOBRA), OBRA '87, the Medicare Catastrophic Coverage Act of 1988, the Family Support Act of 1988, and OBRA '89, Congress expanded Medicaid coverage to first-time pregnant women, women in two-parent homes, children up to five years of age in families which would not otherwise qualify for Medicaid, and working families leaving AFDC for six months, and also expanded CHAP to cover children up to eight years of age. While no single measure abruptly changed the landscape of Medicaid coverage, the group of them together substantially increased the pool of eligible recipients and guaranteed care to many more pregnant women. And while the focus of these expansions was clearly on pregnant women and children, men and married couples benefited as well from the provisions in the Family Support

Act of 1988, which allowed working families to continue receiving Medicaid benefits even after leaving the AFDC rolls.[6]

The expansions in Medicaid eligibility served to raise the number of children in the program by 2 percent by 1990, and the number of pregnant women by almost as much, and greatly increased the number of elderly who were able to qualify for the program (see discussion below). However, the changes disproportionately aided the marginally poor without granting the poorest of the poor the one benefit they most needed—more generous reimbursement for doctors. Thus, although by 1990 the Medicaid rolls were expanding, poor people living in inner cities or in isolated rural areas still had great difficulty finding a physician willing to take Medicaid payment.

The Budget Buster: Long-Term Care

Less obvious than the budget cuts, but ultimately more deleterious to the state of Medicaid in the 1980s, was the growing demand which nursing home reimbursement made on the program. Although poor elderly, blind, and permanently disabled persons had been covered by Medicaid since the program's inception, these patients had drawn a relatively small amount of total funds disbursed during the first decade. Starting in the mid-1970s, however, all three of these categories of patients, particularly the poor elderly, drew an increasing share of the program's funds. By 1983 these three groups, which constituted only 30 percent of all Medicaid recipients, drew over 75 percent of all Medicaid funds, of which over a third went for nursing home care—over 25 percent of total Medicaid funds spent.[7] Noting this trend, the American Hospital Association announced in 1987 that Medicaid had largely become a "secondary insurance program for the elderly, blind and disabled," rather than a "primary insurance program for the poor."[8] Given the falling proportion of the nation's poor covered by Medicaid, and the rising proportion of total program dollars going to the aged and disabled, the conclusion bore weight.

The result of this skewed distribution was an expected discrepancy between average spending on disabled patients and spending on poor patients. By 1986 disabled, blind, and elderly recipients received $4,000 a year from the program on average, while poor children received $400 a year and poor adults $800 a year. Skilled nursing and intermediate care facilities (SNFs and ICFs) accounted for nearly 45 percent of all Medicaid payments, yet treated only 7 percent of all Medicaid patients. In total, Medicaid paid for nearly the same portion of the nation's nursing home bill as it did for the nation's charity health care bill—about 50 percent.[9]

Two parallel trends accounted for the growing prominence of the elderly within the Medicaid program: aging demographics and personal mobility. The first was obvious and measurable; as better nutrition and health care had increased average life expectancy by some thirty years over the previous century, the number of citizens requiring assistance and institutional care had risen commensurately. This trend was expected to continue. The six million Americans aged sixty-five and over in 1980 were expected to more than double to fifteen million by 2050, while the 1.5 million octogenarians were expected to quadruple in number during the same period.[10] At the same time, adult children were showing themselves less willing both to take aging parents under their own roofs and to spend their patrimony on institutional care for their parents. Explanations for this unwillingness ranged from the greater number of women in the work force to increased mobility on the part of all Americans, but the results were clearly observable. Thus, the nation found itself in the odd position of using taxpayer funds to pay nursing home bills for the elderly parents of middle-class and upper-middle-class children.

To make matters worse, elderly persons were increasingly likely to transfer all or most of their assets to their children, and then qualify for Medicaid reimbursement for nursing home services. Although this practice was outlawed in 1982, savvy individuals could manipulate their financial records and cheat the system into paying their nursing home bills. "Medicaid has always found it hard to distinguish the honest poor from the phony poor," Jane Bryant Quinn wrote in *Newsweek* in 1983.[11] The growing financial burden of caring for an aging population could be borne only by individuals, their families, or taxpayers, and taxpayers had the least concerted interest in fighting the bills.

Not all families eschewed responsibility, of course. Studies showed that a significant share of elderly Americans, perhaps three quarters, lived within thirty minutes of at least one child and saw that child at least once a week. Furthermore, trends toward declining family size and childless-ness among women presaged greater involvement of children with their aging parents. Nonetheless, by 1985 Americans generally preferred seeing their elderly parents cared for either in institutions or by paid profes-sional caretakers, so long as the government was willing to pay a sizable portion of the bill.[12]

Long-term care raised troubling issues for the Medicaid program in that it usually involved *caretaking* services rather than fundamentally *medical* services. While residents of nursing homes did require help with medication and oxygen, and walking, and did draw on the services of nearby nurses and emergency medical technicians more frequently than the nonelderly did, the basic service supplied by nursing homes was assistance with the activities of daily living (ADLS). ADLS ranged from dressing and bathing to cooking, eating, and cleaning. The elderly moved into nursing homes (or were moved into them by children or other relatives) primarily because they lacked the ability to continue to care for themselves in the most mundane ways. Children frequently moved their parents into homes when they realized that their parents had grown thin from malnutrition, or when they saw their parents wearing soiled cloth-ing or living in unsanitary conditions. Payment for long-term care thus called into question the underlying focus of the Medicaid program. By 1986 Medicaid was as much a nursing program as a medical one. Witness-ing this, the AHA called for dividing the program into three sections providing acute care for the poor, chronic nonmedical care for the el-derly, and chronic medical care for the permanently disabled. Doing so would allow both federal and state governments to construct bureau-cracies and payment mechanisms appropriate to different types of care.[13]

While the Reagan administration did not seriously consider the AHA's proposition, it did respond to the incongruity of having a medical care program paying for ADL assistance by creating a waiver program within OBRA '81. Known as the section 2176 waiver, the program allowed states to apply for permission to pay for home care for the elderly and perma-nently disabled with Medicaid funds, thus providing nonmedical services more cost-effectively. The program was exploited by twenty-two states within three years, and by 1990 nearly one million Medicaid recipients were receiving home-based and community-based care courtesy of the program. Nonetheless, double this many Medicaid recipients were still being cared for in nursing homes by 1991, leading one scholar of Medicaid to observe that home-based care required a "substantial philosophical shift" which was not easily made by state-level Medicaid officers.[14]

Medicaid's shift toward long-term and chronic care of the nonpoor was somewhat invisible to many poor care advocates, but easily visible within state Medicaid bureaus. Although the shift allowed the program to fund services necessary to a population specified as eligible under the original Medicaid legislation, that population had not been intended as the primary target of the program, and in fact the expansion of its weight within the program had been unplanned and largely unacknowledged by either Congress or federal officials. While the shift was hardly perfidious, it did undermine the cost-cutting efforts of the first Reagan administration and consumed much of the savings made at the expense of the poor.

Dumping and Indigent Care

Cuts in Medicaid eligibility and reimbursement rates in the early 1980s, coupled with state and local tax rollbacks, increased the amount of uncompensated care demanded of private hospitals, both in patient volume and in absolute dollars. Unsponsored care at private, nonprofit hospitals nationally rose from 3.7 percent of total expenses in 1980 to 4.8 percent in 1986, while uncompensated care (which could not be shifted onto private, paying patients) rose from $4.6 billion to $11.7 billion during that same period.[15] At the same time the proportion of community hospitals allocating more than 5 percent of their expenses to uncompensated care rose from 25 percent to 60 percent, and of those allocating more than 7.5 percent from 11 percent to 33 percent. While some of the uncompensated care resulted from a greater number of Americans losing private insurance coverage, at least a fourth of it resulted from Medicaid cuts.[16]

The rise in uncompensated care in community hospitals led directly to an increase in "dumping," the purposeful transfer of nonpaying patients to public hospitals for fiscal reasons. While dumping had existed for many years, public hospitals reported a sharp increase in the practice in the four years after the passage of OBRA '81. Parkland Memorial Hospital in Dallas, for example, reported that transfers of patients from private hospitals rose from 70 a month in 1982 to 200 a month in 1983, while the number rose from 15 to 77 at General Hospital in Washington, and from 107 to 470 at Cook County in Chicago. Moreover, public hospitals found that the transferred patients had disproportionately high rates of expensive and unprofitable diagnoses, such as HIV and complicated pregnancies.[17] Although a federal law enacted in 1986 prohibited dumping that could jeopardize a patient's health, the measure failed to ameliorate the financial threat to the nation's public hospitals. Arnold Relman, editor of the *New England Journal of Medicine*, expostulated on the situation: "Who will pay for the medical care of the poor? How should health services for the uninsured be financed in an increasingly price-sensitive and commercialized system which leaves no room for charity or cross subsidization?"[18]

Not surprisingly, the surge of transfers led to a crisis in bad debt for many public hospitals. Although Medicaid had never paid as generously as private payers, it had been a source of substantial revenues for virtually all public hospitals nationwide since its inception. With the rise in dumping, however, the proportion of Medicaid patients in public hospitals declined, while the proportion of patients with no insurance at all increased. As a result, the bad debt held by public hospitals rose sharply in the mid-1980s. By 1985 public hospitals, with 5 percent of all hospital beds, held over 20 percent of all bad debt, and in California, where cuts in Medi-Cal had been particularly harsh, public hospitals held over 60 percent of all bad debt in those counties which had public hospitals.[19] Moreover, dumping led to such increased crowding in public facilities that many operated at or above capacity and began triaging patients to ensure beds for the most critical cases. "The public hospital serves as the last resort for the desperate, who are being dumped by other faculties," wrote the public health scholar Henrik Blum in 1987, "and now those patients can't even get dumped! I can't think of anything more awful."[20]

The dumping phenomenon called into question the basic financing mechanism for public hospitals. Always possessing an ambiguous role in a nation of charitable private hospitals, public hospitals had long existed as part of a "strange symbiosis between the public and private sectors," in the words of the medical historian Charles Rosenberg.[21] Private hospitals received nonprofit status (and its concomitant tax protection) in exchange for caring for at least a portion of the uninsured and indigent, while public hospitals picked up the remainder of the indigent who generally lived close by. The role of public hospitals had not changed appreciably after the implementation of Medicaid, although Medicaid itself essentially moved a substantial part of the financial burden of running the public hospitals from local and county governments to state and federal governments. Certainly the need for public hospitals had not been diminished. Private hospitals generally did not seek out poor patients with greater alacrity once they came insured with Medicaid policies, while public hospitals continued to play a central role in the nation's medical education system. But the torrent of wholly uninsured patients which flooded the wards of the nation's public hospitals in 1983 and 1984 exposed the weaknesses in the informal system of patient sharing and indigent financing by which public and private hospitals had been dividing up the indigent care population for twenty years.

Not everyone viewed dumping as bad. At least a few physicians and hospital administrators asked why private professionals and facilities should be volunteering their time and resources to care for patients for whom appropriate tax-funded public facilities existed. While no one suggested that private hospitals should turn away patients in critical condition because of their insurance status, some administrators did question why private hospitals should treat able-bodied and medically stable uninsured patients if public hospital beds were available. After Texas passed an antidumping law in 1986, one physician, Mohsin Shah, observed that the new law made available free private hospital care to anybody who demanded it. "Some Texans must now wonder why they are still buying health insurance," he wrote.[22] Similarly, a physician in Dallas, Tillman Hein, demanded, "Why do we have to pay the hospital bill for somebody who decided to spend his or her money on consumption rather than on health insurance?"[23] And an irate physician in Missouri, Ellison Weaver, wrote, "You say that in medicine today there is 'the obligation to serve the poor without pay' . . . Let me tell you, buddy, I don't do *anything* in this business without financial remuneration."[24]

Most physicians, nurses, administrators, and planners, by contrast, found the transfers troubling. To one administrator they were "inexcusable," to another a "cowardly abdication of professionalism."[25] Nearly

80 percent of all internists in fee-for-service practices offered free or reduced-rate care in 1986, and a similar proportion of pediatricians offered care to Medicaid patients. Writing in the *Journal of the American Medical Association*, James Davis declared that physicians had an "inherent, basic responsibility for the health requirements of the needy," and that they must provide for "all in our society who are in need of medical care."[26] Paradoxically, it was Medicaid itself which had called this fundamental tenet of medical practice into question. The existence of Medicaid had given license to many doctors to dispense with the commitment toward the poor that they had felt hitherto, and to many private hospitals to expand their capital bases without adequately budgeting for uncompensated care.

Dumping was troubling not so much because it reduced the quality of care for the nation's poor, but because it exemplified the troubled and ill-defined relationship between private and public hospitals, particularly in light of a diminished Medicaid system. Should public hospitals simply close their doors and allow states and municipalities to divert funds toward private institutions to care for the poor? Conversely, should private hospitals cease to take all noninsured patients (except in critical cases in which the patient was not stable enough to be moved), and admit that theirs was not fundamentally an eleemosynary mission? Or should the two systems maintain an ill-defined coexistence, with public institutions taking the poorest of the poor while private ones took on the more interesting, less costly cases in an effort to retain a steady supply of teaching material for their residency programs and justify their nonprofit status? Few planners or politicians offered a clear response to the question, other than decrying the overcrowding in the public hospitals and pleading for a greater social commitment from the privates.

Minorities, the Mentally Ill, and the Rural Poor

Cities faced particular challenges in providing charity care in the late 1980s, because they harbored a large share not only of the nation's poor but also of its African American population, which disproportionately lacked private health insurance. Although as recently as 1930 nearly 80 percent of blacks in the United States had lived in the rural South, the succeeding decades had brought substantial black migration to northern cities for industrial jobs, turning blacks from the most rural ethnic group in the country to its most urban.[27] Although the initial movement of blacks into industrial jobs lifted the economic fortunes of the population, later declines in industrial employment left many blacks unemployed and bereft of the social and religious institutions which had long sustained them in the South.[28] The movement of blacks into the middle and professional classes in the decades after the passage of the Civil Rights Act of 1965 created a net outflow of wealthier and more accomplished blacks to the suburbs, leaving a core of impoverished blacks in the inner cities. Urban black communities, dependent on welfare and Medicaid, came to symbolize the greatest failure of the American system for many social observers and critics in the 1970s and 1980s. President Carter visited what was perhaps the epicenter of the urban social welfare scourge—the South Bronx in New York City—in 1977, promising to rebuild and rejuvenate, but true solutions to the problems were elusive or absent altogether. Most of America simply stayed away from inner cities, or at least the most blighted neighborhoods.

Social dysfunction naturally bred ill-health, and blacks continued to lag behind whites in health and longevity. Whether measured by infant mortality; life expectancy; rates of infectious disease, smoking, obesity, hypertension, and heart disease; use of prenatal health care; or incidence of low-birth-weight babies, blacks trailed whites significantly throughout all income and age groups. (The one exception was in rates of depression, anxiety, and affective disorders, where blacks did slightly better, resulting concomitantly in lower suicide rates.) By 1984 black infant mortality stood at 18.4 deaths per 1,000 live births, while the rate of white infant mortality stood at little more than half—9.4 deaths per 1,000.[29]

Oddly, after Reagan's Medicaid cuts infant mortality in general, and black infant mortality in particular, improved. The gap between white and black babies, for example, slightly decreased. Black declines in post-natal mortality rates exceeded those of whites from 1960 to 1984 (60 percent versus 43 percent), and black declines in the number of low-birth-weight babies nearly matched those of whites.[30] "Our feeling is that the gap is no bigger now than it has always been," said Shellie Lengel of the Public Health Service in January 1984.[31] Furthermore, gains for the nation as a whole had accelerated under Reagan's watch. During President Carter's final year in office, 1980, the nation posted 45,526 infant deaths. The figure dropped each year during Reagan's first term, and by 1984 there were only 39,200 infant deaths nationwide. And while black American teenagers posted the highest pregnancy rate of any population or subpopulation in any developed country in the world, the teenage pregnancy rate for the United States as a whole was also extremely high— 83 per 1,000—far exceeding the posted rates for any other industrialized nation.[32] Although the United States had more pronounced, extreme, and widespread poverty than most industrialized countries, under Reagan the health of the poor was improving for all races.[33]

Some public health officials and health watchers saw racism and bigotry underlying the health disparities. The president of the National Medical Association, Edith Jones, called for a fight against "hopelessness, joblessness" rather than for greater health resources for blacks.[34] People who viewed the health deficiencies of minorities through this lens would blame persistent racism in the nation's businesses and educational institutions. Fix society, the argument went, and the black problem would fix itself. Not everyone agreed, even among black intellectuals and scholars. A growing number of sociologists, public health professionals, and social workers had begun to suspect by 1985 that while black social pathology might have originated in slavery, racism, and sanctioned legal discrimination, with emancipation and the advent of civil rights protections it was managing to survive quite nicely on its own. Some observers believed that blacks, not whites, held the keys to the black future, and that repeated harkening back to the injustices of the past was counterproductive. As Harry Schwartz, professor of medicine at Columbia, wrote in 1984, "The violence of ghetto life is a good place to begin for anyone who wants to correct the conditions that now make black males the shortest-lived race-sex group."[35]

Perhaps no statistic was more disturbing than the 47 percent of black children born to unwed mothers in 1985. By contrast, only 15 percent of white babies were born out of wedlock that year. As recently as 1960, Eleanor Holmes Norton pointed out, over three fourths of black families were intact nuclear families headed by a husband and a wife, and evidence suggested that even under slavery most black slave children were born within the confines of marriage.[36] Pierre deVise, an urban studies scholar at Roosevelt University, called the social dissolution of the black community "the most important and alarming demographic development of our time . . . welfare motherhood has become the role model for girls, and drug dealing and pimping the role models for boys."[37] William Raspberry wrote in the *Washington Post*, "Middle-class blacks will either undertake an unprecedented and enormously difficult salvage operation—or else run for our lives."[38] Most notably, Jesse Jackson during his presidential campaigns called on blacks to solve their own problems, and support for this view began to build among such traditional bulwarks of the black community as the NAACP, the Urban League, and the sorority Delta Sigma Theta.

Although life patterns were somewhat to blame, lack of access to health care also explained the poor health status of blacks. Despite disproportionate use of the Medicaid program, blacks—particularly urban blacks—received preventive care and necessary intervention at lower rates than whites, even controlling for income. By the mid-1980s nearly 40 percent of pregnant black women began prenatal care after the first trimester had ended (at which point several correctable gestational defects were already unresponsive to treatment), as opposed to 20 percent of white pregnant women.[39] By contrast, under Sweden's socialized medical care system 99 percent of pregnant women had received some prenatal care by the end of the first trimester. Among persons reporting a history of hypertension, 30 percent of blacks had not had a blood pressure check in the previous year, as opposed to 19 percent of whites. While blacks were less likely than whites to carry any sort of health insurance (including Medicaid), the gap was especially wide with regard to private insurance—72 percent versus 85 percent. And even when blacks did qualify for Medicaid, their benefits under the program lagged behind the benefits accorded to white Medicaid recipients, mostly because they resided disproportionately in rural, southern states with poorly funded Medicaid programs.[40]

As has previously been discussed, blacks suffered particularly from lack of access to black physicians, who were in short supply. By 1986 blacks averaged only 3.4 physician visits a year, compared to 4.4 for whites. Black patients tended to be most comfortable with black physicians, and the number of black students in medical schools, apart from the two that were traditionally black, had fallen since the early 1970s, while the number of students at those two schools—Howard and Meharry—had remained stagnant.[41] While some black doctors opened practices in the inner cities to serve a poor clientele, the majority, like their white colleagues, located their practices in the suburbs to serve educated, middle- and upper-middle-class patients who had private insurance and could pay the requisite co-payments and deductibles. The situation did not begin to improve until immigrant physicians, predominantly trained in India, Pakistan, and Nigeria, began arriving in large numbers in the late 1980s and setting up inner-city practices.

The shortage of private primary-care physicians in inner cities led quite naturally to overuse of hospital emergency rooms and inpatient services by black patients. By the mid-1980s blacks were using 50 percent more hospital care than whites, although one study in Michigan found that the bulk of this discrepancy could be explained by income disparities.[42] An even more pronounced overuse of hospital facilities could be found in the nation's growing Hispanic community, whose annual hospital use exceeded that of the general population by a full day, and who drove up emergency room usage in public hospitals which served predominantly Hispanic communities. Not surprisingly, insurance coverage for this group, whether from private companies, Medicaid, or Medicare, trailed that of blacks by a significant margin, with fewer than two thirds of all individuals covered.[43]

Lack of access to health care for blacks and Hispanics, whether due to the absence of proximate private physicians or third-party coverage, or some unknown reason, exacerbated the already poor health profiles of these populations.[44] Clearly government had a role to play. More generous funding for urban community health clinics, for public health doctors, or for special urban nursing corps could at least bring more health professionals into the neighborhoods and communities where they were most needed. Additionally, adjustments to Medicaid eligibility limits could expand the umbrella of coverage available to minority communities (and to poor whites as well) and thus allow greater use of existing private providers. But research suggested that government could solve only part of the problem. Changing habits of use of medical care, and encouraging prevention, proper nutrition, and salubrious activities, could be as elusive for the insured as the uninsured, and a broader change in cultural patterns would probably bring more change than simply increasing the physician force or the capacities of hospital emergency rooms.

Among children too, blacks and Hispanics fared worse than whites. Nearly half of all black children lived in impoverished families, versus 30 percent of Hispanic children and 17 percent of white children. And for children living in households headed by women, these rates skyrocketed to 68.5 percent, 70.5 percent, and 47.6 percent.[45] "The average black child can expect to spend more than five years of his childhood in poverty; the average white child, less than 10 months," one report read.[46] From 1968 to 1983 the total number of poor children in the country increased by three million, even as the total number of children dropped by nine million, and families who were defined as poor received proportionately less government support than they had twenty years previously.

Other subpopulations experiencing declining health status in the 1980s included the chronically mentally ill and the rural poor. Psychiatric patients, released from state mental hospitals en masse in the 1970s, had visibly reemerged as "street people" by 1985.[47] Begging on the sidewalks of the nation's metropolises, and sleeping in train and bus depots, homeless people seemed to multiply during this time even as urban residents grew increasingly numb to their supplications. While cutbacks in federal housing grants explained part of the phenomenon, the majority of the new homeless were deinstitutionalized schizophrenics, devoid of family and community support, unstable, and often noncogent. Estimates placed the proportion who were severely mentally ill at between one third and two thirds of the total homeless population, but these were just guesses.[48] Similarly, advocacy groups placed the total number of mentally ill homeless nationwide at between 250,000 and 3 million—the former estimate from the U.S. Department of Housing and Urban Development, the latter from the nonprofit homeless advocacy group the Community for Creative Non-Violence.[49]

Beyond the obvious health needs associated with their mental illness, the homeless mentally ill exhibited a plethora of physical ailments which often went untreated. Skin lesions and ulcers, systemic sepsis, malnutrition, untreated sexually transmitted diseases, and alcoholism frequently made living on the street for prolonged periods fatal. Homeless people often suffered from severe edema due to their practice of sleeping while sitting propped against walls, which in turn led to phlebitis and further infection and ulceration. A growing number of the homeless suffered from tuberculosis during the 1980s (some from antibiotic-resistant strains), and many suffered from scabies and body lice, which they contracted from sharing "camps," cots, and public shelters. Lacking a permanent address, supportive family members, or social service advocates, the homeless mentally ill rarely qualified for Medicaid. The community mental health centers which had been established in part to serve the discharged population in practice often treated working- and middle-class patients, while state psychiatric hospitals tended to medicate patients and return them to the streets. Not surprisingly, discharged schizophrenics lacking family or community support often died in their forties, or sooner.[50]

Though better positioned than urban ghetto dwellers or deinstitutionalized mental patients, the rural poor also continued to suffer in the 1980s. Lacking the strong cadre of urban poverty advocates who lobbied for and attended to the needs of the impoverished minorities in the inner cities, poor rural patients tended to go without care entirely, lacking both insurance and accessible providers. The National Health Service Corps, which by 1988 had temporarily placed over thirteen thousand recent medical graduates in rural communities throughout the nation, had seen its funding sharply cut back under the Reagan administration (from $100 million in 1978 to $2 million in 1988), although this reduction was mitigated to some degree by an increase in the federally funded loan forgiveness program for young doctors who chose to practice in impoverished areas. While the Public Health Service responded to the shortages by designating Health Manpower Shortage Areas and Medically Underserved Areas, the structuring of these grant programs around matching funds to local tax revenues undermined their ultimate effectiveness. Federal officials tinkered with the mandated matching rates throughout the late 1980s, but rural communities continued to experience severe shortages of qualified physicians, nurses, paramedics, and mental health workers.[51]

Despite the decrease in funding for poor-care programs, however, the medical fortunes of marginal communities—ethnic and racial minorities, the mentally ill, the rural poor—improved during the 1980s, despite cuts to many of the programs which served them. In general, however, they improved at rates slower than mainstream populations, and existing gaps in health status narrowed only slightly, if at all. Whether poor health within minority groups resulted from inadequate government efforts or was merely an ancillary symptom of more profound social dysfunction became a question germane to health planning. As a consequence, public health officials and policy planners began to question the efficacy of the many social welfare programs which had been implemented under President Johnson's Great Society. Such skepticism was new, and promised to increase over time. America continued to exhibit sympathy for the poor and vulnerable, but it seemed no longer sure of an appropriate course.

Children

The high infant mortality rate in the United States continued to trouble health policy makers during the 1980s, even as planners of differing political proclivities continued to argue about its exact causes. The basic facts were not in dispute: infant mortality nationwide had dropped from 47 (per 1,000 live births) in 1940 to 13.1 in 1979. The decline continued at a rate of 4.6 percent a year until 1983, then slowed to 2.7 percent in 1984. The Public Health Service had set a national goal of 9 deaths per 1,000 for 1985, but given the slowed decline this rate would not be achieved until 1990. By 1985 the rate stood at 10.6, well behind the world's leaders— Japan, Finland, and Sweden—which maintained rates of just below 7.

Policy planners were puzzled by the oddly high rate relative to other wealthy countries, and could not pinpoint the exact cause. Certainly the United States had unique challenges which other industrialized nations did not have, including large-scale immigration, racial disparities in education and income, a large rural population, and a more porous social safety net. Different studies pointed to a lack of adequate prenatal care, pediatric care for minority populations, hygiene education for recent immigrants, and nutrition and fitness programs in the public schools. The most important epidemiological insight into the problem in the early 1980s was that among babies of common birth weight the United States fared no worse than other nations; rather, too many American babies were simply born small. Natality statistics bore this argument out: nearly 7 percent of all babies born in the United States weighed less than 2,500 grams at birth (the official cutoff for low birth weight), and nearly 13 percent of black babies did so.[52]

Recognition of America's birth-weight deficit was both comforting, because it indicated that the nation's neonatal and pediatric systems were equal to those of other nations in keeping babies alive once they were born, and disquieting, because an elevated number of low-birth-weight babies indicated problems in the nation's social welfare system. The route to raising birth weight was well known by 1985: a healthy prenatal diet; prenatal avoidance of tobacco, alcohol, narcotics, and prescription medicine; and routine prenatal obstetrical care. The solution was within the reach of nearly all Americans, regardless of income or residence, so long as they possessed a reasonable degree of medical knowledge and situated themselves within an informed and supportive community. But this was precisely what was missing for a high number of American mothers. American women were getting pregnant with greater frequency in adolescence or within communities which lacked tight social networks and support systems, and remained ignorant of basic rules of hygiene and health. America's infant mortality problem was not so much a medical problem as a social one.

This point was made in a disturbing fashion by the health economists Michael Grossman and Steven Jacobowitz, who discovered that the single most important factor in reducing infant mortality by 1985 was an increase in legal abortions, suggesting that the ultimate solution to the problem was not in more widely disseminating prenatal care but in helping prevent pregnancies from happening in the first place for young unmarried women.[53] This conjecture was confirmed in studies showing that even poor countries, such as Sri Lanka and Portugal, could sharply reduce infant mortality by making available family planning services and abortions. Reducing the incidence of poverty would help as well, insofar as illiteracy, truancy, and out-of-wedlock pregnancy were all correlated with poverty. A slight correlation between expansion of the WIC program and decline in low-birth-weight infants lent credence to this line of thinking.[54]

The Reagan administration viewed the problem with jaundiced eyes. For one, it questioned whether further investments in public health and social services should come from the federal government at all, regardless of the eventual form they might take, for the bulwark of the Reagan revolution was devolution and local control.[55] Beyond this, conservative pundits and administration staffers questioned whether a declining drop in the *rate* of decrease represented so much a public health problem as simply "good news at a somewhat slower rate" (in the words of the conservative policy scholar Ben Wattenberg).[56] Furthermore, domestic policy advisors in the Reagan White House operated from the assumption that large Great Society social welfare programs had frequently failed because they were attempting to impel broad changes in human behavior by essentially giving away money and services, rather than by creating financial inducements for people to change their behavior on their own. Such thinking was personified in the ideas of Jack Kemp, secretary of housing and urban development, who aggressively turned to tax-protected "Urban Enterprise Zones" and other free-market techniques to alleviate urban poverty.[57]

Under Reagan federal efforts in pediatric care continued to be delivered primarily through Medicaid, and specifically through the EPSDT components of the programs.[58] Unfortunately, nearly two thirds of all impoverished children in the country were not covered by Medicaid in any given year, and supplementary pediatric medical programs such as state Crippled Children programs, maternal and child block grants, and Community and Migrant Health Center programs failed to bring the remainder under the EPSDT umbrella. Part of the problem was the wildly divergent eligibility standards in the programs, which persisted despite congressional tinkering in the early 1980s. In 1986, for example, a female-headed family of three in Alaska could qualify for Medicaid as soon as its income fell below $719 a month, while in Alabama that same family needed to earn less than $118 a month to be eligible. (This last figure was extreme, even with the low cost of living in Alabama: it represented only 16 percent of the federal poverty threshold.) Because EPSDT eligibility was identical to general Medicaid eligibility, the divergent and sometimes bizarre Medicaid eligibility standards were the greatest barrier to more comprehensive pediatric care and immunization nationwide. Overall, poorly adjusted AFDC eligibility levels (which drove the Medicaid eligibility levels), coupled with the cuts of the early 1980s, prevented millions of children from receiving Medicaid and EPSDT coverage, and alternative programs could not compensate adequately.[59]

Medicaid and Managed Care

Although certain HMOs had been willing to enroll Medicaid recipients from the program's inception, the total numbers of such enrollees stayed quite low until the early 1980s. A dearth of willing HMOs, along with widespread ignorance of the mechanics of managed care on the part of both Medicaid recipients and Medicaid program officers, kept HMO membership to just 1.4 percent of all Medicaid recipients in 1981. New contracting rules written into OBRA '81, however, helped to facilitate Medicaid capitation contracting, just as states began to seriously look into mechanisms to cut costs in the Medicaid programs. By 1984 twenty-eight states were experimenting with regional Medicaid HMO contracting, and Arizona and California had implemented statewide capitation contracting rules. At the same time, the Robert Wood Johnson Foundation announced a $15.6 million program to enroll nearly half a million Medicaid patients into prepaid health plans in ten states.[60]

Experiments with Medicaid contracting came about just as private-sector managed care was burgeoning. Managed-care companies were partly responsible for reducing medical care inflation from 12 to 15 percent annually (which had been common in the late 1970s and early 1980s) to 3 to 6 percent by the early 1990s. Although some prescient industry analysts warned that these abnormally low inflation rates could not be sustained, most employers were delighted, and began to more aggressively push their remaining employees into the new plans. Over the next half-dozen years managed-care plans spun off a variety of new products—IPAS, PPOS, POSS—in an effort to make managed care more palatable to both subscribers and physicians.

Managed care could not promise the same level of inflation reduction for Medicare and Medicaid. Medicare, serving an old and sick population, would have a difficult time realizing the same savings from managed care as plans serving younger groups did. Moreover, the prospect of forcing millions of elderly voters into HMOs that offered them only limited health care choices was politically unappealing both to members of Congress and to HCFA officials. Initial efforts relied on inducing Medicare beneficiaries to join by reducing their co-pays substantially, and by providing all or part of a subscription drug plan which was not included under the existing part B program. Despite such allurements, few of the elderly enrolled in the programs in the 1980s, and many of those who did disenrolled within two years of joining, once they realized that the membership in an HMO precluded them from consulting specialists in the manner to which they had grown accustomed. Simultaneously, many managed-care organizations began to drop Medicare enrollees when they realized that they could not make money (or even cover costs) with this population under HCFA reimbursement guidelines.[61]

Managed care for Medicaid patients held both lesser and greater promise than it did for Medicare patients. On the down side, Medicaid contracting rates were so low that most managed-care executives doubted whether they could make a profit from enrolling the recipients. Additionally, Medicaid patients often delayed going to physicians until their conditions were quite advanced, making them poor insurance risks. On the plus side, Medicaid patients were younger than average, unlikely to complain about lack of choice, and not acclimated to a world of indemnified specialty care. Moreover, since one of the great failings of Medicaid historically had been its inability to provide preventive care, Medicaid managed care offered the promise of regular physician care for the first time to many Medicaid recipients.

Although it would be a decade before most states began moving Medicaid patients into managed care on a large scale, early regional results conducted under waiver dispensation were promising. Medicaid patients did go to the doctor more frequently when co-pays were minimal, and early intervention appeared to cut down on some emergency room abuse. In addition, physicians who had long maintained a predominantly Medicaid practice found that their incomes were actually rising under managed care, as they were able to count on regular capitation payments while referring out patients for specialty needs. If privately insured patients were finding that health care was less convenient and less pleasant under managed care, Medicaid patients were finding just the opposite.

The only questions were whether the intermediary agencies doing the contracting could break even under the programs, and whether state Medicaid agencies were saving any money.[62]

Comprehensive Reform

By the mid-1980s the health system was plagued with a catalogue of challenges, including growing costs, declining quality, diminished choice wrought by managed care, an increasing number of Americans who lacked any sort of health insurance (either public or private), and a growing concern over the "job lock" which employment-based health insurance often imposed on workers seeking to change jobs. In response, various political and professional leaders, as well as scholars of health care delivery and professional health planners, began to favor some sort of comprehensive reform effort toward medical service payment and delivery. While ideas ranged from expanding Medicaid and amending the tax code to adopting a national health insurance program, the notable fact of this ideation was its relatively broad acceptance. Polls conducted in the late 1980s by the Public Agenda Foundation, as well as by CBS and the *New York Times*, found that at least 55 percent of Americans expressed a willingness to fund expanded Medicaid and Medicare coverage through increased taxes, and 82 percent believed that everyone had a right to health care and that the federal government had an obligation to guarantee it.[63]

One obvious approach to comprehensive reform was simply to expand the Medicaid program to cover a larger portion of the poor, dual-parent families, and nonpoor families who were deemed medically needy. This approach appealed particularly to both the American Hospital Association and the Catholic Hospital Association (CHA), whose members were bearing the brunt of the growth in the uninsured population, as well as the reimbursement cuts brought about by the expansion of managed care. Both associations delineated specific adjustments to AFDC, SSI, and Medicaid enrollment guidelines which would enable their constituents to continue to meet their historic obligation to the needy.[64] Of particular concern to the AHA was the increase in "Ribicoff Children"—impoverished minors excluded from Medicaid coverage because their parents were maintaining an intact marriage. These children could offer zero reimbursement to a hospital, yet for political and ethical reasons they were nearly impossible to transfer to a public facility.

Beyond simply expanding the Medicaid program, planners and scholars suggested such options as federalizing it, combining it with Medicare, or making it available to those whose incomes exceeded eligibility limits by allowing them to "buy in" on a sliding scale. Each of these options had proponents; Michael Whitcomb, a professor at the University of Missouri School of Medicine, favored placing each of the fifty state Medicaid programs under the jurisdiction of the federal government in an effort to avoid "piecemeal" reform efforts which would be time-consuming and probably ineffective. Senator John Chafee (R., R.I.) favored a buy-in plan that would make Medicaid coverage available for purchase to those with incomes up to 200 percent of the poverty line.[65] The problem with most of these ideas was that they were prohibitively expensive. In addition, none would guarantee universal coverage, which was often a stated goal of those who favored comprehensive reform. Chafee's Medicaid expansion bill would still leave 26.2 million people uninsured, and most buy-in proposals being debated in Congress would leave 10–15 million people uninsured.[66]

A second approach to comprehensive reform would be to adopt a national health insurance program along Canadian lines. This approach appealed to a few reform-minded physicians, as well as professional health planners. Physicians felt slightly more comfortable with the Canadian system than almost any other, first because they viewed Canadian medical training as more similar to American training than that offered elsewhere, and second because Canadian doctors retained their professional autonomy and independence under their nation's national insurance plan, as well as their hospital admitting privileges. The AMA actually went as far as endorsing Senator Edward Kennedy's All Workers Act of 1987 (S. 1265), which would have created a limited form of the Canadian model.[67] Professional health planners also liked the approach for its imposition of a regional planning authority on hospital expansion and purchasing, giving government some ability to limit the wasteful overbuilding and technological redundancies which plagued the system.[68]

For many planners, legislators, and reform advocates, a Canadian approach was a near perfect solution to America's health care dilemma. Canadians reported themselves to be very pleased with their system: they spent 20 percent less per capita on health care than Americans, their life expectancy exceeded that of the United States by several years, and they delivered the system through a scheme of provincially based health authorities which could easily be transferred to the American states. Health reform advocates had been pointing to the Canadian example almost from the day Saskatchewan inaugurated the first of the provincial plans in 1955, and scholars of health care delivery and public policy never tired of pointing northward for the perfect example of a public-private compromise in delivering universally accessible care.

Unfortunately, several substantial barriers dissuaded most legislators from emulating the Canadian example. For one, the establishment of a similar system would mean the demise of existing private health insurance companies in the United States (both nonprofit and for-profit), which stood united in their opposition. For another, Americans had indicated repeatedly throughout the twentieth century (in 1914, 1939, 1941–49, and 1977) a reluctance to allow government to expand substantially into the delivery of or payment for private medical care.[69] Voters had historically opposed congressional candidates who proclaimed their support for it, and in the 1950 midterm elections had rejected nearly every member of Congress who had too visibly supported Truman's national health insurance proposals.[70] Third, by 1987 cracks had begun to appear in the Canadian system, as reports of queuing and "cross-border" hospital shopping trickled out. A few Canadian physicians emigrated to the United States and reported declining investment in hospital infrastructure and medical technology in Canada, as well as diminishing standards in specialty training. While mortality statistics did not confirm the assertion that Canadian medicine was on the wane, the anecdotes dissuaded many Americans from supporting a movement toward the Canadian model.

A promising third way to comprehensive reform was exemplified by a plan conceived in Oregon in 1989 by State Senator John Kitzhaber. The plan ranked some seven hundred medical and surgical procedures and professional interactions according to their cost-benefit ratio, favoring inexpensive procedures which promised a large payoff in medical outcome or improved quality of life, and disfavoring expensive ones which promised little. The idea was to take the existing Oregon Medicaid budget, supplanted by additional funding, and apply it to as many procedures on the list as possible. "They may not all eat steak," Kitzhaber stated in an interview, "but they will eat."[71]

The plan, which earned Kitzhaber the sobriquet "Dr. Death," brought strong condemnation from a variety of bioethicists, as well as civil liberty advocates and defenders of patients' rights. "To withhold proven, efficacious treatment from someone who needs it does not seem ethical," stated the bioethicist Arthur Caplan, and many legislators rejected any sort of rationing whatsoever as unfair. Despite support for the program from professional health planners and some politicians—"Oregon is trying to say, 'Let's ration rationally,'" said Governor Richard Lamm of Colorado—most Americans felt distinctly uneasy with the proposal.[72] For a nation accustomed to unimpeded access to specialized procedures and interventions, the mere existence of sanctioned rationing threatened the continued generosity of their own private plans. Ultimately, the Oregon plan was successfully challenged in court by the American Civil Liberties Union on the ground that it deprived disabled Medicaid recipients of due process under the Americans with Disabilities Act (ADA) by denying them medical care.[73]

The last approach to comprehensive reform actively discussed in the mid-1980s was a "consumer choice" universal health plan conceived by Alain Enthoven, an economist at Stanford University. Capitalizing on the potential of HMOs to reduce administrative overhead as well as the "specialization" of the system, Enthoven proposed using general tax revenues to grant each American the option of buying into the HMO of his or her choice in a transaction which would be heavily regulated by the federal government. The government would ensure that multiple private HMOs would bid for each policy (and thus keep prices competitive through market pressure), while at the same time mandating a minimum benefit menu to avoid the problems of the Oregon plan. By requiring employers to participate (or, as it was phrased at the time, using "employer mandates" the government would ensure that individual managed-care companies would have a proportionate share of expensive and inexpensive members. Supporters of the idea emphasized that it would enable the nation to guarantee universal coverage for an aggregate cost no higher that that which the present system was incurring.[74] Unfortunately, experience with managed-care plans over the following decade demonstrated their limited ability to reduce health care inflation over the long term.

For poverty care, the late 1980s were defined by the restoration of some of the Medicaid cuts of the early 1980s, managed care, and debate over comprehensive reform. Although expansions under various OBRA and COBRA bills did restore access to health care for some of the nation's poor (particularly very young children, pregnant women, and poor children of intact marriages), other fiscal demands more than absorbed the funds added for this purpose. Private hospitals found themselves facing unprecedented budgetary pressures, which spilled over to public hospitals. Public hospitals in turn, facing depleted municipal coffers, looked to Medicaid to absorb even more of their costs. Another drain on the newly increased Medicaid funds was an expanding program of long-term care for the Medicaid-eligible elderly.

As had been true for most of the twentieth century, comprehensive reform (in the guise of either national health insurance, an expanded Medicaid program, employer mandates, or an optional Medicaid buy-in) seemed to offer a solution to both the challenges of poor care and the threats of a burgeoning population of the uninsured. Such a panacea attracted the attention of professional planners, scholars, and even members of Congress, but the broad American middle was far more reserved in its endorsement. Any government solution to a "problem" that beset a system with which nearly 80 percent of Americans were basically satisfied had always been bound to fail. Although Americans were grumbling about their health care more in 1985 than they had in the past, they still preferred their system over virtually any other to be found, either abroad or in the minds of economists and legislators.

11

Managed Medicaid, AIDS, and
the Clinton Health Bill

The Uninsured in the Early 1990s

By 1990 33 million Americans, nearly 15 percent of the total population, lacked health insurance of any sort, and the number was growing. As recently as 1980 the uninsured had numbered only 23.4 million (12.3 percent), but this number had grown by nearly a million a year for the past decade, and the trend gave no indication of abating. With Senator Edward Kennedy declaring that the situation was a crisis which threatened the "health and well being of every American family," and no obvious solution to the problem in sight, the growth of the uninsured stood as one of the great challenges to both state and federal governments at the start of the decade.[1] Always a source of some national embarrassment, the existence of such a large group of uninsured citizens threatened to overtax the nation's charity care infrastructure and bankrupt public hospitals and clinics.

The uninsured were not uniformly distributed throughout the population. Young adults, aged eighteen to twenty-four, were more likely than any other age group to be uninsured, with 25 percent lacking coverage. By contrast, only 10 percent of adults between thirty-five and sixty-five were uninsured, and because of Medicare virtually none over sixty-five were. Poor households were far more likely than middle-class or rich ones to be uninsured, despite the presence of Medicaid: 30 percent of families with incomes below the poverty level were uninsured, versus 23 percent of the near poor (incomes below 200 percent of the poverty level), and only 6 percent of the middle-class and wealthy (incomes above 300 percent of the poverty level). Families in which the primary earner worked less than thirty-five hours a week were also disproportionately likely to be uninsured, as were single-parent families, families in which at least one adult was unemployed and seeking work, and families in which the parents had been recently separated. In fact, access to private coverage created a compelling argument for the primacy of the traditional family, as only 8 percent of households in which married parents lived together with children lacked insurance.[2]

The crisis hit minority groups worse than the general population. While only 12.5 percent of whites were uninsured, 19 percent of blacks were, as were over 20 percent of Latinos. It also hit select parts of the country, particularly the Deep South, worse than the country as a whole. Moreover, the severity of the situation varied between states, largely depending on Medicaid eligibility rates. New York, for example, was able to insure 83 percent of all poor residents, while Texas insured only 42 percent. Nationwide, part-time workers, young adults, unmarried adults, and workers with less than a high school education were all far more likely to lack insurance than the population as a whole. And while expanded Medicaid eligibility could rectify the problem for some of the poor, many others—seasonal and part-time workers, the unemployed, the underskilled, and the uneducated—would still lack insurance in large numbers no matter how inclusive Medicaid became.

Lack of insurance posed more than a fiscal challenge or a health threat to the uninsured: it also affected their confidence in themselves, and in the future. The uninsured were far more likely than the insured to feel ambivalence toward pregnancy and to consider having abortions. They were twice as likely to admit to depression, to lack adequate food, and to feel ostracized by family and community. And they were far less likely to discuss health problems with friends and neighbors.[3] Living without health insurance in the United States in 1990 meant living on the edge— surviving from day to day, but feeling threatened that an illness, an accident, or a pregnancy could upset the structure of life and leave a person outcast, impoverished, and helpless. Health insurance was not only a guarantor of reasonable medical care; it was a guarantor of continuity, stability, and place.

Of particular concern to health planners was the rise in the ranks of uninsured children. Making up over a quarter of all of the nation's uninsured, children lacking insurance came, not surprisingly, from poor families, but also from families in which one or both parents were working part time or full time. Nearly half the children of the working poor were uninsured, and fewer than 15 percent of uninsured children came from families with unemployed parents. While Medicaid, and to a much lesser degree Medicare and military health plans, prevented many more children from being uninsured, the quirky holes in the Medicaid programs allowed over nine million children to go uninsured each year.[4]

As was true for adults, lack of insurance affected children's health adversely. Children without insurance were far less likely than the insured to be in good or excellent health, less likely to be immunized against polio, diphtheria, pertussis, tetanus, and smallpox, more likely to be infected with HIV, and more likely to have untreated emotional disorders. While a number of correlates of lack of insurance, including poverty and the greater likelihood of living in a single-parent home, were also at least partly responsible for these children's poor health profiles, insurance status alone accounted for some of the problem, irrespective of other indicators.[5]

The rise in uninsured children mirrored the rise in poor children in the United States since 1970, which in turn was highly correlated with the explosion in out-of-wedlock teenage births. Out-of-wedlock births in the United States had grown from 13 percent of teenage births in 1955 to an extraordinary 53 percent by 1990. This sharp rise, coupled with declining industrial employment after 1970, was responsible for much of the growth in the number of juveniles lacking insurance. The percentage of children living in poverty had grown by nearly a third since 1970, so that by 1990 over 16 percent of non-Hispanic white children, 40 percent of Hispanic children, and 46 percent of black children lived in poverty. Lack of insurance was both a consequence and a cause of this trend, as poorer access to health professionals led to less knowledge of hygiene and higher rates of teen pregnancy, smoking, drug use, and obesity.[6]

Although black children exceeded Latino children in rates of non-insurance, among adults, Latinos outstripped all other groups. Nearly 40 percent of adult Latinos were uncovered in 1990, compared with 24 percent of blacks and 12 percent of whites. And although there was substantial variation in rates of insurance between Latino subgroups—42 percent of Mexicans were uninsured, for example, as opposed to only 22 percent of Cubans—recent arrivals from Central and South America, Puerto Rico, and Cuba generally adhered to life patterns which excluded them from the employer-provided insurance infrastructure. Latino immigrants worked disproportionately as day laborers in agriculture and construction, two industries which provided little insurance coverage for employees. They also were frequently self-employed, or owned or worked in small businesses—all situations, again, which were associated disproportionately with lack of coverage. And because they frequently earned too much to qualify for Medicaid, or held immigration status which precluded their applying, they had no public program on which to fall back. Indeed, the Mexican immigrant paradigm of little formal education and a highly developed work ethic, coupled with tight family and community allegiances and a strong entrepreneurial spirit, seemed almost a perfect recipe for exclusion from private health insurance. In addition, Latino immigrants were the youngest, and most heavily male, subpopulation in the country—both characteristics associated with lack of insurance.[7]

Although the problem of the uninsured reached all parts of the population by 1990, it was disproportionately a problem of the poor, the unmarried, blacks and Latinos, and young adult men. More specifically, the problem pervaded the ranks of employees of small businesses, migrant and seasonal workers, and the recently unemployed. The wholly destitute, particularly single women with children and no apparent sources of income, were shielded by Medicaid, as was the broad swath of middle- and upper-class employees of large and mid-sized corporations, governmental and nonprofit entities, and the professions. Given the strong association of private insurance with employment in traditional concerns, the shifting nature of American work since 1970 had exacerbated the problem of the uninsured. America's large-scale shedding of industrial jobs and movement toward a more service-based economy underlay the rise in the uninsured population, and the trend would therefore continue in the absence of substantial reforms in the nation's health care system.

Medicaid in the Early 1990s

Despite substantial growth in the Medicaid programs over the previous decade, poor people continued to face substantial difficulties in gaining access to care. While various laws had loosened Medicaid eligibility standards during the 1980s and raised reimbursement to "safety net" hospitals, low reimbursement rates, and declining interest in general practice and primary-care medicine among young physicians, served to severely limit the number of physicians attending to Medicaid patients. Studies in Michigan and North Carolina found that nearly 25 percent of pediatricians in each state restricted Medicaid access to their practices, and other studies demonstrated similarly high rates of restriction in adult primary care.[8] When pressed, doctors quickly pointed to declining reimbursement rates as the reason for withdrawing from the program, or at least limiting their exposure to it, in addition to bureaucratic barriers to payment, and the generally less-than-cooperative attitude of many Medicaid patients. For example, reimbursement for a basic office consultation under Medicaid in New York had increased only 30 cents over twenty-four years, to a stunningly low $7.50 a visit, compared with a regular private reimbursement of $45. No doctor could take on many patients at this level of pay and "stay in practice for any length of time," wrote J. E. Pipas, a physician in Syracuse.[9]

Private hospitals also continued to resist treating Medicaid patients, transferring them to public hospitals when possible, or refusing outright to give them any but the most basic treatment. One irate mother watched as her son, who had Down's syndrome and was Medicaid-eligible, was turned away from several private hospitals, even while shaking with fever, vomiting, and exhibiting signs of severe dehydration. "Adrift in a sea of white coats," the mother wrote, "the only mercy we were shown was a towel to catch the vomitus."[10] The son was ultimately treated, successfully, at the local public hospital.

Patients who were able to qualify for Medicaid benefited greatly from the program, despite its shortcomings. Medicaid patients saw private doctors more frequently than the indigent uninsured did, received better preventive care, visited the hospital less frequently, and exhibited generally better health. Children covered by Medicaid received their primary care in physicians' offices 56 percent of the time, compared to 47 percent for poor children who did not qualify for Medicaid. (Pediatric patients insured with a private carrier received 81 percent of their primary care in a physician's office.)[11] And poor geriatric patients who qualified for Medicaid (which reimbursed their co-payments, prescription drugs, and part B premiums) stayed away from nursing homes and hospitals at substantially higher rates than those elderly who did not qualify for the program.[12] Thus, Medicaid programs were much better than nothing, despite their underfunding, quirky loopholes, and uncooperative bureaucracies. Acknowledging this, few critics of the program aspired to reinvent a poor-care program from scratch. Rather, the route to improvement for poor care seemed to lie in incremental advances in reimbursement rates and procedures.

The expansion in eligibility which Congress had embarked on in the early 1980s had continued in 1989 with a regulation requiring states to cover all pregnant women and children (under the age of seven) with family incomes below 133 percent of the poverty level. Medicaid enrollment, which had stood at 22 million in 1988, had increased to 30 million by 1991, with further increases likely.[13] As a result, the proportion of the poor covered under Medicaid had risen by 4 percentage points, and that of the near poor by 2.5 points since 1980, even as a decreasing number of the poor and near poor were covered by private insurance.[14] Despite the expansion, however, a large number of eligible families were refusing Medicaid coverage, sometimes because of existing coverage from a private policy, but more often because of procedural snags in the application process which thwarted thousands of applicants from receiving benefits.[15] Procedural barriers, ranging from presentation of inappropriate tax documents, wage statements, and birth certificates to improper residency, lack of proper receipts for child care and tuition, or unpaid doctor's and dentist's bills, were responsible for over half of all denials for Medicaid coverage in the early 1990s. One odd consequence was the hiring of professional application specialists by many hospitals. Leslie Aronovits, an analyst for the GAO, wrote in 1994: "Quick identification and enrollment of eligible Medicaid patients is of paramount importance to hospitals."[16]

Inadequate Medicaid reimbursement to physicians was hardly the result of miserly appropriations by state and federal legislatures. Indeed, Medicaid expenditures had increased tremendously since the mid-1980s, and were threatening to overwhelm state budgets. Aggregate spending on all of the nation's Medicaid programs from federal and state agencies had grown from $53.5 billion in 1988 to $120 billion in 1992, for an average annual growth rate of nearly 23 percent. The group accounting for the greatest growth was poor families (whose budgeted allowance had grown nearly 24 percent a year during this time), but programs for the elderly and for the blind and disabled grew at more than 15 percent a year as well.[17] The increased funds went to paying hospital inpatient billings, which had more than tripled since 1988; to private practitioners, whose billings had more than doubled; and for prescription drugs, whose costs to the program had doubled as well.[18] And while increases in administrative fees had been limited (only 50 percent growth over five years), the cost of treating AIDS had gone from a nearly trivial amount in 1985 to $2.1 billion by 1991, with every indication of increasing further. And because AIDS was gradually shifting from a disease of homosexuals, who held private insurance policies at a rate similar to that of the general population, to one of IV drug users and their partners, who relied on Medicaid at a disproportionately high rate, not only would the disease continue to absorb a larger portion of the Medicaid budget, but its rate of growth was likely to increase precipitously in the next half-decade. For many urban Medicaid and charity care programs, AIDS was a financial time bomb.[19]

Spending among the different state programs was not uniform, and even after the growth of the late 1980s and early 1990s it tended to mirror the discrepancies which had existed between the programs since their inception. New York continued to spend the most in the nation, at $7,286 per recipient, while New Hampshire spent $5,264, Vermont $3,171, and Mississippi $2,372. California, which had historically funded its Medicaid program quite generously, had pulled back during the 1980s, so that by 1992 it was spending only $2,801 per recipient, and antitax sentiment among the state's citizens precluded further growth in the program.[20] These disparities in spending meant that the quality of care available to Medicaid recipients varied tremendously, and as a result so did the ensuing health outcomes for Medicaid populations in different states.

Per capita spending did not tell the whole story, however. Although New York led the nation in its expenditures per recipient, the high cost of physicians and hospital services there meant that Medicaid patients there were not necessarily the best off in the nation. By some measures New Hampshire held that honor, for there average Medicaid payments to hospitals averaged 231 percent of average patient costs to hospitals, meaning that to a typical community hospital in the state, accepting a Medicaid patient effectively meant receiving double billing. Other states whose Medicaid hospital payments greatly exceeded typical patient costs were Tennessee (131 percent), South Carolina (124 percent), Texas (117 percent), and Maine (116 percent). By this measure, New York came out in the middle of the pack, with hospital payments which averaged 101 percent of costs (compared to the national average of 93 percent)—barely ahead of California's 96 percent. And some wealthy states such as Connecticut, Kansas, Massachusetts, and Pennsylvania reimbursed hospitals at rates of less than 80 percent of average patient costs.[21] While increased expenditures did not necessarily improve the quality of hospital care, they did facilitate access to hospitals, which was a prerequisite to superior care.[22]

Similarly, physician reimbursement by different states emerged in a different light when compared to the average Medicare reimbursement per patient, which was generally adjusted to account for differing costs of living in different areas. By this measure, Washington, Alaska, Arizona, and South Dakota all came in quite high—with average physician reimbursements substantially higher than those paid by Medicare in those states—while Louisiana, Vermont, Rhode Island, and New York all reimbursed physicians at 50 percent, or even less, of Medicare rates. There was little sense to the relative generosity of physician reimbursement by the states. While several states in the Deep South, such as Louisiana, Mississippi, and Alabama, reimbursed parsimoniously, so too did Rhode Island, Massachusetts, New York, and Maine. Arkansas, one of the poorest states in the country, which ranked near last in spending on roads, schools, and social services, reimbursed for physician Medicaid services as well as any state in the country (120 percent of Medicare rates). At the other extreme, New York, which made hefty payments to hospitals, felt ill-disposed to its doctors, who earned only 20 cents per patient for each dollar they earned from Medicare patients. Perhaps the only trend which explained some of the decisions about reimbursement levels was the relative power of states' hospital associations, medical association, and hired lobbyists.[23]

To fund these tremendous increases in the programs, states turned to general tax revenues, greater cost sharing with counties and municipalities, public bond issues, and, with increasing frequency in the early 1990s, financial shenanigans which bordered on fraud. The schemes took a variety of forms, but generally they relied on creating a special "tax" on hospital services so that hospitals sent part of their patient billings back to the state. This money was then returned to the hospitals in the form of higher Medicaid payments, but as such it qualified for federal matching funds. The hospitals came out the same, but the state was able to foist a larger portion of its Medicaid hospital expenses on the federal government. The General Accounting Office investigated these schemes in 1994 and recommended closing the legislative loopholes which allowed them, but states protested.[24] "Medicaid is quite literally driving states to the verge of bankruptcy," said Nelson Sabatini, Medicaid director of Maryland, in justifying the "creative" financing approaches.[25] Further investigations in the early 1990s revealed that nearly all states were participating in some sort of payment improprieties, often having to do with applying for Medicaid payment for some patient billings before private insurance and other payment options had been exhausted.[26]

Although changes in Medicaid eligibility and reimbursement were the principal factors driving the cost of poor-care coverage, other programs influenced the ability of the poor to get reasonable medical care as well. The National Health Service Corps, for example, offered medical school scholarships in exchange for a promise by the recipients to offer primary care in rural areas for some time afterward. The program succeeded in its first two decades in providing primary care to many rural residents, as well as in inducing the program's graduates to choose careers in primary care. Declining support for the program in the late 1980s, however, curtailed the effectiveness of the program on both fronts, as was reflected in the declining proportion of graduating medical students who chose primary-care specialties: 40 percent in 1980, 25 percent by 1990. And while not all primary-care doctors ultimately served Medicaid patients, the Medicaid program relied more than privately insured medicine did on primary-care gatekeepers, to screen Medicaid patients and refer them to appropriate specialists, hospitals, and clinics. Any decline in the ranks of primary-care doctors (among either allopaths or osteopaths) disproportionately affected the ability of the nation's poorest to gain access to medical care.[27]

Medicaid in 1991 was in a state of flux, with tremendous growth which threatened to overwhelm state budgets, but reimbursements too low to guarantee that an adequate number of primary-care doctors chose to participate in the program. Where was all the money going, if not to reasonably compensating physicians? Probably a quarter of the increase in the programs' costs was accounted for by general health care inflation. Another third could be accounted for by the increased enrollment spurred by the expansion in eligibility guidelines in the late 1980s, and perhaps another quarter to paying for greater technology in the hospital sector. But at least part of the money went to paying for more services for each enrolled recipient in Medicaid, suggesting that the average Medicaid patient in 1991 was receiving better medical care relative to the general population than twenty years previous. That a greater proportion of Medicaid patients were receiving care in private, rather than municipal, hospitals by this time supported this claim, as did the greater frequency with which domestically trained doctors (as opposed to foreign medical graduates) treated Medicaid patients. And although many critics pointed to the burgeoning administrative costs of the programs, and bloated bureaucracies, these alone accounted for no more than 1 percent of the total increase. Health care was simply getting more expensive, and this was true for the poor as well as for everybody else.

State and Local Reform

The twin phenomena of increasing Medicaid budgets and increasingly numerous uninsured persons led many states, and a few localities, to begin experimenting with reform legislation in the early 1990s. The legislative measures took two forms: an expansion of Medicaid coverage to bring more of a state's citizens under the health insurance umbrella, and the integration of various managed-care mechanisms into the programs to reduce costs. Many states reported at least partial success with both types of programs, although all hit certain pitfalls.

Oregon continued to lead the nation in aggressively working to make its Medicaid program more inclusive. After the setback in its universal care efforts in 1991, the legislature reformulated the code to reduce its impact on disabled persons, resubmitted the plan to the federal government, and received clearance from the Clinton administration in 1993. Under the new plan, 100 percent of impoverished families qualified for Medicaid benefits as delivered through thirteen managed-care organizations which contracted with the state. Oregon's rate of uninsured dropped from 14 to 12 percent after the program's implementation, even while the national rate of uninsured rose to 15 percent. At the same time, however, the state's Medicaid budget increased by 36 percent over the following three years, whereas national increases hovered around 30 percent over the same period. Most Oregonians approved of the tradeoff, and in 1994 they elected John Kitzhaber, the program's primary author, governor of the state.[28]

Oregon's program continued to arouse controversy after its passage. While budget experts, public administrators, political scientists, and health economists supported and indeed welcomed it as greatly overdue, many medical ethicists and leading physicians, not to mention members of the general public, found the program troubling. Most of these critics failed to familiarize themselves with the details of the program but understood it in some vague sense as medical "rationing" imposed unfairly on the poor, and opposed it on principle more than on any specific adverse outcome that it was likely to produce. Some critics viewed the program as a first step toward universal rationing for the broad middle class, as happened frequently under the National Health Service in Great Britain, while others viewed it as an assault on the sanctity of life, the integrity of the medical profession, or the compassionate moral base of America. "In a country that spends as much as we do on health care, there should be no need to deny medically necessary services (including the best of modern technology) to anyone," wrote the editor of the *New England Journal of Medicine*, Arnold Relman.[29]

Relman and other critics reacted to the plan on principle without examining the details. They mistakenly assumed that the plan was predicated on denying expensive procedures and covering inexpensive ones, but this was not so: had they looked more closely, they would have discovered that it was the unnecessary, useless, and superfluous procedures which were being mandated out of the Oregon plan, even as expensive albeit effective procedures, such as dialysis treatment for end-stage renal disease, were being retained. The plan worked by denying ineffective procedures and retaining effective ones, regardless of cost. While it was true that if two effective treatment options were available the plan favored the less expensive one, the emphasis was on outcome more than cost. Few physicians could have found the plan objectionable upon close consideration; its only natural enemies were ethical absolutists who demanded that every available measure be taken for every patient, regardless of prognosis, age, condition, or potential quality of life.

Other states took different tacks in expanding the umbrella of health insurance to their citizens. Hawaii, for example, had taken the bold step in 1974 of implementing its own "pay or play" scheme, requiring most employers in the state to provide insurance for their full-time employees, or else pay into a system which provided a state-sponsored insurance program for most citizens with incomes below 150 percent of the poverty line. The system had worked to provide health insurance to more than 95 percent of the state's population, while at the same time keeping per capita costs at the lowest level in the country. Because of their near universal access to primary and preventive care, Hawaiians spent fewer days hospitalized each year than residents of almost any other state, while posting rates of cancer and heart disease well below the national average. At the same time, the state's health care costs represented just 7 percent of the state's economy, as compared to 13 percent nationally. And Hawaiians liked the system. Fewer than 50 percent looked to the federal government to take a lead role in health planning and reform (compared to 62 percent nationally), while 43 percent believed that health care policy making appropriately took place at the state level, versus 30 percent nationally.[30]

Hawaii's program had existed for over fifteen years by 1991, yet it was rarely viewed as a model for health reform nationwide. Because of its unique geography, Hawaii could afford to enact measures undermining the competitiveness of its business sector without fear that businesses would move elsewhere. There was a substantial cost to relocating a business to the mainland, some three thousand miles away, and many of the state's businesses served markets specific to the state. The tourism industry, for example, had no choice but to operate within Hawaii, as did most of the retail operators, professional services providers, educators, real estate developers, and builders. While large manufacturing concerns would obviously avoid locating a plant in an area where the cost of labor was artificially inflated by mandated health benefits, few manufacturing concerns had ever sited plants in the islands, because of other unique expenses. Thus the implementation of Hawaii's Prepaid Health Care Act in 1974 had little effect on the state's business environment. The same would hardly be true in manufacturing states along the Great Lakes, or in states laden with light industry such as the Carolinas, Tennessee, New Jersey, California, Pennsylvania, New York, Massachusetts, and Delaware. Indeed, many of the northeastern states had already lost many jobs over the preceding decades, primarily because of their high labor costs, to the southern states and nonindustrialized countries.[31]

Minnesota took a different approach in creating MinnesotaCare in 1992, a health insurance program available to all residents with incomes up to 275 percent of the poverty level. The program required that its beneficiaries pay premiums on a sliding scale, with poor families paying as little as 1.8 percent of their income in premiums and those at the top paying nearly 9 percent. Even those families paying the most, however, paid for less than 50 percent of the true cost of the premiums; the remainder was paid for out of general state revenues supplemented by new taxes on cigarettes and hospital and physician services, and new surcharges on medical licenses. Physicians were willing to support the measures for the promise of higher patient billings in the future and less time spent on nonreimbursable care. In theory, future billing increases would more than offset the increased taxes and fees.[32]

Other states emulated the Minnesota model. Between 1988 and 1993 Massachusetts, Vermont, Florida, Maryland, Colorado, Washington, New York, and California all dabbled in legislation creating public insurance programs for subsets of the uninsured population.[33] All were subsidized through general tax revenues, used some sort of small-group market reform, and leveraged managed-care mechanisms to restrict spending. Vermont and Florida looked to pay-or-play templates; Colorado used a novel mandatory contribution approach; Minnesota, Vermont, and Washington raised revenues through increased cigarette taxes; California, Maryland, Oregon, and Florida looked to insurance reform and small-group purchasing regulation to allow or require small businesses to purchase private insurance plans for their full-time employees; and Vermont purported to move toward a universal access model by 1994. All the plans were bound by their incrementalist approach to the problem. Whereas the great federal reform efforts of the 1930s and 1940s had always modeled themselves on comprehensive programs like those in effect in Europe (Medicare was firmly in this lineage), the state plans of the early 1990s all tried to make fixes for the most needy in the most politically acceptable manner (thus the cigarette taxes rather than increased general income taxes). The goal of these efforts was to include the largest portion of the uninsured population with the least constraining regulation, using the least intrusive bureaucracies and agencies. They eschewed radical change, and focused instead on sliding-scale contributions, limited population targets, and managed-care cost-control mechanisms.[34]

Cities and counties too, often in conjunction with local medical societies, developed programs to alleviate the plight of the uninsured. Medical residents at the University of Virginia garnered a $20,000 grant and established the Charlottesville Free Clinic at the university's hospital, which they staffed with local physicians. Elsewhere in the state doctors coalesced to establish at least twenty other free clinics.[35] Doctors in Alachua County, Florida, established the "We Care Physician Referral Network" to coordinate the pro bono services of the area's private practitioners, who each agreed to see one charity patient a month in behalf of the program. In Dover, New Jersey, Robert Zufall operated a free evening clinic to provide primary care, immunizations, and emergency screening to (primarily) local Hispanic residents, while in San Francisco the local medical society, in conjunction with the San Francisco Health Department, created a program by which the city would absorb liability for any doctor willing to serve the city's homeless population gratis. These were but a few examples of the sort of local medical philanthropy which had long defined American medicine, and which enjoyed a resurgence in the early 1990s as a result of of broad gaps in Medicaid and the private health system.

Unfortunately, these programs were not comprehensive. The fundamental challenge of serving the uninsured—to provide *coordinated* and *continuous* care, rather than just critical care in emergencies—was scarcely met by these programs. True, local programs like the Charlottesville Free Clinic could make flu shots, pap smears, prenatal screening, and other basic preventive care more widely available than it might otherwise have been, but they fell short in coordinating complex treatment regimens for patients afflicted with chronic conditions. Whereas a privately insured patient could use his primary-care physician's office as a home base from which to explore treatment options at specialty clinics, teaching hospitals, or private specialists' offices, the beneficiary of a free clinic would draw whoever was on duty on a particular night, with little chance of seeing the same physician on a repeat or follow-up visit.

Moreover, some physicians resented the charity clinics' demand on their time, which was already being partly given over to uncompensated care. Doctors typically wrote off a sizable portion of their billings as uncollectible, and rarely resorted to lawsuits or collection agencies to make themselves whole. One doctor angrily responded to accusations that the medical profession was inadequately committed to pro bono work by citing the $1 million in billings that he and his partners dismissed each year—nearly $50,000 per physician. "As sizable as it is," he wrote, "the financial write-off is only a footnote to the stress, sleep deprivation, health risks, and liability incurred in caring for these patients."[36] Another physician suggested allowing doctors the ability to claim pro bono work as a charitable deduction on their federal income taxes, while another insisted that the city or county should indemnify pro bono practitioners by assuming all liability risk (as had been done in San Francisco). The use of private eleemosynary efforts to alleviate the pains of the uninsured could only be called quixotic.

The other goal of most state reform efforts in the early 1990s was cost control, and most efforts in that direction were pursued under the waiver allowance provided for in section 1115 of the Social Security code, which allowed states to experiment with programs and delivery mechanisms to better serve the client population. While the 1115 stipulations existed from the outset of the Medicaid program (in fact predating it by several years), they had been used primarily by states to experiment with alternative at-home treatments for the elderly. Cost overruns in the late 1980s, however, induced states to begin experimenting with managed-care contracts in an effort to reduce Medicaid costs. Although states had to prove "budget neutrality" in any 1115 demonstration program, as well as guarantee the same basic menu of services to their Medicaid recipients, HCFA proved quite flexible in granting waivers to states so that they could attempt to cap increases by placing segments of their populations in managed-care programs.[37]

Between 1990 and 1995 two dozen states began to move Medicaid patients into managed-care contracts under the 1115 waivers, with Tennessee, Rhode Island, and Maryland leading the way. The managed-care programs appeared to reduce costs, or at least stem inflation, and unlike the Medicare managed-care program they proved quite popular with Medicaid recipients. In Maryland, for example, 120,000 Medicaid recipients requested transfer to an HMO between 1993 and 1995, suggesting that they perceived the quality of care under the managed-care contractors to be superior to that provided by traditional Medicaid providers, or at least more convenient and more consistent.[38] Their perception was probably accurate. The most intrusive components of managed care—gatekeepers, required referrals, and closed networks—provided Medicaid patients with the exact sort of continuity of care and case management which they had always lacked under traditional Medicaid reimbursement. Medicaid patients moving into managed care were assigned a primary-care physician—often the first family doctor the patients had ever known—and given a list of specialists nearby who were committed to caring for the special needs of a Medicaid population. Little wonder that the general health of Medicaid patients actually improved slightly under managed care, contrary to the experience of the rest of the population.[39]

While capitated managed-care contracting was the primary avenue for cost containment efforts in state reform in the early 1990s, a few states experimented with alternative programs. Nevada, for example, worked to reform lab testing procedures by moving Medicaid laboratory work away from facilities owned by physicians and toward state-run facilities, and several states worked to streamline state agencies to reduce administrative overhead.[40] A few states and cities made efforts to reduce the use of municipal hospitals, or close public hospitals altogether, under the theory that private hospitals, subject to the discipline of competition, could provide hospital services to Medicaid patients more cheaply and efficiently. Leading this effort was Mayor Rudolph Giuliani of New York, who ran for office in 1994 partly on a platform of privatizing several of the city's twelve public hospitals. While his proposals ultimately came to naught, the sentiment was indicative of a broader skepticism toward the role of public hospitals in the care of Medicaid patients.

Medicaid Expansion and Comprehensive Reform

A half-decade of growth in the ranks of the uninsured, coupled with two decades of double-digit health care inflation, compelled lawmakers in the early 1990s to consider more substantial changes to government's role in health care. Of the many plans proposed by members of Congress and agency officials, the least intrusive was a straightforward expansion of Medicaid. Since Congress had already been loosening eligibility requirements for Medicaid for a decade, this approach had the appeal of a proven record, political acceptability, and relative ease of implementation. A plan described by the Congressional Budget Office in 1991 proposed to expand Medicaid to all U.S. citizens and legal residents with household incomes below the federal poverty level, and to allow any citizens or legal residents with household incomes below 200 percent of the poverty level to buy into the program by paying a sliding-scale premium.[41]

Such a plan would greatly expand the Medicaid program, adding some 25 million recipients to the current 14 million, of whom about half would receive benefits for free, another fourth would pay less than $25 per month, and the remaining fourth would pay up to one-third the actuarial value of the program. In addition, nearly 7 million people would receive secondary coverage through Medicaid under the plan, and 300,000 veterans receiving VA benefits would probably shift to Medicaid. Overall, the number of uninsured people would drop from 33 million to about 13 million—a decline of over 60 percent—while federal and state outlays would grow by about $28 billion (although states would save $3 billion on indigent care).[42]

A drop of 60 percent in the number of uninsured in the country would register as an extraordinary success by most measures, and the use of Medicaid as a vehicle for accomplishing this guaranteed a manageable level of bureaucratic growth, as virtually all state Medicaid agencies could grow to accommodate the increased numbers. The plan required no fundamentally new institutions, boards, or executive officers; it left both the organizations of medical professionals and private hospitals virtually untouched; and it offered little threat to the existing private insurance industry. To its detriment, the program would still leave 13 million persons (5 percent of all Americans) uninsured; it would require substantial tax increases by both the federal and state governments; and it offered little promise of reducing health care inflation. Moreover, Medicaid's reputation for providing second-rate medical care in second-rate venues discouraged many politicians from endorsing a substantial expansion of the program.[43]

Competing with Medicaid expansion was a series of comprehensive reform proposals emanating from various members of Congress, congressional committees, health policy analysts, and professional groups. These plans took the form of pay-or-play proposals, universal mandates, private insurance subsidies, and managed competition—the last being an approach to health reform which purported to play competing managed-care organizations against each other in an effort to reduce prices, improve quality, and minimize regulation. At one point in 1992 at least fifteen competing plans were being debated on Capitol Hill, with numerous others circulating among physicians' groups, political scientists, and staff members of the competing presidential campaigns. All looked to expand access, contain costs, and guarantee quality, but they used quite different mechanisms to accomplish these goals.

The first type of plan was that which expanded the private employer-sponsored insurance market (through either federal regulation or tax incentives) while maintaining a program resembling Medicaid for the poor and near poor. This type of approach recognized the political barriers to superseding private health insurance, yet at the same time acknowledged that government had a role, perhaps a large role, to play in guaranteeing health insurance for a large swath of the American population. Such a plan was first proposed by the U.S. Bipartisan Commission on Comprehensive Health Care, chaired by Representative Claude Pepper (D., Fla.), and incorporated into a bill drafted by Senator John D. Rockefeller IV (D., W.Va.).[44]

One of the most comprehensive proposals based on the Pepper Commission's template came out of the Conservative Democratic Forum's Task Force on Health Care Reform, which essentially became the health care plan for the Democratic party platform in 1992. This plan would have replaced Medicaid with a federal indigent care plan to cover all people with incomes below the poverty line, while encouraging employers to purchase private health insurance for employees. To make private health insurance more accessible to small businesses (which traditionally had the most difficult time negotiating reasonable rates with insurance companies), the Democratic plan proposed to consolidate small businesses (those with fewer than forty employees) into Health Insurance Purchasing Cooperatives (HIPCs), which would then negotiate with managed-care plans on their behalf. To better control costs, the plan created Community Health Partnerships (CHPs)—tax-advantaged managed-care plans which agreed to forgo experience ratings, ignore preexisting conditions, require substantial co-pays and deductibles for hospital and physicians' services, and refrain from offering benefit packages more generous than those prescribed by the federal government. Framers of the plan hoped that existing managed-care organizations would be forced to compete on price and quality for private clients, who would take advantage of the community rating standard and uniform benefit packages. Because the plan preserved private insurance companies, and actually played them against each other, the plan also fell vaguely under the rubric of managed competition.

The Democratic plan was ambitious but problematic. In establishing two wholly new institutions, HIPICs and CHPs, the plan would have created huge new bureaucracies charged with carrying out rather sophisticated tasks, for which no model or template currently existed. Moreover, requiring private carriers to forgo all experience ratings seemed quixotic to many observers. It could not be long before managed-care organizations began to game the system, regardless of the federal requirements. Nonetheless, the plan recognized the political necessity of maintaining a private insurance industry, and retained a two-tier medical system which would appeal to private employers: one for the gainfully employed, the other for everyone else.[45]

A second type of reform proposal, the "pay-or-play" scheme, would have required all private employers with over a minimum number of full-time employees to either purchase private insurance for their employees or pay a substantial tax, which would go to providing insurance through a new government program. This type of proposal would provide universal coverage, but it would integrate many middle-class employees of small firms into a federal program which would probably be dominated by the existing Medicaid population. While those yet uninsured would welcome the new coverage, many employees of small firms who had employer-sponsored private insurance would probably lose that private coverage and be forced into the federal program, which they might resent. Also, small businesses would have a strong incentive to game the system (shedding full-time employees through the use of contract workers and consultants to get below the stated minimum number of full-time equivalents), while insurance companies would continue to apply experience ratings to small groups which would have difficulty buying into the private insurance market.

The third type of reform plan was known as single-payer. Plans of this type would terminate private insurance markets as well as the existing Medicaid program, and create a comprehensive federal insurance program for all Americans, regardless of employment status, income, or wealth. The plans would be financed out of general tax revenues (which would obviously require a greatly enhanced base through higher marginal rates), and would be administered either through a central office in Washington or through states or regions (as were the Canadian, Australian, and New Zealand plans). While both doctors and hospitals would remain private, the payer function would become wholly public, or nearly so. The government could use managed-care mechanisms such as gatekeepers, co-payments, and capitation to reduce costs, and end any vestige of a two-tier system. In a sense these plans just expanded Medicare to all Americans. Plans proposed by Physicians for a National Health

Program, the Committee for National Health Insurance, and the American Public Health Association were of this type.

Single-payer plans were utopian. A huge and powerful private insurance industry would obviously fight against its own demise; physicians would resist such expansive governmental powers; and hospitals would fight for a continuing relationship with private payers. Most Americans as well resisted such large-scale governmental intrusion into their lives, and polls conducted in the early 1990s revealed that while Americans looked favorably upon Medicare, they did not tend to associate the success of that program with a similar success in a universal plan. While people familiar with the Canadian system found American resistance to it hard to explain, the resistance was firmly established, regardless of the growing number of people lacking any insurance at all.[46] "For Americans angered by self-serving politicians," wrote one editorialist in the *Atlanta Journal*, "the idea of Congress and bureaucrats controlling a family's health-care benefits is bound to be a disturbing prospect."[47]

Comprehensive health reform became a prominent topic in the presidential race in 1992 after the little-known candidate Harris Wofford defeated Richard Thornburgh, a popular ex-governor who had also served as attorney general of the United States, in a special U.S. Senate race in Pennsylvania. Wofford's victory was credited largely to his willingness to address the issue of declining health coverage, and to his promise to work toward health reform with mandated universal coverage. His victory prompted all presidential candidates to develop or reconstruct their own health reform plans, and elevated the plans to positions of higher prominence in their campaigns.

Governor Bill Clinton of Arkansas initially toyed with a single-payer plan, dismissed it as politically unfeasible, and turned to a classic pay-or-play scheme with enforced community rating and HIPICs for small market reform. His plan guaranteed nearly universal coverage, the end of "job lock," and at least some effort toward cost control. A critical President Bush predicted that the plan would have the "efficiency of the House Post Office and the compassion of the KGB."[48] Bush, by contrast, shied away from any sort of government mandate, and turned instead to a series of tax reform proposals designed to place more money in the hands of the poor and middle class so that they could buy their own private insurance. Under Bush's plan, low-income families would receive up to $3,750 in tax credits to purchase health plans, while small businesses and independent contractors would be able to deduct the full cost of any insurance that they purchased. Additionally, Bush's plan promised malpractice reform, administrative streamlining, a ban on screening for preexisting conditions, and the creation of small business purchasing pools along the lines of HIPCs termed "Health Insurance Networks."[49] The price for the whole program was estimated at a rather low $35 billion, making it by far the least expensive of all programs proposed by the candidates, and Bush's secretary of health and human services, Louis Sullivan, lauded it for maintaining the "viability and integrity of the private sector."[50]

The weakness in the president's reform plan was its failure to end the problem of the uninsured, and its lack of strong cost controls. At most, only half of those uninsured would gain insurance under the plan, and it proposed no new expansion of Medicaid. Additionally, the plan relied on optimistic assumptions about the ability of the middle class to purchase family policies with little more than tax deductions, and small businesses were unlikely to leap into the health insurance networks with the alacrity predicted by the plan's drafters. As for cost containment, the plan relied heavily on malpractice reform and administrative streamlining, but most health economists estimated that malpractice litigation was responsible for no more than 3 percent of all health care costs, and administrative streamlining could only produce substantial results if the country moved to a single-payer system.[51] By maintaining a competitive private-sector insurance market, the plan promised to retain the redundancy and inefficiency necessary for competing plans to each develop their own administrative forms, managerial structures, and internal rules.[52]

Clinton's initial inclination toward a pay-or-play model changed substantially after his election in November. Under the leadership of the management consultant Ira Magaziner, the administration produced an enormously complicated plan in the following summer, using the managed-competition template of Alain Enthoven and Paul Ellwood as its base but incorporating as well a universal mandate, price controls, and a host of proposals to expand public health. The health care task force employed the talents of nearly five hundred professional health policy analysts, economists, political scientists, and health care administrators over months, and produced a twelve-hundred-page bill so byzantine that few lawmakers (or their staffers) actually managed to read it.[53] The Health Insurance Association of America launched an effective ad campaign to defeat the bill, in which two actors playing the fictional, upper-middle-class characters "Harry" and "Louise" perused a description of the bill and expressed appropriate dismay at its length, complexity, and mandates for government expansion. The campaign particularly emphasized that most Americans would be forced into HIPICs and then into HMOs, which would by necessity constrain their choice of physicians. Combined with an effective floor assault by the Senate minority leader Bob Dole (R., Kan.), the bill was defeated that fall.[54]

Clinton's health plan proposed several profound changes in the American health system, any one of which could have been radical enough, and frightening enough, to force defeat of the entire package. The creation of a national network of HIPCs (called "health alliances") cost it support, since few Americans understood what these new institutions were or what their function would be. ("People are not going to be marching around the reflecting pool in Washington shouting 'HIPICs Now!,'" reflected an executive with the Kaiser Family Foundation, Mark Smith.)[55] The mandated use of managed-care plans discouraged supporters who feared loss of choice and quality. And although within five years of the plan's demise over 85 percent of all insured Americans would receive care through managed-care organizations, in 1993 this was not yet so, and most Americans continued to assume that they would receive care through traditional indemnity plans. Furthermore, since the reform plan would supersede Medicaid, public hospitals feared the loss of a principal revenue source, as did municipal clinics and physicians with large Medicaid practices.[56]

But beyond generating fear born of ignorance, Clinton's plan contained several substantial flaws which even the least intimidated and most knowledgeable health care consumer might find troubling.[57] The health alliances would need to be created entirely anew and staffed with professionals highly experienced in insurance purchasing, government contracts, and public affairs communication. Scholars of bureaucracy doubted that a nationwide system of such complex agencies could be created quickly without substantial delay and error.[58] More troubling was the plan designers' almost religious faith in the power of managed-care organizations to restrain cost increases and provide adequate medical care. Managed care in any form could only function in areas with high enough patient density to sustain comprehensive physician and hospital networks, and thus was an inappropriate form of care delivery for rural areas. And given that the plan's cost-containment scheme was based on establishing competition between managed-care plans in the same area, it would be unworkable for large swaths of the Midwest and the Rocky Mountain region, where scattered populations could hardly support one managed-care plan, much less several. Last, the end of Medicaid would mean the end of federal subsidies to the public hospitals and clinics, which provided care to the many illegal residents who would not qualify for Clinton's new plan. Bruce Goldman, for one, executive director of Harlem Hospital Center, declared that the plan would leave the community "in a worse situation than [it] had in the first place."[59]

But above all, Clinton's health plan failed because America simply was not ready for it. In 1993 Americans still retained the illusion that for all but a small minority of self-employed and seasonal workers, health care of the highest quality was an entitlement of citizenship, with little or no deductible or co-payment, no limits on specialty consultations or diagnostic tests, and no hindrance to the patient's free choice of provider. Clinton's plan would conclusively end this system. Americans were not rejecting any specific component of the plan (in fact, few Americans were knowledgeable about its precise details) but rather were rejecting the idea of health reform at all. Wofford's victory had misled political pundits into believing that there was a groundswell of support for comprehensive reform, but in fact Pennsylvania, with declining rust belt industries and lagging unions, was not representative of the country.[60] Ironically, had the plan been proposed five years later, after managed care had made sweeping inroads into employer-sponsored health programs, the public might have been more willing to entertain the idea of a government-sponsored program. By that time, however, comprehensive insurance reform had become so politically tainted as to be untouchable by any member of Congress, no matter how foresighted or strongly committed to the cause.[61]

AIDS

Diagnosed AIDS cases had grown from virtually nil in 1980 to over 100,000 by 1992, and many epidemiologists suspected that half again as many infected persons were circulating undiagnosed in the general population. By 1993 the disease had become an $8 billion public health problem, and the cost could only grow as newly diagnosed cases ran their course over the next five years. And while the antiretroviral drug AZT could prolong life for the few patients who could afford it, most patients would decline into a mess of opportunistic infections, pneumonias, and cancers.[62] Statistical models showed no evidence that the growth curve was leveling off, and no vaccine or effective treatment was even in the testing stages.[63] A report of the National Commission on AIDS in 1991 warned that without clear progress on prevention and treatment, the country would face "relentless, expanding tragedy."[64]

AIDS did not remain confined to the gay community where it had started, however, but neither did it appear to be making inroads in the larger heterosexual community by 1991. The disease's spread out of the gay community was almost exclusively into the ranks of those using intravenous drugs and sharing needles, usually at "shooting galleries" in slum neighborhoods. Although the virus died quickly upon exposure to air, syringes seemed almost designed to spread it. Nearly airtight, the cylinders continued even after being cleaned to hold small amounts of virus-laden fluid, which was then injected directly into the bloodstream of the next user. A study of shooting galleries in Miami in 1990 found that 20 percent of syringes with visible blood in the chamber contained HIV— a startling finding considering that most users injected themselves several times daily.[65] As a result of these practices, and given the declining speed of transmission among gay men, over 50 percent of all new AIDS cases by 1991 occurred among intravenous drug users.

As AIDS infected intravenous drug users, the face of the epidemic became more black and Hispanic. Black Americans had long posted higher rates of sexually transmitted diseases than whites, and the spread of AIDS into the black community was consistent with these higher rates, but it also reflected the disproportionate representation of blacks among habitual heroin users.[66] The Hispanic population also had higher rates of sexually transmitted diseases than whites, but among Hispanics the rapid spread of AIDS was at least partly attributable to language barriers in educating the community about safe-sex practices.[67] By 1992 blacks accounted for 28 percent of all AIDS cases (and only 12 percent of the general population), and Hispanics for 17 percent (7 percent of the general population).[68] Community leaders began to refer to the disease as a new black holocaust, and at least one black minister preached that AIDS had been created by genocidal white scientists with the specific intent of destroying young black men. While the assertion was absurd and invidious, it did reflect the fear and bewilderment which the new, untreatable malady was instilling in the black community.

The shift of the disease from gay men to intravenous drug users meant a shift in financing as well. While gay men had private insurance policies at rates consistent with the general population, drug users overwhelmingly lacked private coverage, and relied instead on Medicaid or indigent care delivered by public hospitals. The shift was reflected in the rising proportion of all AIDS hospital bills paid for by Medicaid: from 17 percent in 1983 to nearly 40 percent in 1992 in New York and San Francisco.[69] (Los Angeles, another city with a large number of AIDS patients, had proportionally fewer Medicaid patients, since so many infected Hispanic persons could not qualify for Medicaid, or failed to apply.) As neither the general growth of the epidemic nor its specific growth in impoverished drug-using patients was expected to abate, AIDS loomed as a growing drain on Medicaid, and as a potentially catastrophic drain on municipal hospital systems.

Responding to the potential fiscal crisis, Congress passed the Ryan White AIDS Care Act in 1990, to funnel emergency money to states and cities which had been badly affected by the epidemic. The program delivered funds under four titles to badly affected municipal areas, state agencies, and pediatric infectious disease programs. Title I, which targeted the most heavily infected urban areas, drew most of the funding, to be spent on virtually any services demanded for AIDS patients. These services were likely to be nonmedical: as municipal AIDS planning boards queried patients for their service needs, they found a more acute demand for housing and transportation subsidies, emergency food and funds, social services, and child care than for medication, medical attention, or hospital care. The patients, accustomed to receiving free medical and hospital care through indigent care programs and Medicaid, gave higher priority to their other, nonmedical needs even as the cities desperately needed to shunt the federal funds over to their own hospitals and Medicaid programs. The planning process pitted patients' representatives and community activists against agency officials, and the legislation favored the patients. Thus Ryan White money, while helpful, did little to alleviate the pressure being placed on public hospitals and urban Medicaid programs. For those, the burden fell to local and state taxpayers.[70]

Over the next several years, education programs, greater acceptance of the use of condoms, and better anti-retroviral drugs combined to stabilize the AIDS epidemic. In 1996 the number of deaths from AIDS declined to 31,000 (from 38,000 the previous year), and new "combination" therapies offered the promise of substantially prolonging life in patients infected with HIV. Contrary to the most pessimistic prognoses of statistical modelers, AIDS had failed to widely penetrate the general heterosexual population, female-to-male transmission had proved rarer than expected, and a declining number of sex partners in the population limited the opportunities for the infection to spread. Despite reports of regression to unsafe sex practices in the gay community, the bathhouses where unsafe activity had been rampant remained closed, and deaths from AIDS among gay men leveled off and then declined. Only among intravenous drug users did the epidemic rage unabated. Intravenous drug users tended toward self-destructive habits, and were thus precluded from using combination therapies because of their reluctance to follow carefully structured prescription regimens. Although the epidemic continued to pose a long-term challenge for municipal health systems, the crisis was on the wane.[71]

Expansion of Managed Medicaid

In June 1991 the New York legislature adopted an initiative aimed at placing 50 percent (1.25 million) of the state's Medicaid population in managed care within the decade. With managed-care membership by Medicaid recipients then at a nearly trivial level (75,000 in 1990), the initiative indicated an altogether new level of commitment by a major state to Medicaid managed care. Various forces had previously dissuaded most states from wholeheartedly moving toward Medicaid managed care—foremost among them the unwillingness of new HMOs to enter the New York market, the relative dominance of academic medical centers in New York City, and the unwillingness of existing HMOs to insure Medicaid recipients—but by 1991 the bias against managed care was weakening. The Medicaid scholar Michael Sparer writes, "Anyone who clearly contemplated the state's fiscal crisis, the political precariousness of Medicaid, the loss of confidence in the status quo, the abstract appeals of managed care, and the reassuring record of managed care initiatives to date could hardly deny that, in 1991 in New York State, Medicaid managed care was an idea whose time had come."[72]

Medicaid programs had been placing recipients in managed-care plans since at least the late 1960s, when California began enrolling select patients into staff-model HMOs (the most rigid type of managed-care plan, in which patients are limited to seeing physicians in the full-time employ of the HMO), but complaints about inferior care and limited access to physicians prompted Congress to tighten HMO contracting regulations in 1976. Under the "50/50" law passed that year, states were allowed to enroll Medicaid recipients in HMOs, provided that at least 50 percent of an HMO's membership consisted of non-Medicaid subscribers. While this restriction was eased to 25 percent in 1981, it was largely inoperable in any event, as many Medicaid recipients lived in neighborhoods where substantial majorities (over 90 percent) of the patients were Medicaid subscribers. HMOs skirted the problem by applying for congressional waivers, or by locating in wealthier neighborhoods and busing Medicaid patients to their facilities.[73] Ultimately, the rule was repealed under the Balanced Budget Act of 1997, which devolved HMO licensing to the states.

States tended to adopt managed-care contracting gradually. To induce potential patients to join, Managed Care Organizations (MCOs) often resorted to heavy-handed sales tactics (some verging on fraud), including promises to Medicaid recipients of fully rescindable trial memberships which turned out to lock patients in for a year or more. In the words of Nell Whitman of the Campaign for Better Health Care, "They're being lied to, coerced, and harassed by people who are paid commissions to sign them up."[74] Not all HMOs adopted such shady practices, though, and many Medicaid recipients welcomed the comprehensive services available to them without long waiting lines, trips to inconveniently located physicians' offices, or relying on local emergency rooms. By 1997 nearly 50 percent of all Medicaid recipients nationwide were members of MCOs, and many states were moving to implement mandatory capitation programs under which Medicaid patients no longer had a choice as to what sort of coverage they received. Paradoxically, the loss of choice probably improved the quality of the MCOs contracting with Medicaid plans, as little advantage would accrue to the lower-grade MCOs which had aggressively courted the patients a few years earlier.[75]

For both patients and states, Medicaid capitation brought mixed results. For the patients, membership in an MCO reduced acute-case physician visits (suggesting that patients were seeking more appropriate prophylactic care), but did not reduce their visits to emergency rooms (meaning that Medicaid patients used the emergency rooms in atypical ways, irrespective of access to primary care).[76] For states, managed care reduced costs, but not as much as had been hoped. By 1997 state reporting data showed that managed-care contracting reduced costs by 5 to 10 percent, but these savings were somewhat illusory given the greater amount of charity and other forms of uncompensated care which states were being forced to provide as financially strapped hospitals reduced the free care they had traditionally provided.[77] A study by the Urban Institute called the Medicaid managed-care revolution "more of a skirmish than a revolution," one that had produced limited success in expanding Medicaid recipients' access to physicians and in saving money for the states.[78] After reaching a low of 3.8 percent in 1997, Medicaid inflation revived in the late 1990s, and this time state legislatures seemed to have lost the political will to force parsimonious plans and systems on the patients.[79]

The nation's experience with Medicaid managed care in the 1990s could not be wholly separated from its experience with managed care in general, which was producing decidedly tepid reactions by 1997. The early cost reductions of 1993–95 were giving way to resurging inflation by 1998 (suggesting that savings had resulted from an early selection bias in plan enrollment); patients with fee-for-service or at least PPO options were exercising them in greater numbers, regardless of the higher co-payments and deductibles; and plans, having failed to earn profits in Medicaid and Medicare contracts, were deserting the programs in droves.[80] Physicians as well derided the new system, which they considered "meaner" than the old, inadequate to the needs of the population, and generally doomed to failure.[81]

Public Hospitals, Disproportionate Share
Hospitals, and Academic Medical Centers

Managed Medicaid harshly affected public hospitals, certain urban academic medical centers, and other disproportionate share hospitals (DSHS). Although Congress had released special funds to DSHS through Medicaid reimbursement under a law enacted in 1987, these funds tended to be absorbed into managed-care contracts, which were then funneled to regular (non-DSH) private hospitals. Additionally, the growth of the DSH funds paradoxically created a political "ricochet" in which state budget officials and consumer watchdog groups protested the endless increase in federal spending on the hospitals, much of which required matching by the states. Ultimately, the anti-spending forces persuaded Congress to cap growth in the program at 2.7 percent after 1995—this, combined with the shunting of DSH funds to the non-DSH hospitals, eroded the revenue streams of many public hospitals, which began to close their doors en masse in the late 1980s. The number of public hospitals nationwide fell from 1,800 in 1980 to 1,390 in 1993, leading the health system expert Jerome Kassirer to note that the nation was witnessing a "rapid and chaotic dismantling of an important source of care."[82]

Private managed care also took its toll on public hospitals. As managed-care companies negotiated progressively lower reimbursement rates to private hospitals throughout the 1990s, private hospitals began to aggressively court Medicaid patients, whose reimbursement was now often a welcome source of revenue. Private hospitals in many cities began to advertise for Medicaid patients, purchase physician practices which were made up predominantly of Medicaid recipients, and in certain instances even bribe ambulance drivers to divert patients away from the traditional public hospital emergency rooms. Bellevue Hospital in New York, which was public, faced a looming financial crisis by 1995 along with many other major urban medical centers, as it continued to maintain its traditional open-door policy even as revenues declined substantially through the decade. "People come from Russia to Kennedy airport and show up at our triage desk with luggage and say, 'I need an operation,'" recalled Brian Miluszusky, an administrator at Bellevue. "That's money that ain't coming in, but we have an open-door policy."[83]

The financial difficulties of public hospitals, combined with private hospitals' newfound willingness to serve Medicaid patients, caused many people to reconsider the role of public hospitals. Although a few planners had predicted their demise in 1965 when Medicaid was first enacted, uncompetitive Medicaid reimbursement rates and a steady flow of uninsured patients guaranteed public hospitals a place in the system. But the mass closings of public hospitals in the early 1990s raised new questions about their relevance to modern health care delivery. The system's harshest critics asserted that these old institutions had simply outlived their usefulness—that they were superfluous, and inefficient as well. "What's so terrific about the system we have now?," demanded Maria Mitchell, a mayoral health advisor in New York City. "We spend more money per capita than anyplace else in the country, and we don't have a single health outcome that tells us we've gotten more for our money."[84] Moreover, private hospitals continued to have empty beds, suggesting that the public system was playing an unnecessary role in picking up overflow patients.

Others argued that the public hospitals continued to have a special role within the system, as guarantors of care for everyone, regardless of insurance or financial status, nationality, or personal attractiveness. For these advocates, occupancy rates in the private sector were irrelevant in defining a role for the public, much as excess space in private colleges was no argument for closing public campuses. "You don't close a soup kitchen because there are empty tables in restaurants," stated Mark Finucane, director of health services for Los Angeles County. "We don't serve the same stuff to the same people."[85] Such sentiments were lent credibility by the tendency of many private hospitals, under the pressures of managed care, to provide less rather than more charity care, regardless of their eleemosynary charters.[86] One particularly stark bit of investigative reporting in Chicago revealed that the University of Chicago Hospitals— the dominant medical system of the city's generally impoverished South Side—scheduled appointments by telephone in wildly disparate fashion depending on the callers' insurance status, in some cases delaying appointments for over a month, even when the callers described their symptoms and problems identically. Further, Medicaid and uninsured patients were urged to try the local osteopathic hospital and were required to go to an evaluation clinic before being admitted to an outpatient service, while privately insured patients were admitted immediately to various services, with a minimum of wait and fuss.[87]

The role of public hospitals (and select disproportionate share private hospitals) remained ambiguous in the late 1990s, as it had been since Medicaid's inception in 1966. Although managed care in both the Medicaid program and the private insurance markets had changed the status of public hospitals, only the most simplistic anti-government crusader could have asserted by 1997 that public hospitals no longer had a role to play. A rising number of uninsured working-class men (and their dependents) continually demanded ever more outpatient and emergency room services from the hospitals, even as traditional Medicaid patients fled to financially hurting private hospitals. For municipal and county officials, the hospitals continued to represent a terrible drain on local budgets, but they served a disorganized and largely disenfranchised constituency, and closing them entirely invited misery on a wide scale.

Incremental Reform in the Late 1990s

In the late 1990s forty million Americans (14 percent of the nation) continued to lack health insurance—a systemic stasis which seemed largely unaffected by episodic dips in unemployment, interest rates, the profitability of managed care, or hospital closures. While major political parties eschewed large-scale health reform, they did express willingness to experiment with reforms that were incremental. Among those attempted were the Health Insurance Portability and Accountability Act of 1996 (HIPAA) and the State Children's Health Insurance Program (SCHIP). HIPAA was conceived not so much to close the gap on health insurance but to circumvent the job lock which kept so many people tied to unsatisfying jobs merely so they could keep their health insurance. Although since 1986 COBRA had guaranteed eighteen months of access to private health insurance to employees who had left a job with health benefits, HIPAA guaranteed them the right to purchase a wholly new insurance policy, regardless of any preexisting conditions. Unfortunately, the bill was passed without controls on the premiums which could be charged, meaning that many people attempting to exercise their HIPAA rights found that the prices were exorbitant.[88]

SCHIP easily won passage but afterward proved fraught with problems. More than half of all children who should have been eligible for insurance through SCHIP failed to apply in the first few years, and the ones most likely to apply were from families with greater earnings. Conservative observers called the program a potential "entitlement albatross around the state's neck," and a "giveaway program," while liberal governors such as Howard Dean of Vermont and Cecil Underwood of West Virginia embraced the program for its promise of immunizations and pediatric primary care. "In prosperous times, it's easy to forget that the voice of the poor is often the voice of a child," Underwood said, but the political scientist Don Boyd suspected that politics underlay support for the program. "It's pretty simple," he concluded. "These just aren't tight budget times right now, and politicians figured out that voters like kids."[89]

At the same time, states discovered that their Medicaid rolls declined precipitously after welfare reform was enacted in 1996. Georgia led the way with a 50 percent decline in Medicaid recipients between 1996 and 1999, and Texas, Ohio, Florida, Virginia, Louisiana, New Jersey, and North Carolina all posted declines of greater than 30 percent.[90] In southern California, Texas, and Florida, Hispanic immigrants—a group always underrepresented on the Medicaid rolls, if one controlled for income— appeared ready to slip out of the system altogether. In Los Angeles welfare reform left nearly half of all Hispanic residents who were eligible for Medicaid uncovered by 1997.[91] A number of economists and health policy scholars who examined the declining Medicaid enrollment found that low physician reimbursement was the primary culprit. In the absence of competitive pay, doctors refused to treat Medicaid patients, which action dissuaded eligible residents from enrolling. In other words, studies showed that even doctors with large Medicaid practices considered financial gain quite strongly in their professional calculus, and desisted from working when practice ceased to be sufficiently remunerative.[92]

As the 1990s drew to a close, the most talked-about issue in the field of indigent care concerned neither the truly poor, nor the working poor, nor recipients of Temporary Assistance for Needy Families (TANF), nor public hospitals, but rather nursing home payments. Medicaid had always reimbursed for nursing home care once a patient's assets fell below a certain level, but creative financing schemes—including Medicaid trust accounts, asset transfers, and education trusts—had allowed a growing number of well-to-do elderly to retain some control over their funds while qualifying for Medicaid. The federal government cracked down on many of these schemes starting in 1996, provoking near violent opposition from the elderly lobby, retiree groups, and nursing home owners. As the population was growing substantially older, and as long-term care would clearly be a central financial challenge for most American families for the foreseeable future, many Americans began to view long-term care as the foremost health financing challenge of the twenty-first century. Even as private insurance companies began to offer long-term care insurance and nursing home developers created novel financing mechanisms, many Americans began to demand that government step into the gap. Social Security's old age insurance program was simply inadequate in a world in which people routinely lived until their late eighties, miles away from the children. As of early 2005, neither the states nor the federal government had taken substantial legislative action in this area.[93]

As George W. Bush began his second term, health reform maintained an ambiguous hold on the nation's consciousness. While few Americans supported any sort of comprehensive reform, many elderly Americans lobbied strongly for Medicare prescription drug privileges, and state budget officers pressed hard for further rollbacks of the most stringent reimbursement caps mandated by the Balanced Budget Act of 1997. Bush himself seemed generally uninterested in health care. As governor of Texas he had shown little concern with state health issues, and his primary area of domestic policy interest as president was education. While the president did oversee the enactment of a limited prescription drug program for Medicare beneficiaries late in his first term, the action seemed designed more to assuage the concerns of his elderly voters going into his reelection campaign than to alleviate systemic pressures on the system. Whatever reforms were to come from Washington would continue to be incremental.

Medicaid appeared to have reached a sort of stasis. The SCHIP efforts had been only partly successful, yet had met with widespread support in state legislative chambers.[94] The number of Americans who lacked health insurance seemed to be neither increasing nor decreasing, although the recession which began in the spring of 2001 promised to force many Americans off their employer-sponsored plans and onto COBRA, at least temporarily. Public hospitals and clinics continued to limp along, chronically short of funds yet miraculously carrying out their charge to provide care to all who needed it. Both private hospitals and physicians in private practice continued their reluctant dispensing of charity care; the tap had not been closed entirely, but eleemosynary care now came with a grimace rather than a smile. The medical world of charity and indigency was neither appreciably better nor worse than it had been a decade previous; it had merely shifted slightly.

12

Afterword

What can we conclude? At first glance, the history of charity care over the past forty years seems bereft of simple lessons or themes. Rather, we seem to have stumbled repeatedly into byzantine fights over eligibility, professional autonomy, and relationships between the states and the federal government. Forty years of experimentation and amendments have left us with a great many uninsured persons, relatively high infant mortality rates, a near bankrupt public hospital sector, and a dwindling commitment from private hospitals and physicians to provide uncompensated care. If progress has been made, it has been over a circuitous path.

Yet several themes do emerge from this history. Among them are the omnipresent search for appropriate venues for charity care, the general commitment of government to be involved in providing it, the central role of the Medicaid program as the vehicle for government involvement, and the repeated efforts of lawmakers to amend Medicaid. These themes exist within the general matrix of ambivalence that Americans have shown toward social insurance, as discussed in the Preface. I will discuss each of these themes in turn.

The effort to provide charity care is old, universal, and constant. Charity care has existed as long as efforts to heal the sick have existed, and has been codified at least since the time of Hippocrates. Throughout the history of medicine, physicians have dedicated part of their time and energy to serving patients who could not pay prevailing fees. Communities in the United States have built institutions to serve poor patients since before the nation's founding. Although these institutions have evolved over time—from almshouses, to public dispensaries, to public hospitals, to community health centers—the public has never fundamentally questioned their existence. Additionally, private hospitals have viewed charity care in some form as central to their mission for most of their history. Although private hospitals are less willing today than in the past to treat nonpaying patients, most continue to provide charity care of some sort.

An accompanying trend to most of these historical efforts to provide charity care has been a lack of coordination between different professionals and institutions in providing that care. This has always been a pivotal distinction between charity care and privately purchased medical care. Doctors, hospitals, and clinics have served patients within their means, but have frequently failed to follow up and provide referrals. Thus poor patients have often received care at a more advanced state of illness than private patients have, and have been treated in less-than-ideal venues.

The disadvantages resulting from lack of coordination became more acute in the 1950s. As medicine grew in complexity and cost in that decade, and as more and more Americans financed their purchase of medical care with private health insurance policies, the system (or nonsystem) of poor care began to seem less adequate, *relative to the quickly progressing private system*. Thus by 1960 the plight of the poor in acquiring health services became more desperate, not because their own health status had slipped but because the rest of the nation had advanced. A haphazard system of pro bono efforts by physicians and public and private hospitals was inadequate to provide the sort of sophisticated medicine newly available to private patients. The United States was able to pass substantial health insurance programs in the early 1960s (the Kerr-Mills program, and later Medicare), having failed repeatedly to do so in the past. This success came about at least in part because more sophisticated, scientific medicine highlighted the inability of the existing charity care system to provide adequately for the old and poor.

The modern provision of charity care belongs, most naturally, with government. The move made in 1965, from uncoordinated eleemosynary efforts at charity care to government-provided insurance, appears to be irreversible. Although Medicaid has been subject to critiques and amendments over the past forty years, virtually no serious policy analyst or lawmaker has suggested returning to a system of voluntarily funded and donated charity care.

This can be explained on two grounds: the greater complexity and accompanying cost of modern medicine, and a more expansive public view of social welfare. Medicine is substantially more expensive today than in 1965, relative to per capita earnings, national earnings, and the cost of other consumable goods and services. Our national medical bill now exceeds 15 percent of GDP—over triple that of forty years ago. The expense has been driven largely by innovations in biomedical research and technology, and by specialization within the medical profession. Both developments have allowed modern medicine to produce novel cures and procedures, but have necessitated a high degree of coordination if they are to be effectively delivered. Both providing and coordinating these services is expensive.

In social welfare provision too, the nation seems unwilling to return to the more laissez-faire attitudes of yesteryear. The public strongly supported the welfare revisions of 1996, but it did not advocate ending welfare altogether. As charity care has long been closely associated with social welfare programs, the public's general sympathy toward funding these programs has expanded to include supporting Medicaid and other government-funded charity care programs.

Moreover, private physicians and hospitals have not expressed interest, as a group, in taking greater responsibility for charity care. Although both private physicians and hospitals continue to play a central role in delivering health care to the poor, they are generally *agents* of the government, rather than competitors with it. Doctors have debated among themselves the level of care which they should be obligated to provide to the poor, and their ethical and professional obligations to serving the poor, but few have suggested that they could replace the government. Similarly, private hospitals have eagerly sought Medicaid patients over the past decade, and higher Medicaid reimbursement rates, yet they have not expressed a desire to supplant Medicaid. Generally, the nonprofit and private individuals and institutions which provided most charity care in this country for its first two hundred years have comfortably ceded responsibility to the government.

Government efforts at charity care are inextricably associated with efforts to provide national health insurance, or some other comprehensive system of health services. A consistent presence in both the creation of Medicaid and its evolution has been a debate over its relationship to a broader national health program. As discussed in chapter 2, some government watchers suspected at the outset that the program was shoddily conceived because it was meant to be superseded by a national health insurance program. This may or may not have been true, but many observers have questioned the ethical propriety of having a charity care program coexist with a privately insured health care delivery system, rather than having a unified national health insurance program. So long as the poor receive their care through a different process from that which serves the rest of the population, such observers argue, the care that they receive will be inferior. The ultimate solution to this inequity, they argue, is the implementation of a national health insurance program.

Debate over national health insurance has been nearly omnipresent in domestic policy debate throughout the last forty years. In that time at least twenty-five bills have been introduced in Congress proposing national health insurance, and two presidents—Carter and Clinton—have made comprehensive health payment reform a cornerstone of their domestic agenda. The debate continues today. Almost by definition, a national health insurance program would obviate a national charity care program (or set of programs). Thus the continuing existence of Medicaid is a constant reminder to some health planners of a larger failing in the health care delivery and payment system. The American public does not appear to have been won over to this line of thinking. Voters have repeatedly placed their confidence in incremental rather than comprehensive reform. Additionally, few voters have favored national health insurance legislation to correct inequities in the private health insurance market, instead preferring small-scale insurance regulation and correction. The nation seems fairly comfortable with a separate and inferior national charity care program coexisting with a private insurance program, along with a national health insurance program for the elderly.

Medicaid is a flawed program, and has always been. Readers of this book will have concluded on their own that Medicaid has had systemic problems which have never been wholly corrected. For most of its history, the program did not reimburse providers at rates competitive with private insurance and Medicare; it never covered all of the nation's poor; and it failed to produce consistent standards between the different states' Medicaid plans. The reader will also note that all three of these flaws can be traced back to the original design of the program. The federal government, in an effort to devolve authority to the states, allowed states to design and implement their own programs, funding them at different levels. Few states committed themselves to funding the program at levels competitive with private insurers, and most states justified this policy on the grounds that their programs would exploit existing public hospitals and physicians who were willing to work at below-market rates. Further, most states accepted an obligation to provide for only certain poor people—single mothers and children, the chronically disabled—rather than for all of the poor.

These choices resulted in a second-tier charity care program. Although some lawmakers in the 1960s hoped that Medicaid would give the nation's poor access to the private health care system, the program never achieved this. Most states, and the federal government, conceded that the poor would continue to receive different care under Medicaid from the care that the middle class and rich received through private insurance. Given its lack of popular support for national health insurance proposals, the electorate seems comfortable with this disparity.

Much has changed in Medicaid over the years, and this book documents how some of these changes ameliorated the worst weaknesses of Medicaid. The program now covers a greater proportion of poor children, poor families, and pregnant women than it did at its inception. Further, the program now places most recipients under the care of primary-care physicians as a result of the move toward managed-care contracting. Last, more and more Medicaid recipients are receiving hospital care in private, rather than public, hospitals, although that is due as much to changes in the private insurance market as to legislative actions affecting Medicaid. Nonetheless, even after all these changes and amendments, the program provides the poor with medical care different from that available to most privately insured citizens.

Medicaid has relied on the existence of other charity care providers, even if not intending to do so. Throughout the history of Medicaid, its patients have been forced to use public hospitals, community and neighborhood health centers, and rural health clinics to receive their care. The program was not designed to force recipients to use these sources, yet recipients did, using Medicaid funds, from the beginning. This was due in part to a lack of private physicians' practices in areas proximate to poor people, and in part to the unwillingness of private hospitals to accept Medicaid reimbursement. In any event, the program was never purposefully amended to end these practices.

Today, most Medicaid patients receive their care from private doctors and hospitals, yet this development has little to do with changes in the program. Rather, the widespread use of managed care by private health insurance companies has made Medicaid reimbursement rates competitive with private ones, and Medicaid managed contracting has made primary-care capitation attractive for some private physicians.

Public hospitals and community health centers were not central to the design of Medicaid, yet they quickly became important components of the Medicaid delivery system. Public hospitals found themselves well positioned to take advantage of the newly available Medicaid funds starting in 1966, and they did. Community health centers, by contrast, were created anew in the late 1960s, but not to supplement Medicaid. Rather, the centers grew out of a social conception of community health. Once the centers were created, they became natural adjuncts to state Medicaid programs. Thus the use of public hospitals and community health centers in the Medicaid program was more historical accident than design. Once the accident occurred, few legislators attempted to undo it.

Despite all of its flaws, Medicaid has been highly successful. We should not forget that poor people are in better health today, and receive better health care, than had Medicaid not been created. Throughout this book I have documented the state of health of the nation's poor in several historical periods, and the reader may note that that state has been steadily improving. By almost any measure—infant mortality, maternal mortality, life expectancy, incidence of contagious disease—Medicaid has improved the health of the poor. Similarly, almost all measures of health care access for the poor—physician visits per year, dental visits per year, hospital days per year—have shown continuous improvement. Despite the weaknesses in the program, Medicaid has done much good.

Even the spread of AIDS has not stymied this march toward improvement. Many Medicaid recipients have their drug "cocktails" wholly paid for. Medicaid has paid for the majority of AIDS care in public hospitals over the past decade. Despite the financial stress which the epidemic has placed on Medicaid, the program has responded competently and effectively. Although Medicaid cannot provide a permanent solution to the AIDS epidemic in the form of an effective vaccine, it has been able to provide stopgap remedies and palliative treatment.

Under managed Medicaid contracting, the program has shown unexpected success. Poor people in the United States are now receiving regular primary care for the first time in the nation's history, and this has translated into fewer days of hospitalization and lower infant mortality rates. Certain flaws remain, among them the large number of eligible children who have not registered for SCHIP. We should not, however, discount the program's many accomplishments as we debate its failings.

We continue to have a two-tier system of care today, despite all efforts to make it uniform. A number of public hospitals have closed over the past two decades, yet the majority stay open. Most Medicaid recipients continue to receive care from physicians whose practices are disproportionately made up of Medicaid patients. Medicaid continues to pay below-market reimbursement for most hospital procedures (often substantially so), and many Medicaid recipients report difficulties in finding primary-care doctors.

Coupled with these challenges in charity care are deep flaws in our medical system as a whole. The nation has nearly 45 million residents who lack any health insurance; workers continue to take undesirable jobs simply to qualify for insurance; and many patients express dissatisfaction with the present state of managed care. Health care inflation has returned to the levels of the 1970s, employees are paying for a larger portion of their insurance premiums, and doctors complain about the oversight to which they are subjected by managed-care corporations.

There is little support for comprehensive reform. The present state of charity care will most likely continue, with minor changes, into the foreseeable future. This may not be altogether bad. Federalism has been preserved, and local control remains an important part of the Medicaid system. The United States has never promised its citizens equity in most of life's prizes; health care, it seems, is no exception.

Notes

Abbreviations Used in Notes

AHA	American Hospital Association, Chicago
AJPH	*American Journal of Public Health*
DC	Douglas Cater Papers, Johnson Library
DPS	Domestic Policy Staff Files, Carter Library
JAMA	*Journal of the American Medical Association*
JG	James Gaither Papers, Johnson Library
MMFQ	*Milbank Memorial Fund Quarterly* (continued by *Milbank Quarterly*)
NEJM	*New England Journal of Medicine*
PHR	*Public Health Reports*
RC	Robert Carleson Papers, Reagan Library
SSB	Social Security Bulletin
WHCF (JC)	White House Central Files, Carter Library
WHCF (LBJ)	White House Central Files, Johnson Library
WR	William Roper Papers, Reagan Library

Preface

1 Robert Pear, "Rising Costs Prompt States to Reduce Medicaid Further," *New York Times*, 23 September 2003, § A, 18.
2 Rothman, *The Discovery of the Asylum*, 7.
3 Ibid., xviii.
4 The extant scholarship on the history of American hospitals is rich. A brief listing would include Vogel, *The Invention of the Modern Hospital*; Rosner, *A Once Charitable Enterprise*; Dowling, *City Hospitals*; Charles Rosenberg, *The Care of Strangers: The Rise of America's Hospital System* (Baltimore: Johns Hopkins

University Press, 1987); and Stevens, *In Sickness and in Wealth*. Many histories of individual hospitals exist as well.

5   A single most readable comparative study of health systems in a number of industrialized nations is Laurene A. Graig, *The Health of Nations: An International Perspective on U.S. Health Care Reform* (Washington: Congressional Quarterly Press, 1999). See also Joseph White, *Comparative Advantages* (Washington: Brookings Institution, 1995).

6   Skocpol, *Protecting Soldiers and Mothers*, 45.

7   Noble, *Welfare as We Knew It*, 23.

8   Skocpol, *Protecting Soldiers and Mothers*, 7–8. See also Hacker, *The Divided Welfare State*, 221.

9   Skocpol, *Protecting Solders and Mothers*, 506.

10 Ibid., 481.

11 See Mary Jo Bane, "Politics and Policies of the Feminization of Poverty," *The Politics of Social Policy in the United States*, ed. Weir, Skocpol, and Orloff, 382–83.

12 Noble, *Welfare as We Knew It*, 23–24.

13 Ibid., 16–17.

14 Ibid., 28.

15 Skocpol, *Protecting Soldiers and Mothers*, 5.

16 A huge literature exists on the history of national health insurance efforts in the United States. See, for starters, Monte Poen, *Harry S. Truman versus the Medical Lobby*; Hacker, *The Divided Welfare State*; Ronald Numbers, *Almost Persuaded: American Physicians and Compulsory Health Insurance, 1912–1920* (Baltimore: Johns Hopkins University Press, 1978); Daniel Hirshfield, *The Lost Reform: The Campaign for Compulsory Health Insurance* (Cambridge: Harvard University Press, 1970); and Jonathan Engel, *Doctors and Reformers: Discussion and Debate over Health Policy, 1925–1950* (Columbia: University of South Carolina Press, 2002).

17 Hacker, *The Divided Welfare State*, 190.

18 See Starr, *The Social Transformation of American Medicine*.

Chapter 1: Antecedents

1   See John Burnham, "American Medicine's Golden Age: What Happened to It?," *Science* 215 (1982): 1474–79. See also Stevens, "Health Care in the Early 1960s," for an account of the broader context of health care delivery during this period.

2   As quoted in Stevens, "Health Care in the Early 1960s," 16.

3   White House Memo, Wilbur Cohen to S. Douglass Cater Jr., 28 October 1964, WHCF (LBJ), box HE-1, folder: 22 November 1963–25 September 1965.

4   Luther Terry, "The Economics of National Health," PHR 79 (1964): 773.

5   For statistics on per capita health spending in 1962 see Louis Reed and Dorothy Rice, "National Health Expenditures: Object of Expenditures and Source of Funds, 1962," SSB, August 1964, 11–21.

6   Ibid., 15, 19.

7 Margaret Klem, "Physician Services Received in an Urban Community in Relation to Health Insurance Coverage," *AJPH* 55 (1965): 1699–1716.

8 Ibid., 1703.

9 Herbert Klarman, "Effect of Prepaid Group Practice on Hospital Use," *PHR* 78 (1963): 956. Readers savvy in the use of statistics will understand that at least part of this discrepancy was the result of endogeneity—that is, individuals who were members of health cooperatives or covered under Blue Cross were people who were more likely to be healthier, regardless of health insurance status. Statistical analysis was less sophisticated in 1960 than it is today, and I have found no studies controlling for these endogenous factors. Still, we know from more recent studies (using more sophisticated statistical techniques) that access to private health coverage is positively correlated with decreased lengths of hospital stay, regardless of income bracket or employment status. The uninsured tend to wait longer before seeking medical attention, and thus are sicker by the time they enter the system.

10 Klem, "Physician Services Received in an Urban Community in Relation to Health Insurance Coverage," 1704.

11 Charlotte Muller, "Income and the Receipt of Medical Care," *AJPH* 55 (1965): 520.

12 Ibid., 511.

13 Wilbur Cohen, "Economic Problems in the Distribution of Medical Care," *American Medicine: The Forensic Quarterly* 37 (1963): 5.

14 Ibid., 6.

15 As quoted in Stevens, "Health Care in the Early 1960s," 12.

16 Nelson Rockefeller, "The Effective Use of Our Resources, Governmental and Private," *AJPH* 55 (1965): 1779–80.

17 An excellent discussion of nineteenth-century charity care may be found in David Rosner, "Health Care for the 'Truly Needy': Nineteenth Century Origins of the Concept," *MMFQ* 60 (1982): 355–83.

18 A rich literature exists on theories of nineteenth-century poverty and charity care. See, among others, Rothman, "The Hospital as Caretaker"; Stevens, *In Sickness and in Wealth*; Vogel, *The Invention of the Modern Hospital*; Rosner, *A Once Charitable Enterprise*; Rothman, *The Discovery of the Asylum*; Carol Smith-Rosenberg, *Religion and the Rise of the American City: The New York Mission Movement* (Ithaca: Cornell University Press, 1971); and Charles Rosenberg, *The Care of Strangers* (Baltimore: Johns Hopkins University Press, 1987).

19 The most comprehensive study of America's shifting view of the poor through the nineteenth century is in Katz, *Poverty and Policy in American History*, particularly part II, chapter 2, "Poorhouses, Paupers, and Tramps."

20 Chinese Hospital Association (New York City), *First Annual Report*, 1892, as quoted in Rosner, "Social Control and Social Service," 185.

21 C. R. Henderson, "How to Care for the Poor without Creating Pauperism," *Charities Review* 5 (1896), as quoted in Rosner, "Health Care for the 'Truly Needy,' " 367.

22 R. Hunter, *Poverty* (New York: Macmillan, 1904), as quoted in Rosner, "Health Care for the 'Truly Needy,'" 365.

23 "In a Modern Hospital," *New York Times*, 6 December 1896, as quoted in Rosner, "Social Control and Social Service," 191.

24 See Rothman, "The Hospital as Caretaker," for a lengthy discussion of the evolution of mission in sectarian hospitals.

25 Chas. Gordon Heyd, "The Medical Society of the State of New York: Our Responsibilities and Our Obligations," *New York State Journal of Medicine*, 15 April 1933, 493.

26 See for example Edward Stockwell, "Infant Mortality and Socio-Economic Status: A Changing Relationship," MMFQ 40, no. 1 (1962): 1, for a detailed comparison of infant mortality rates in differing income groups over time. Until the widespread availability of antibiotics, differences between income groups were minimal.

27 See John Harley Warner, *The Therapeutic Perspective* (Cambridge: Harvard University Press, 1986), for an extended treatment of the evolution of nineteenth-century medical therapeutics. For more on the sliding scale in medicine see Jonathan Engel, *Doctors and Reformers: Discussion and Debate Over Health Policy 1925–1950* (Columbia: University of South Carolina Press, 2002), particularly chapter 3. For vivid descriptions of the heroic therapies of the nineteenth century see the opening chapters of William Rothstein's *American Physicians in the Nineteenth Century* (Baltimore: Johns Hopkins University Press, 1972).

28 Some of the best exposés of quacks were written by Morris Fishbein, who later edited the *Journal of the American Medical Association* for twenty-five years. See for example *The New Medical Follies* (New York: Boni and Liveright, 1927) for an elucidating, and amusing, description of the charlatans who plied their trade in turn-of-the-century America.

29 A very good history of immigrant health is available in Howard Markel, *Quarantine! East European Jewish Immigrants and the New York City Epidemics of 1892* (Baltimore: Johns Hopkins University Press, 1997), especially the descriptions of concerns of the medical inspection officers on Ellis Island, and the reaction of many of the immigrants upon first confronting an ambassador of modern medicine.

30 Louis I. Dublin, address before the American Public Health Association, 1920, as quoted in *American Labor Legislation Review* 10 (1920): 251.

31 *Illinois Medical Journal* 39 (1921): 143, as quoted in Kristine Siefert, "An Exemplar of Primary Prevention in Social Work: The Sheppard-Towner Act," *Social Work in Health Care* 9, no. 1 (1983): 94–95.

32 Hearings on HR 12634, House Committee on Interstate and Foreign Commerce (20–29 December), as quoted in Siefert, "An Exemplar of Primary Prevention in Social Work," 93.

33 Siefert, "An Exemplar of Primary Prevention in Social Work," 100. See also Edward Schlesinger, "The Sheppard-Towner Era: A Prototype Case Study in Federal-State Relationships," AJPH 57, no. 6 (1967), as well as Theda Skocpol, *Protecting Soldiers and Mothers*, chapter 9, for more nuanced discussions of the politics underlying the program's rise and demise.

34 Of note here is the absence of a national health insurance program under the

Social Security Act. Although the original proposals by the Committee on Economic Security included provisions for NHI, they were removed from the bill for fear of political opposition. See Engel, *Doctors and Reformers*, chapter 3.

35 For a detailed history of the FSA cooperatives see Michael Grey, *New Deal Medicine* (Baltimore: Johns Hopkins University Press, 1999).

36 U.S. Department of Health, Education and Welfare, *Health of Children of School Age* (Washington, 1964), 27–28.

37 American Public Health Association, *Services for Children with Emotional Disturbances* (1961).

38 U.S. Department of Health, Education and Welfare, *Health of Children of School Age*, 8.

39 Ibid., i.

40 George James, "Poverty as an Obstacle to Health Progress in Our Cities," *AJPH* 55 (1965): 1765.

41 Ibid., 1757.

42 As quoted in ibid. For a more extensive description of changing perceptions of poverty see Joel Handler, *Reforming the Poor: Welfare Policy, Federalism, and Morality* (New York: Basic Books, 1972), particularly chapter 2.

43 As quoted in Handler, *Reforming the Poor*, 8.

44 Cohen, "Economic Problems in the Distribution of Medical Care," 9.

45 Handler, *Reforming the Poor*, 10.

46 All poverty statistics are from Mollie Orshansky, "Who's Who among the Poor: A Demographic View of Poverty," *SSB*, July 1965.

47 All statistics concerning southern poverty are drawn from Mollie Orshansky, "More About the Poor in 1964," *SSB*, May 1966.

48 U.S. Department of Health, Education and Welfare, *Health of Children of School Age*, 25–26.

49 James, "Poverty as an Obstacle to Health Progress in our Cities," 1759.

50 Edward Suchman, "Social Factors in Medical Deprivation," *AJPH* 55 (1965): 11.

51 Alonzo Yerby, "The Disadvantaged and Health Care," *AJPH* 56 (1966): 6.

52 Edward Cooper, "Aspects of Medical Education and Research," *JAMA* 56, no. 3 (1964): 263–64.

53 Handler, *Reforming the Poor*, 18.

54 Gunnar Myrdal, "The War on Poverty," *New Republic*, 8 February 1964, 15.

55 John Kenneth Galbraith, "Let Us Begin: An Invitation to Action on Poverty," *Harper's Magazine*, March 1964, 21.

Chapter 2: Precursors to Medicare and Medicaid

1 See Stevens and Stevens, *Welfare Medicine in America*, 15–17, for the role of the PHS in the broader context of the historical development of charity care. For a general introduction to the history of public health in America see John Duffy, *The Sanitarians: A History of American Public Health* (Urbana: University of Illinois Press, 1990).

2 Extensive literature exists on the history of national health insurance legislation,

and the interested reader is referred to any of the texts listed here: Starr, *The Social Transformation of American Medicine*; Ronald Numbers, *Almost Persuaded* (Baltimore: Johns Hopkins University Press, 1978), which details the AALL health insurance drives of the second decade of the twentieth century; Daniel Hirshfield, *The Lost Reform* (Cambridge: Harvard University Press, 1970), on New Deal efforts in health reform; Monte Poen, *Harry S. Truman versus the Medical Lobby*; and Jonathan Engel, *Doctors and Reformers: Discussion and Debate Over Health Policy, 1925–1950* (Columbia: University of South Carolina Press, 2002).

3   Jonathan Oberlander argues that a significant impetus to the provision of government-sponsored insurance to the elderly was the concern of the middle class over simultaneously funding both their parents' health care needs and their children's college tuition. His detailed political analysis of the birth of Medicare can be found in Oberlander, *The Political Life of Medicare*, 22–26.

4   For a detailed discussion of the political origins of the Forand Bill see David, *With Dignity*, chapter 1. See also Antonia Maioni, "The Development of Health Insurance in Canada and the United States, 1940–1965," *Comparative Politics* 29 (1997): 411–31.

5   For detailed discussion of the political alliances contracted in the fight over Medicare and its predecessor bills see Marmor, *The Politics of Medicare*; Jacobs, *The Health of Nations*; and Morone, *The Democratic Wish*, particularly chapter 6. Both Morone and Marmor parse the legislative debates over Medicare in far greater detail than is presented here.

6   Cohen, "Reflections on the Enactment of Medicare and Medicaid," 3.

7   David, *With Dignity*, 10.

8   As quoted in ibid., 12.

9   Peterson, "How Good Is Government Medical Care?," 30.

10 The anecdote is found in David, *With Dignity*, 34.

11 Testimony before the House Ways and Means Committee, 31 July 1961.

12 Testimony of Walter McNerney, "Proceedings of the House of Delegates of the American Hospital Association," January–April 1962 (Chicago), 19.

13 Testimony before the House Ways and Means Committee, 31 July 1961.

14 From "Proceedings of the House of Delegates of the American Hospital Association," 26–28 September 1961 (Atlantic City), 32.

15 From "Proceedings of the AHA House of Delegates," 27–29 August 1963 (New York), 55, 57.

16 For an enumeration of the flaws in Kerr-Mills reimbursement, and an exposition of the concerns of the hospital community, see "Proceedings of the House of Delegates of the American Hospital Association," 18–20 September 1962 (Chicago), 31–33.

17 Charlotte Muller, "Income and the Receipt of Medical Care," *AJPH* 55 (1965): 513.

18 For example, by 1980, when there were supposed to be over 2,500 CMHCs in the United States, only 600 had been established, and these tended to treat patients who had never been in the state hospitals to begin with. For a rich history of mental health policy during these years see Gerald Grob, *From Asylum to Com-*

munity (Princeton: Princeton University Press, 1991). For an early, optimistic assessment of the CMHC program see Lucy Ozarin, "The Community Mental Health Center: A Public Health Facility," *AJPH* 56, no. 1 (1966).

19 Abraham Ribicoff, "Pro: Should Congress Approve the Administration's OASD Medical Care Proposal?," *Congressional Digest*, January 1962, 10.

20 Edward Annis, "Con: Should Congress Approve the Administration's OASD Medical Care Proposal?," *Congressional Digest*, January 1962, 11.

21 Morone analyzes the legislative history of the King-Anderson bill at length in its passage through both committee and full assembly. Substantial Democratic infighting in committee between ensconced southerners (particularly the chairman Wilbur Mills) and other members led to prolonged debate, despite the large Democratic majority. Interested readers are rerferred to Morone, *The Democratic Wish*, 39–57.

22 For good statistics on the health expenditures of various government agencies on medical care in the early 1960s see Elmer Staats, "Survey Analysis of Expenditures for Federal Health Programs," *PHR* 78 (1963): 10.

23 Wilbur Cohen to S. Douglass Cater Jr., 28 October 1964, WHCF (LBJ), box HE-1, folder: 22 November 1963–25 September 1965.

24 Robert Strauss, "Poverty as an Obstacle to Health Progress in Our Rural Areas," *AJPH* 55 (1965): 1774–76.

25 Ibid., 1775.

26 Breathitt to LBJ, 14 December 1964, WHCF (LBJ), HE-5 box 16, folder: "Hospital-Medical Care."

27 LBJ to Breathitt, 29 December 1964, WHCF (LBJ), HE-5 box 16, folder: "Hospital-Medical Care."

Chapter 3: War on Poverty

1 Duhl to Moyers, 18 August 1965, WHCF (LBJ), box HE-3, folder: 1 october 1968.

2 See for example minutes from various White House health policy meetings in 1964 and 1965 in JG, box 206, folder: "Health Meeting."

3 "The National Commission Reports," *AJPH* 56, no. 5 (1966).

4 R. Tunley, "America's Unhealthy Children: An Emerging Scandal," *Harper's*, May 1966, 41–46.

5 A great deal of political deal making went into the legislation, led largely by Wilbur Mills. For details of the legislative history see Morone, *The Democratic Wish*, chapter 4.

6 A helpful discussion of the development of the Medicare legislation by two of its central creators can be found in Wilbur Cohen and Robert M. Ball, "Social Security Amendments of 1965: Summary and Legislative History," *SSB*, September 1965, 3–21.

7 "President's Statement on Signing the Social Security Amendments of 1965," Enrolled Legislation collection (LBJ Library), box 22, folder: "P.L. 89-97 H.R. 6675," 1.

8 As quoted in Cohen, "Reflections on the Enactment of Medicare and Medicaid," 4.

9   Wilbur Cohen, "Social Security: The Conservative Approach," WHCF (LBJ), box LE/1S, folder: 11 September 1964–28 February 1965.

10 Harris to LBJ, 1 December 1964, WHCF (LBJ), box LE/1S, folder: 11 September 1964–28 February 1965.

11 As quoted in Cohen, "Reflections on the Enactment of Medicare and Medicaid," 3.

12 Ibid., 9.

13 See Hacker, *The Divided Welfare State*, 246–48.

14 "Report of the Committee on Ways and Means on H.R. 6675," House Report no. 213, 29 March 1965, 80.

15 "Research Memorandum Regarding Effects of Certain Present Provisions of Part 2 (Title XIX)," Citizens' Committee for Children of New York, Inc., 23 April 1965, 2–6, WHCF (LBJ), box LE 151, folder: 1 March 1965–31 May 1965.

16 Friedman, "The Compromise and the Afterthought," 280.

17 As quoted in ibid.

18 "Statement to the Senate Finance Committee," Gardner, 22 August 1967, 23, WHCF (LBJ), box LE/WE-164, folder: "WE/WE 6."

19 Cater to LBJ, 10 September 1966, WHCF (LBJ), box LE/1S, folder: 1 September 1965.

20 Arizona was the holdout, refusing to establish a Medicaid program until 1982.

21 Raymond Lerner and Corinne Kirchner, "Social and Economic Characteristics of Municipal Hospital Outpatients," AJPH 59, no. 1 (1969).

22 See Joseph Hochstein, Demetrios Athanasopoulos, and John Larkins, "Poverty Area under the Microscope," AJPH 58, no. 10 (1968).

23 A number of studies conducted in the early 1960s demonstrated the association between insurance and use of medical resources. See for example Joy Cauffman, Milton Roemer, and Carl Shultz, "The Impact of Health Insurance Coverage on Health Care of School Children," PHR 82 (1967): 4.

24 Eveline Burns, "Policy Decisions Facing the United States in Financing and Organizing Health Care," PHR 81 (1966): 675.

25 William Willard, "Report of the National Commission on Community Health Services: Next Steps," AJPH 56 (1966): 1835.

26 Theodore Berry, "Recent Federal Legislation: Its Meaning for Public Health," AJPH 56 (1966): 585.

27 Lisbeth Bamberger, "Project Planning and Development by Official Health Agencies," AJPH 56 (1966): 597.

28 Herbert Domke and Gladys Coffey, "The Neighborhood-Based Public Health Worker: Additional Manpower for Community Health Services," AJPH 56 (1966): 603.

29 Ibid., 604.

30 Berry, "Recent Federal Legislation," 583.

31 See for example Cauffman, Roemer, and Shultz, "The Impact of Health Insurance Coverage on Health Care of School Children."

32 Johnson, *The Vantage Point*, 71.

33 Noble, *Welfare as We Knew It*, 93.

34 "The Problem of Poverty in America," *Economic Report of the President* (Wash-

ington: Government Printing Office, 1964), as quoted in Patterson, *America's Struggle Against Poverty in the Twentieth Century*, 112.

35 Coles, "What Poverty Does to the Mind," 747.

36 Academic sociologists such as Herbert Gans, Lloyd Ohlin, Richard Cloward, and Oscar Lewis also took a heightened interest in explanations of poverty, proposing variants on the idea of a "culture" of poverty spread intergenerationally, which produced a wholly separate and alien culture isolated from mainstream societal values. See Patterson, *America's Struggle against Poverty in the Twentieth Century*, 113–17.

37 As quoted in Bernstein, *Guns or Butter*, 97.

38 See Patterson, *America's Struggle against Poverty in the Twentieth Century*, 113–16.

39 Wilbur Cohen, "Ten-Point Program to Abolish Poverty," *SSB*, December 1968, 12.

40 Johnson, *The Vantage Point*, 75.

41 Ibid., 218.

42 Hacker, *The Divided Welfare State*, 243.

43 Carolyn Jackson and Terri Velten, "Residence, Race, and Age of Poor Families in 1966," *SSB*, June 1969.

44 Nicholas Lemann, "The Unfinished War," *Atlantic Monthly*, January 1989, 61.

45 Stevens and Stevens, *Welfare Medicine in America*, 96–99, 100–102. See Stevens and Stevens generally for detailed discussion of the genesis of the Medicaid programs in New York, California, and Illinois.

46 C. J. Conover, "Medicaid in Kentucky," *Journal of the Kentucky Medical Association* 79 (1981): 156–67.

47 Greenfield, *MEDI-CAL*, 9.

48 "Medicaid in Michigan: Its Modest Beginnings," *Michigan Hospitals*, October 1978, 4–5.

49 As quoted in David Gardner, "Running Out of Money, Not Patients," *New Republic*, 17 February 1968.

50 Appell to Cater, 25 August 1965, DC, box 1965, folder: "AMA Meeting with LBJ."

51 Cohen to Cater, 26 July 1965, DC, box 1965, folder: "AMA Meeting with LBJ."

52 James Boland, "Evaluation of Medicaid," *NEJM*, 20 January 1972.

53 "Proceedings of the AHA House of Delegates," 31 August–2 September 1965 (San Francisco), 63.

54 "Proceedings of the AHA House of Delegates," 21 May 1966 (Chicago), 33.

55 "Proceedings of the AHA House of Delegates," 17–19 February 1970, 138–39.

Chapter 4: Hard-to-Reach Groups

1 Statistics from M. Alfred Haynes and Michael McGarvey, "Physicians, Hospitals, and Patients in the Inner City," *Medicine in the Ghetto*, ed. Norman, 117–19.

2 Ibid., 118.

3 Ibid., 117.

4 Mark Lepper et al., "Approaches to Meeting Health Needs of Large Poverty Populations," *AJPH* 57 (1967): 1155.

5 Commission on the Delivery of Personal Health Services (Gerald Piel, chair-

man), "Comprehensive Community Health Services for New York City" (1967), 6–8.

6 Statistics are from Sager, "Why Urban Voluntary Hospitals Close," 454. See also Martin Cherkasky, "A Hospital Administrator Says That the City Should Get Out of the Hospital Business," *New York Times Magazine*, 8 October 1967, as well as Dowling, *City Hospitals*, 185.

7 "Impact of Governmental Programs on Public Hospitals," PHR 83 (1968): 54–59.

8 An analysis of the decline of philanthropy to private hospitals in the 1960s can be found in Sloan et al., "The Demise of Hospital Philanthropy."

9 Godfrey Hodgson, "The Politics of American Health Care," 53.

10 Eveline Burns, "Social Policy and the Health Services: The Choices Ahead," AJPH 57, no. 2 (1967).

11 David Steinman, "Health in Rural Poverty: Some Lessons in Theory and from Experience," AJPH 60, no. 9 (1970).

12 Joseph Brenner et al., "Children in Mississippi: A Report to the Field Foundation," June 1967, 3, WHCF (LBJ), box HE-2, folder: 1 May 1967–31 July 1967.

13 Ibid., 4.

14 Earl Lomon Koos, *The Health of Regionville: What the People Thought and Did about It* (New York: Columbia University Press, 1954).

15 See S. Polgar, "Health and Human Behavior: Areas of Interest Common to the Social and Medical Sciences," *Current Anthropology* 3 (1962): 2.

16 M. W. Susser and W. Watson, *Sociology in Medicine* (New York: Oxford University Press, 1963). See also R. Strauss, "Sociological Determinants of Health Beliefs and Behavior," AJPH 51, no. 10 (1961).

17 Ann DeHuff Peters and Charles L. Chase, "Patterns of Health Care in Infancy in a Rural Southern County," AJPH 57, no. 3 (1967). See also J. David Richardson and F. Douglas Scutchfield, "Priorities in Health Care: The Consumer's Viewpoint in an Appalachian Community," AJPH 63, no. 1 (1973).

18 Peters and Chase, "Patterns of Health Care in Infancy in a Rural Southern County," 421.

19 Brenner et al., "Children in Mississippi," 7.

20 Donald Hochstrasser, G. S. Nickerson, and Kurt Deuschle, "Sociomedical Approaches to Community Health Programs," MMFQ 44, no. 3 (1966): 351. See also Kenneth Welsh, "Initiating Community Health Development in an Appalachian County," AJPH 58, no. 7 (1968).

21 Thomas Rice and Roger Jeyer, "Raising the Level of Child Health in a Rural Community: A Model," AJPH 60 (1970): 2284. Original data from *Report of the National Advisory Commission on Health Manpower* (Washington: Government Printing Office, 1967).

22 See Howard Bost, "A New Outlook upon the Problem of Poverty and Health in Eastern Kentucky," AJPH 56, no. 4 (1966).

23 Bill McCullough, "The Demise of Rural Medicine," delivered to the West Texas Press Association, 20 February 1971, as reprinted in *Vital Speeches*, 15 June 1971, 517–18.

24   Preston Valien, "Overview of Demographic Trends and Characteristics by Color,"
      MMFQ, 48, no. 2, part 2 (1970): 36.
25   For statistics see ibid., as well as Leonard Rubin, "Economic Status of Black
      Persons: Findings From Survey of Newly Entitled Beneficiaries," *SSB*, September
      1974, 16–35.
26   See Valien, "Overview of Demographic Trends and Characteristics by Color," 31.
27   See Rubin, "Economic Status of Black Persons," 23.
28   Paul Cornely, "The Health Status of the Negro Today and in the Future," *AJPH* 58
      (1968): 649.
29   Interestingly, blacks have constituted just about 12 percent of the population of
      the United States since the antebellum era. The proportion fell slightly in the
      1920s and 1930s because of an influx of immigrants, but then rose back to 12
      percent by 1950. It continues to be the same today, although many demographers
      predict a gradual decline as more blacks move into the middle class (with con-
      comitant decline in birth rates) and as the United States continues to welcome
      unprecedented numbers of immigrants.
30   Nancy Milio, "A Neighborhood Approach to Maternal and Child Health in the
      Negro Ghetto," *AJPH* 57 (1967): 618.
31   Cornely, "The Health Status of the Negro Today and in the Future," 648.
32   Ibid., 653.
33   See George Foster, "Problems in Intercultural Health Programs," memorandum
      to the Committee on Preventive Medicine and Social Science Research (New
      York: Social Science Research Council, 1958).
34   Milio, "A Neighborhood Approach to Maternal and Child Health in the Negro
      Ghetto," 618.
35   Leonard Lawrence, "On the Role of the Black Mental Health Professional," *AJPH*
      62 (1972): 58.
36   Nathan Hare, "Does Separatism in Medical Care Offer Advantages for the
      Ghetto?," *Medicine in the Ghetto*, ed. Norman, 45.
37   Price Cobbs, *Black Rage* (New York: Basic Books, 1968), as quoted in ibid., 45–46.
38   See Elizabeth Watkins, "Low-Income Negro Mothers: Their Decision to Seek
      Prenatal Care," *AJPH* 58, no. 4 (1968).
39   Edward Cooper, "Talent Recruitment: the Most Important New Task of the
      National Medical Association," *Journal of the National Medical Association* 57
      (1965): 184.
40   The benchmark was set by the American Association of Medical Colleges in 1970.
41   Arguably the decline in academic quality was directly related to the increasing
      numbers of blacks attending college. The talent pool could not expand signifi-
      cantly in a mere five years, and thus college admissions committees were forced
      to reach deeper into the pool of applicants. See Ruth Hanft and Catherine White,
      "Constraining the Supply of Physicians: Effects on Black Physicians," *Milbank
      Quarterly* 65, supp. 2 (1987).
42   The Charles Drew Postgraduate School was later folded into the University of
      California at Los Angeles and effectively ceased to be a black medical college. By

1985 only six medical schools in the country had enrollments more than 12 percent black: Morehouse College, the University of Illinois, New Jersey Medical School of the College of Medicine and Dentistry of New Jersey (CMDNJ), Michigan State, Southern Illinois, and East Carolina. Ibid., 257–58.

43 Cornely, "The Health Status of the Negro Today and in the Future," 650.

44 J. G. Hughes, "President's Address to the American Academy of Pediatrics," *Pediatrics* 39 (1967): 139–41.

45 Ibid., I.1–2.

46 Lester Breslow, "Some Essentials in a National Program for Child Health," 11, Task Force Reports, Johnson Library, box 27, folder: "Interagency 1968 Task Force."

47 H. S. Scrimshaw, "Infant Malnutrition and Adult Learning," *Saturday Review*, 16 March 1968, 64–66.

48 For example, M. B. Stoch and P. M. Smythe, "Does Undernutrition during Infancy Inhibit Brain Growth and Subsequent Intellectual Development?," *Archives of Diseases of Childhood* 38 (1963): 546–52; J. Cravioto, E. R. DeLicardie, and H. G. Birch, "Nutrition, Growth, and Neurointegrative Development: An Experimental and Ecologic Study," *Pediatrics* 38, no. 2 (1966); and A. S. Yerby, "The Disadvantaged and Health Care," *AJPH* 56, no. 1 (1966).

49 See U.S. Department of Agriculture, "Incidence and Location of Serious Hunger and Malnutrition and Health Problems Incident Thereto" (Washington: Government Printing Office, 1968).

50 An early planning document for the CHIP program may be found in "Ten Year Program to Fulfill a Child's Bill of Rights," 1967, WHCF (LBJ), box LE/WE-164, folder: "LE/WE 6." The capitation provision was quite unusual in an age of indemnity health insurance, and spoke to an expressed concern that additional federal health care programs could have an inflationary effect on the health system.

51 See Wirtz to LBJ, "Memorandum for the President," 19 January 1967, WHCF (LBJ), box HE-1, folder: 1 November 1966–24 January 1967. The health manpower program had been started with the formation of a National Advisory Commission on Health Manpower, chaired by J. Irwin Miller. See "Statement by the President on Health Manpower Shortage," 29 September 1966, JG, box 353, folder: "Health."

52 Schultze to LBJ, "Insured Medical Care for Mothers and Children," 3 January 1968, WHCF (LBJ), box LE/WE-164, folder: "LE/WE 6."

53 Ibid., 2.

54 LBJ, "Health in America," 4 March 1968, 15, DC, box 65, folder: "AMA Meeting with LBJ."

Chapter 5: Redefining Health

1 As quoted in Elizabeth Connell, Edwin Gold, and Martin Stone, "Growth and Development of a Family Planning Service at a large Municipal Hospital," *AJPH* 57 (1967): 1315.

2   L. J. Duhl, "Health Research and the University," *AJPH* 59 (1969): 21, as quoted in Herbert Abrams, "Neighborhood Health Centers," *AJPH* 61 (1971): 2237.

3   Ibid.

4   Edmund Muskie, "Health Services at All Levels of Government," *AJPH* 58 (1968): 2201.

5   Hubert Humphrey, "The Future of Health Services for the Poor," *PHR* 83 (1968): 1.

6   Abrams, "Neighborhood Health Centers," 2238.

7   Elliot Segal, "A Slum Landlord Program: An Essential Ingredient in a Housing Code Enforcement Program," *AJPH* 58 (1968): 450.

8   Kerr White, "Organization and Delivery of Personal Health Services: Public Policy Issues," 4, WHCF (LBJ), box 4E-1, file 24 April 1966—11 June 1966.

9   Glick and Thomson, letter to the editor, *NEJM*, 10 September 1970. See also Glick and Thomson, "Patient Care in Municipal Hospitals," *NEJM* 282 (1970): 977–78.

10 As quoted in Humphrey, "The Future of Health Services for the Poor," 2.

11 Peter Poulos Jr., letter to the editor, *NEJM*, 10 September 1970.

12 For a readable history of public health in America see John Duffy, *The Sanitarians* (Urbana: University of Illinois Press, 1990).

13 Dwight Metzler, "Public Health in a Troubled World," *AJPH* 56 (1966): 164, 166.

14 Celia Deschin, "The Need to Extend Medical Services beyond the Hospital If Maternal and Infant Care Is to Become Comprehensive," *AJPH* 58 (1968): 1232–33.

15 Humphrey, "The Future of Health Services for the Poor," 9.

16 Milton Terris, "A Social Policy for Health," *AJPH* 58 (1968): 6.

17 James Cavanaugh, "Comprehensive Health Services," *PHR* 82 (1967): 399.

18 William Stewart, "Partnership for Planning," *PHR* 82 (1967): 395.

19 William Stewart, "Comprehensive Health Planning," 8, Fred Bohen Papers, Johnson Library, box 4, folder: "Comprehensive Health Planning,"

20 William Stewart, "Manpower for Better Health Services," *PHR* 81 (1966): 393.

21 White House Press Release, 17 November 1967, WHCF (LBJ), FG 775, box 413, folder: 1 January 1968.

22 For a good summary of the National Commission's recommendations see Walter McNerney, "Comprehensive Personal Health Care Services: A Management Challenge to the Health Professions," *AJPH* 57, no. 10 (1967).

23 As quoted in McNerney, "Comprehensive Personal Health Care Services," 1718.

24 Lisbeth Bamberger Schorr and Joseph English, "Background, Context and Significant Issues in Neighborhood Health Center Programs," *MMFQ* 46, no. 3, part 1 (1968): 291.

25 William Stewart, "Community Medicine: An American Concept of Comprehensive Care," *PHR* 78 (1963): 97.

26 Alice Sardell, *The U.S. Experiment in Social Medicine*, 58.

27 White House documents attest to the debate over the health centers in 1964 and 1965, with various questions raised over the effects of the centers on market-driven health care, and aspirations for the centers for the social transformation which they could potentially effect. See handwritten notes on the topic in JG, box 206, folder: "Health Meeting," as well as the report of the Community Action

Program, "Community Action: Health Programs," July 1966, JG, box 361, folder: "Health."

28 Both quoted in Sardell, *The U.S. Experiment in Social Medicine*, 61, 63.

29 See Reuel Waldrop, Margaret Guy, and David Cowgill, "Health Priorities in Lubbock, Texas, According to Socioeconomic Groups," *Health Services Reports* 89, no. 2 (1974).

30 David Cowen, "Denver's Neighborhood Health Program," PHR 84 (1969): 1030.

31 See Marion Sanders, "The Doctors Meet the People," *Harper's*, January 1968, 61.

32 See Daniel Zwick, "Some Accomplishments and Findings of Neighborhood Health Centers," MMFQ 50, no. 4 (1972).

33 See Philip Lee to James Gaither, "Report on the 1969 Task Force on Health," JG, box 232, folder: "1968 Task Force on Health."

34 The community mental health center movement was closely associated with a period of deinstitutionalization of the nation's large state psychiatric hospitals, in which inpatient populations fell 80 percent from 1957 to 1970. The causes were multiple, ranging from the move toward community mental health, to the discovery of more effective psychotropic medications (such as Thorazine), to the advent of Medicaid, which allowed states to place chronically mentally ill patients in nursing homes and charge back much of the cost to the federal government. See Gerald Grob's study of the period, *From Asylum to Community* (Princeton: Princeton University Press, 1991).

35 For a good discussion of the political changes within the psychiatric community which accompanied the genesis of CMHCs see ibid., particularly 30–35.

36 John Ritter, "A Short Sad Clinical Note," JAMA 218 (1971): 888.

37 "Good Psychiatric Squabble," *Rocky Mountain News*, 6 May 1970, as quoted in Leighton Whitaker, "Social Reform and the Comprehensive Community Mental Health Center," AJPH 62 (1972): 218.

38 An influential work in mental health policy in the mid-1970s was Franklin Chu and Sharland Trotter, *The Madness Establishment* (New York: Grossman, 1974), the resultant report of a study group under the auspices of Ralph Nader. Chu and Trotter concluded that the CMHCs were treating patients other than those who had been released from state hospitals, and that recently released inpatients were going largely untreated or undertreated.

Chapter 6: Charity Care and Comprehensive Reform

1 Statistics are from Lewis, "Government Investment in Health Care."

2 Klaus Roghmann, Robert Jaggerty, and Rodney Lorenz, "Anticipated and Actual Effects of Medicaid on the Medical Care Pattern of Children," NEJM, 4 November 1971.

3 Ibid., 108.

4 See Earl Brian, "Government Control of Hospital Utilization: A California Experience," NEJM, 22 June 1972.

5 Statistics from Lewis, "Government Investment in Health Care," 22.

6   Ronald Reagan, "Excerpts of Remarks," American College of Surgeons Annual Meeting, 5 October 1972, 5, RC, box OA 9600, file "Cabinet Council on Human Resources 1/6."

7   Reagan, "Excerpts of Remarks," 4.

8   Arthur Burns to Nixon, 1 April 1969, John Ehrlichman Papers, Nixon Presidential Papers Project, box 31, folder: "Domestic Policy."

9   See Mary Alice Norman, "Fees under Medicaid," *NEJM*, 8 February 1968.

10 Ellen Winston, "Health-Welfare Partnership in Programs for Low Income Groups," *AJPH* 57 (1967): 1102.

11 Lusterman, "Medicaid," 560.

12 See U.S. Department of Health, Education and Welfare, *Recommendations of the Task Force on Medicaid and Related Programs* (Washington: Government Printing Office, 1970).

13 As quoted in Hoff, *Nixon Reconsidered*, 1.

14 "All the Philosopher King's Men," *Harper's*, February 2000, 22. The quote was preceded by the statement: "We're going to [put] more of these little Negro bastards on the welfare rolls at $2,400 a family—let people like Pat Moynihan and Leonard Garment and others believe in all that crap. But I don't believe in it." From a White House discussion with Ehrlichman and H. R. Haldeman, 13 May 1971.

15 As quoted in Hoff, *Nixon Reconsidered*, 116.

16 Richard Nixon, "Food, Nutrition and Health," delivered before the White House Conference on Food, Nutrition and Health, 2 December 1969, *Vital Speeches*, 1 January 1970, 163.

17 Statistics are from "Health Care Financing: Background Paper," 5 November 1970, Egil Krogh Papers, Nixon Presidential Papers Project, box 13, folder: "Health."

18 In the president's words, "Only as people are aware of costs will they be motivated to reduce them. When consumers pay virtually nothing for services, and when, at the same time, those who provide services know that all of their costs will also be met, then neither the consumer nor the provider has an incentive to use the system efficiently." From Castelli, "Will Health Beat Nixon in '72?," 109.

19 For details of the initial FHIP plans see "Report of the Domestic Council Health Policy Review Group," 8 December 1970, White House Central Files, Nixon Presidential Papers Project, DC, FG-6-5, box 2, folder: 1 December 1970–31 December 70.

20 Hodgson, "The Politics of American Health Care," 45.

21 As quoted in ibid., 53.

22 Herbert Somers, "Hospital Utilization Controls: What Is the Way?," *NEJM* 286 (1972): 1362.

23 "Health," John Ehrlichman Papers, Nixon Presidential Papers Project, box 41, folder: "Messages to Congress, 1970/Human Resources."

24 TRB, "It Can't Last for Long," *New Republic*.

25 Watson, "Health Service," 250.

26 See Herman, "The Poor."

27 Rashi Fein, "How Can Medical Care in the Ghetto Be Financed?," *Medicine in the Ghetto*, ed. Norman.

28 Statistics from Marjorie Smith Mueller, "Private Health Insurance in 1969: A Review," *SSB*, February 1971, 18.

29 Newman, "Medicaid and National Health Insurance," 23.

30 Kerr White, "Organization and Delivery of Personal Health Services," presented at the Seminar on Health Policy, Institute for Policy Studies, 31 May 1966, 4, WHCF (LBJ), box 4E-1, folder: 24 April 1966–11 June 1966.

31 Thomas Bodenheimer, "The Hoax of National Health Insurance," *AJPH* 62 (1972): 1325.

32 James Cain, "The Doctor of Medicine: A Critical Federal Resource," read at the meeting of the Association of Military Surgeons of the United States, Washington, 20–23 October 1968, 6, WHCF (LBJ), box HE-3, folder: 1 October 1968.

Chapter 7: Health Planning and Community Medicine

1 Karen Davis, "Achievements and Problems of Medicaid," *Public Health Reports* 91, no. 4 (1976), as reprinted in *The Medicaid Experience*, ed. Spiegel, 335.

2 Derks, "Sort of Dampens Your Spirits," 675.

3 Beverly Myers, "Health Care for the Poor," *Proceedings of the Academy of Political Science* 32 (1977): 78.

4 Davis, "Achievements and Problems of Medicaid," 355. See also Congressional Budget Office, *Health Differentials between White and Nonwhite Americans* (Washington: CBO, 1976), for detailed analysis of the state of black health and health care.

5 See Nora Piore, Purlaine Lieberman, and James Linnane, "Public Expenditures and Private Control? Health Care Dilemmas in New York City," *MMFQ*, winter 1977.

6 Dowling, *City Hospitals*, 185–87.

7 James Studnicki, Robert Saywell, and Walter Wiechert, "Foreign Medical Graduates and Maryland Medicaid," *NEJM*, 20 May 1976; Barry Perlman, Arthur Schwartz, John Thornton, Ronna Weber, Kenneth Schmidt, Harton Smith, Steven Nagleberg, and Martin Paris, "Medicaid-Funded Private Psychiatric Care in New York City," *NEJM*, 3 August 1978.

8 Jane Mitchell and Jerry Cromwell, "Medicaid Mills: Fact or Fiction," *Health Care Financing Review* 2, no. 1 (1980); Avedis Donabedian, "Effects of Medicare and Medicaid on Access and Quality of Health Care," *PHR* 91 (1976): 322–31.

9 Buchberger, "Medicaid," 23.

10 On the issue of patients' noncompliance see Frederick Brand, Richard Smith, and Peter Brand, "Effect of Economic Barriers to Medical Care on Patients' Noncompliance," *PHR* 92, no. 1 (1977).

11 Jack Hadley, "Physician Participation in Medicaid: Evidence from California," *Health Services Research*, winter 1979; also Frank Sloan, Jerry Cromwell, and Janet Mitchell, *Private Physicians and Public Programs* (New York: Lexington, 1978).

12 Buchberger, "Medicaid," 28. For a comprehensive discussion of the role of Medicaid in changing nursing home rosters see Bruce Vladeck, *Unloving Care: The Nursing Home Tragedy* (New York: Basic Books, 1980), particularly chapter 4, "Paying the Piper."

13 See Helen Wallace, Herman Goldstein, and Allan Oglesby, "The Health and Medical Care of Children under Title 19," *AJPH* 64, no. 5 (1974); Edward Schlesinger, "The Impact of Federal Legislation on Maternal and Child Health Services in the United States," *MMFQ*, winter 1974; and M. Keith Weikel and Nancy Leamond, "A Decade of Medicaid," *PHR*, 91, no. 4 (1976).

14 U.S. Bureau of Labor Statistics, cited in Davis and Schoen, *Health and the War on Poverty*, 4.

15 See James Callison, "Early Experience under the Supplemental Security Income Program," *SSB*, June 1974, 3–12.

16 By some measures, rates of chronic disease actually increased during this time, as a result of fewer deaths from infectious disease and ever-increasing life expectancy. Controlling for these phenomena, however, chronic disease rates declined along with acute infectious ones.

17 See Victor Fuchs, "The Growing Demand for Medical Care," *NEJM* 279, no. 4 (1968), and David Mechanic, "Approaches to Controlling the Costs of Medical Care: Short-Range and Long-Range Alternatives," *NEJM*, 2 February 1978.

18 As quoted in Courtney Wood et al., "An Experiment to Reverse Health-Related Problems in Slum Housing Maintenance," *AJPH* 64 (1974): 474.

19 Ibid., 475.

20 Arthur Okun, *Equality and Efficiency: The Big Tradeoff* (Washington: Brookings Institution, 1975), 17, and Davis and Schoen, *Health and the War on Poverty*, 9.

21 Mark Siegler, "A Physician's Perspective on a Right to Health Care," *JAMA* 244 (1980): 1591. See also P. R. Lee and A. R. Jonsen, "The Right to Health Care," *American Review of Respiratory Diseases* 109 (1974): 591–93.

22 George Pickett, "The Basics of Health Policy: Rights and Privileges," *AJPH* 68, no. 3 (1978): 237.

23 See Anthony Robbins, "Who Should Make Public Policy for Health?," *AJPH* 66, no. 5 (1976).

24 A. Daniel Rubenstein, "Another View of the Certificate-of-Need Laws," *NEJM*, 15 May 1975.

25 Bruce Vladeck, "Interest-Group Representations and the HSAs: Health Planning and Political Theory," *AJPH* 67 (1977): 23. See also Harry P. Cain, ed., "Health Planning in Action: Accounts and Anecdotes," *PHR* 93, no. 1 (1978), for interesting (and amusing) anecdotes from the experiences of the HSAs.

26 Michael Eliastam, "The Emergency Medical Systems Act of 1973," *JAMA* 232 (1975): 135. For a more positive view of the medical systems act see John Harvey, "The Emergency Medical Service Systems Act of 1973," *JAMA*, 25 November 1974.

27 Robert Corbett, "Some Legal and Political Implications of Comprehensive Health Planning," *AJPH* 64, February 1974, 138.

28 Vladeck, "Interest-Group Representations and the HSAs," 27.

29 The number is highly contentious. If all health center program grantees are included—NHCS, CHCS, maternity and infant care projects, children and youth projects, and free clinics—the total is just over four hundred. However, the number of NHCS and CHCS which were actually established (as opposed to simply granted seed funds) was just over one hundred. See Walter Merten and Sylvia Nothman, "Neighborhood Health Center Experience: Implications for Project Grants," *AJPH* 65 (1975): 248, as well as Roger Reynolds, "Improving Access to Health Care among the Poor: The Neighborhood Health Center Experience," *MMFQ*, winter 1976, 51. Less trustworthy is the claim of 150 centers (with 800 by 1980) made by Howard Freeman, K. Jill Kiecolt, and Harris Allen II in "Community Health Centers: An Initiative of Enduring Utility," *MMFQ* 60 (1982): 246. It is unclear from where Freeman, Kiecolt, and Allen drew their figures, but possibly the question is simply one of defining a CHC.

30 A professor of community medicine at Howard University noted, "Patient education is considered part of the medical regimen. It starts with an order, written by the patient's physicians, for patient education." Naomi Chamberlain, "Partners in Teaching Community Health: A Medical School and an Elementary School," *PHR* 91 (1976): 271.

31 The best data I could find on the impact of CHCS on urban communities was generated by a study sponsored by the Office of Economic Opportunity (OEO) of CHCS in five urban and suburban areas—Atlanta, Boston, Charleston, Palo Alto, and Kansas City—in which the CHCS accounted for between 11 and 33 percent of all patient care for the targeted communities. See Freeman, Kiecolt, and Allen, "Community Health Centers," 249.

32 Clark and Huttie, " 'New Federalism' in the Delta," 24.

33 See Louise Okada and Thomas Wan, "Impact of Community Health Centers and Medicaid on the Use of Health Services," *PHR* 95, no. 6 (1980).

34 Gordon Moore and Rosemary Bonanno, "Health Center Impact on Hospital Utilization," *JAMA*, 15 April 1974. Moore and Bonanno found that in Charlestown, Massachusetts, the opening of the Bunker Hill Community Health Center increased admissions from the neighborhood to Massachusetts General Hospital by 56.1 percent over a two-year period.

35 See Reynolds, "Improving Access to Health Care among the Poor," 76–77.

36 Ibid., 79.

37 Freeman, Kiecolt, and Allen, "Community Health Centers," 266.

38 See James Hester and Elliot Sussman, "Medicaid Prepayment: Concept and Implementation," *MMFQ*, fall 1974.

39 As quoted in Carol D'Onofrio and Patricia Dolan Mullen, "Consumer Problems with Prepaid Health Plans in California," *PHR* 92 (1977): 124.

40 David Rabin, Patricia Bush, and Norman Fuller, "Drug Prescription Rates before and after Enrollment of a Medicaid Population in an HMO," *PHR* 93 (1978): 23.

41 Lewis Thomas, "Notes of a Biology Watcher," *NEJM*, 11 December 1975.

42 See Donald Madison, "Community Hospitals and Medical Group Practice," *AJPH* 74, no. 8 (1984), and R. J. Blendon, I. H. Aiken, and D. E. Rogers, "Improving

Health and Medical Care in the United States: A Foundation's Early Experience," *Journal of Ambulatory Care Management* 6 (1983): 1–11.

43   David Rabin, "Breadth of Concerns of Community Medicine," *JAMA* 225 (1973): 312.

44   Ibid., 311.

45   Sidney Klark, "From Medicine in the Community to Community Medicine," *JAMA* 228 (1974): 1585.

46   Maureen Henderson, Robert Berg, Joseph Stokes, and Robert Kane, "Community Medicine," *JAMA* 226 (1973): 354.

47   Statistics are from John McCoy and David Brown, "Health Status among Low-Income Elderly Persons: Rural-Urban Differences," *SSB* 41 (1978): 21.

48   William Kane, "Rural Health Care: Medical Issues," *JAMA* 240 (1978): 2648; Ira Burney, George Schieber, Martha Blaxall, and Jon Gabel, "Geographic Variation in Physicians' Fees: Payments to Physicians under Medicare and Medicaid," *JAMA* 240 (1978): 13.

49   H. Schmidt, *Health of and Health Services for Rural People*, Congressional Research Service, 7 September 1976, and Harold Luft, John Hershey, and Joan Morrell, "Factors Affecting the Use of Physician Services in a Rural Community," *AJPH* 66 (1976): 870.

50   As quoted in Scott and Susan Graber, "Health Care in the Rural South," *Nation*, 26 June 1976, 785.

51   Larry Finch and Jon Christianson, "Rural Hospital Costs: An Analysis with Policy Implications," *PHR* 96, no. 5 (1981).

52   Robert Baumann and Mary Leonidakis, "Neurological Services for Appalachian Children Provided by a Traveling Team," *PHR* 93, no. 3 (1978).

53   Tim Frary, "Rural Health Care," *JAMA* 241 (1979): 2700.

54   See for example Alan Jacobson, Darrel Regier, and Barbara Burns, "Factors Relating to the Use of Mental Health Services in a Neighborhood Health Center," *PHR* 93, no. 3 (1978).

55   Alvin Becker, Herbert Schulberg, "Phasing Out State Hospitals: A Psychiatric Dilemma," *NEJM* 294, no. 5 (1976).

56   President's Commission on Mental Health, "Report to the President," 1 April 1978, 1, President's Commission on Mental Health, box 9, folder: 17 March 1978–19 March 1978 (3).

57   The literature on shortfalls of CMHCs is extensive. See David Musto, "What Ever Happened to Community Mental Health?," *Public Interest*, spring 1975; Gerald Grob, *From Asylum to Community* (Princeton: Princeton University Press, 1991); and Jonathan Engel, "The Lost Way: Community Mental Health in Maryland 1960–75," *Maryland Historical Magazine* 95, no. 4 (2000).

Chapter 8: Health and Welfare Reform

1   Carter to Califano, 29 July 1978, 1, WHCF (JC), box HE-8, folder: 1 January 1978–31 October 1978.

2 Ibid., 2.

3 Ibid., 3.

4 See HEW's proposal, "Hospital Cost Containment," 10 February 1977, DPS (Eizenstat), box 217, folder: "Hospital Cost Containment o/a 36/2."

5 Figures are from the AHA, found in McMahon, Sammons, and Bromberg to Carter, 2 February 1978, WHCF (JC), box IS-2, folder: 9 January 1978–31 March 1978.

6 Joseph Simanis and John Coleman, "Health Care Expenditures in Nine Industrialized Countries, 1960–76," SSB 43, no. 1 (1980).

7 See Mandel to Carter, 9 May 1977, WHCF (JC), box HE-8, folder: 10 January 1977–15 June 1977, and Castro to Carter, 13 July 1977, WHCF (JC), box IS-2, folder: 20 January 1977–20 January 1981.

8 Here I refer the reader to the appropriate chapters in Stevens, In Sickness and in Wealth, as well as Henry Aaron, Serious and Unstable Condition (Washington: Brookings Institution, 1991), chapter 1, both of which describe in detail the burden which technological investment placed on hospital budgets and ultimately on the national health care investment.

9 Vernon Mark, "A Prescription for the Rising Cost of Medical Care," JAMA 237 (1977): 2384.

10 David Mechanic, "Some Dilemmas in Health Care Policy," MMFQ 59 (1981): 4.

11 See the detailed planning memo on the issue of block grants, Bob Berenson to Joe Onek and Bob Havely, 8 September 1977, DPS, box 214, folder: "Health o/a 6 244/2," particularly 7–15.

12 See "FY 77 Medicaid Initiative," WHCF (JC), box IS-2, folder: 1 July 1977–31 October 1977.

13 Ibid., 13.

14 "Hospital Cost Containment System: HEW Proposal," 10 February 1977, DPS (Eizenstat), box 217, folder: "Hospital Cost Containment o/a 36/2," 1, 3, 5.

15 Eizenstat to Carter, 11 February 1977, DPS (Eizenstat), box 217, folder: "Hospital Cost Containment o/a 36/2," 1.

16 See ibid., 2, 3.

17 Jimmy Carter, "To the Congress of the United States," 25 April 1977, WHCF (JC), box HE-8, folder: 20 January 1977–15 June 1977.

18 Michael Bromberg, executive director of the Federation of American Hospitals, had issued a statement saying that there was not "one chance in a thousand" that the goal of a 9 percent cap could be met. From "Promises Aren't Enough to Curb Hospital Costs," Philadelphia Inquirer, 3 January 1979.

19 Press Release, 18 July 1978, "Statement by Secretary Joseph A. Califano, Jr.," WHCF (JC), box HE-8, folder: 1 January 1978–31 October 1978.

20 A nice description of the various amended versions of both bills can be found in "Talking Points and Background Information: Compromise Hospital Cost Containment Legislation," DPS, box 216, folder: "Hospital Cost Containment o/a 634."

21 Bourne to Jordan and Butler, 17 April 1978, WHCF (JC), box IS-2, folder: 1 April 1978–30 June 1978, 1.

22 HEW press release, 3 April 1977, Bunny Mitchell Papers, Carter Library, box 1, folder: "Advisory Board VHI," 1.

23 Bourne to Jordan and Butler, 17 April 1978, 2.

24 Ibid.

25 Paul Starr argues that the administration was never really committed to comprehensive reform, and had to be shamed into supporting the universal coverage plan proposed by Senator Kennedy. Rather, Starr argues, Carter was most concerned with hospital cost containment, and viewed national health insurance as a decidedly lower priority. Bourne's papers and memoirs suggest otherwise. The interested reader should consult Starr, *The Social Transformation of American Medicine*, 411–14.

26 See Califano to Carter, 31 January 1978, DPS, box 214, folder: "Health O/A 6 244/2."

27 On this point see George Pickett, "The Basics of Health Policy: Rights and Privileges," *AJPH* 68, no. 3 (1978). Pickett, president of the American Public Health Association during the mid-1970s, asserted in one rather fatuous address that if a unified single-payer system were socialized medicine, "then we must agree that it is similar to socialized education, and that system has always been accepted as a right" (ibid., 239). Overlooked in the analysis was that the broad distribution of private health insurance (and private health delivery) created a landscape for health reform altogether different from that facing advocates of education reform in the nineteenth century.

28 Eizenstat warned Carter that federalizing Medicaid would not necessarily improve it. "It does not follow that because Medicaid is run badly by the states it will be run well if assumed by the federal government." Eizenstat and Onek to Carter, 29 May 1979, WHCF (JC), box IS-3, folder: 1 May 1979–30 June 1979, 6.

29 See White House press release, "National Health Plan," 15 June 1979, Chief of Staff Files, Carter Library, box 116, folder: NHI 16 April 1976–17 April 1978.

30 Edward Rada, "Medicating the Food Stamp Program," *AJPH* 64 (1974): 479.

31 Statistics are from Henrietta Duvall, Karen Goudreau, and Robert Marsh, "Aid to Families with Dependent Children: Characteristics of Recipients in 1979," *SSB*, April 1982.

32 The best work on this admittedly contentious assertion is Bradbury, Danziger, Smolensky, and Smolensky, "Public Assistance, Female Headship, and Economic Well-Being." The authors observed that from 1968 to 1975, the proportion of female-headed households receiving welfare increased from 25 to 41 percent, and that the rise in welfare distribution accounted for at least 25 percent of this increase.

33 Bethell, "Inciting Poverty," *Harper's*, February 1980, 18.

34 Califano to Carter, 11 April 1977, WHCF (JC), box WE-12, folder: 20 January 1977–30 April 1977.

35 See Alan Brinkley, *The End of Reform: New Deal Liberalism in Recession and War* (New York: Alfred A. Knopf, 1995).

36 Carter, "Address to Congress," 6 August 1977, 9, 10.

37 A good summary of the proposals can be found in Califano, "Welfare Reform

Memorandum," WHCF (JC), box WE-12, folder: 20 January 1977–20 January 1981, particularly 3.

38 Carter, "Address to Congress," 23 May 1979, WHCF (JC), box WE-13, folder: 1 January 1979–30 June 1979, 6.

39 Lenkowsky, "Welfare Reform and the Liberals," 56, 59.

40 As quoted in C. Arden Miller, "Health Care of Children and Youth in America," *AJPH* 65 (1975): 358. A good analysis of the failures of EPSDT may be found in Anne-Marie Foltz, *An Ounce of Prevention*, particularly 167–79.

41 Marian Wright Edelman, "Action for Healthy Children Day to Help Pass CHAP Now," 10/6/80, WHCF (JC), box IS-4, folder: 1 December 1979–20 January 1981.

42 HCFA, series B, descriptive report 4, "Out-of-Pocket Health Expenses for Medicaid Recipients and Other Low-Income Persons, 1980," 4, 6.

43 Toby Cohen, "Medicaid Fraud Reconsidered," *Dissent* 24 (1977): 392.

44 Carter, "Address to Congress," 25 April 1977, WHCF (JC), box HE-8, folder: 20 January 1977–16 June 1977, 6.

Chapter 9: Block Grants and the New Federalism

1 Buchberger, *Medicaid*, 25–28.

2 Ibid., 41.

3 National Center for Health Services Research, *The Politics of Prevention: Child Health and Medicaid* (Washington, 1981).

4 Robert Mare, "Socioeconomic Effects on Child Mortality in the United States," *AJPH* 72, no. 6 (1982).

5 Diana Petitti and Willard Cates, "Restricting Medicaid Funds for Abortions: Projections of Excess Mortality for Women of Childbearing Age," *AJPH* 67 (1977): 860–62.

6 For detailed background on the role of urban teaching hospitals in the provision of Medicaid services see Robert Blendon and Thomas Moloney, "Perspectives on the Medicaid Crisis," *New Approaches to the Medicaid Crisis*, ed. Blendon and Moloney, 15–17.

7 Judith Feder, Jack Hadley, and Ross Mullner, "Falling through the Cracks: Poverty, Insurance Coverage, and Hospital Care for the Poor, 1980 and 1982," *MMFQ* 62 (1984): 545–48. See also Toby Cohen, "The Medicaid Class Struggle," *Nation*, 21 February 1981, 203–4.

8 Jewel Bellush, "Indispensable Facilities: In Defense of Municipal Hospitals," *New York Affairs* 5 (1979): 115.

9 Usdane to Reagan, 16 July 1981, RC, box OA 9587, folder: "Medical/5."

10 For a good general history of the Reagan administration see Haynes Johnson, *Sleepwalking through History: America in the Reagan Years* (New York: W. W. Norton, 1991). Johnson cites one observer of Reagan's first inaugural describing it as a "bacchanalia of the haves" (20), in stark contrast to the austerity of the Carter years.

11 For a detailed analysis of the block grants see Deloitte, Haskins and Sells, "White Paper Prepared for the National Council of Health Centers," 31 August 1981, copy

in RC, box OA 9587, folder: "Medicaid (5)." See also Randall Bovbjerg and Barbara Davis, "State Responses to Federal Health Care 'Block Grants': the First Year," *MMFQ* 61 (1983): 530.

12 See Gilbert Omen and Richard Nathan, "What's behind Those Block Grants in Health?," *NEJM* 306 (1982): 1057–60.

13 Charles Mahoney, "Human Services: Tough Choices Ahead," *Boston Globe*, 9 November 1980, § A, 1. See also Bernard Guyer et al., "Needs Assessment under the Maternal and Child Health Services Block Grant," *AJPH* 74 (1984): 1014–19.

14 For internal administration debate on Medicaid reform in the early months of the Reagan administration see Richard Williamson to James Baker, Michael Deaver, and Edwin Meese, 7 March 1981, RC, box OA 9587, folder: "Medicaid (2)," as well as other documents in the same folder. Very helpful too is Judith Feder et al., "Health Policy under the Reagan Administration" (particularly 24–43), unpublished report of 24 May 1982, in RC, box OA 9594, folder: "Health Policy under Reagan 1/2."

15 A comprehensive overview of changes in Medicaid regulations through the years can be found in "Perspectives: Medicaid at 25: Rising Expectations."

16 A very helpful document in understanding the changes in Medicaid reimbursement wrought by OBRA '81 and TEFRA is Agranoff and Pattakos, "Intergovernmental Management," particularly 71–76.

17 John Iglehart, "The Administration Responds to the Cost Spiral," *NEJM* 305 (1981): 1364.

18 John Iglehart, "Federal Policies and the Poor," *NEJM* 307 (1982): 840. See also Peter Budetti, John Butler, and Peggy McManus, "Federal Health Program Reforms: Implications for Child Health Care," *MMFQ* 60 (1982): 155–81.

19 Tom Joe, "Profiles of Families in Poverty: Effects of the Fiscal Year 1983 Budget Proposals on the Poor" (Washington: Center for Study of Social Policy, 1982), as quoted in Iglehart, "Federal Policies and the Poor," 838.

20 Richard Nathan, "After Researching Early Reaganomics: Bad News for the Poor," *New York Times*, 13 August 1982, as quoted in ibid.

21 In Massachusetts, for example, both Medicaid and AFDC cost $450 million in 1976, whereas by 1981 Medicaid had doubled while AFDC had remained virtually unchanged.

22 Hunt and Quie to Reagan, 27 February 1981, RC, box OA 9587, folder: "Medicaid (2)."

23 King to Schweiker, 10 February 1981, RC, box OA 9587, folder: "Medicaid (1)."

24 Richard Hodes et al. to Robert Carleson, 31 March 1981, RC, box OA 9587, folder: "Medicaid (2)."

25 Sylvia Porter, "Medicare–Medicaid $$ Cruelly Cut," *New York Daily News*, 20 November 1981.

26 Burt Schorr, "Reagan's Medicaid Plan Stirs Fears of Two-Class Health-Care System," *Wall Street Journal*, 24 February 1981.

27 Harry Peterson, "Changing Federal and State Relationships: A New Era in Health?," *JAMA* 245 (1981): 2169–70.

28 James Sammons, "Statement of the American Medical Association to the Task Force on Entitlements, House Budget Committee," 24 February 1983, 2, 3, RC, box OA 9593, folder: "Entitlements."

29 "Options for Improving Economic Incentives and Competition in the Health Care System," 4 December 1981, 2, RC, box OA 9600, folder: "Cabinet Council on Human Resources 2/6."

30 Analysis of the roots of DRGs and their adoption by Medicare can be found in Oberlander, *The Political Life of Medicare*, 121.

31 "Can a Free Market Cut Health Costs?," *New York Times*, 5 March 1982.

32 For a nuanced discussion of the administration's general attitude toward health-care market reform see Thomas Oliver, "Health Care Market Reform in Congress: The Uncertain Path from Proposal to Policy," *Political Science Quarterly* 106 (1991): 453–78.

33 See transcript from a campaign press conference of 4 February 1980, RC, box OA 9600, folder: "Cabinet Council of Human Resources 2/6."

34 On this point see Jahn and Ortiz, "The Texas Medicaid Program," working paper no. 65 of the Policy Research Project on Health Care Cost and Access of the Lyndon Johnson School of Public Affairs (Austin, 1992), particularly 10–13.

35 Deloitte, Haskins and Sells, "White Paper Prepared for the National Council of Health Centers," 11.

36 As quoted in Juan Williams, "Black Children Sliding Backward, Report Finds," *Washington Post*, 4 June 1985, § A, 1.

37 Ronald Strauss, "Sociocultural Influences upon Preventive Health Behavior and Attitudes towards Dentistry," *AJPH* 66 (1976): 375–77.

38 Ernest Harburg et al., "Skin Color, Ethnicity, and Blood Pressure: Detroit Blacks," *AJPH* 68 (1978): 1177–83.

39 Karen Davis et al., "Health Care for Black Americans: The Public Sector Role," *MMFQ* 65, supp. 1 (1987): 215, 218, 235.

40 Lois Gray, "The Geographic and Functional Distribution of Black Physicians: Some Research and Policy Considerations," *AJPH* 67 (1977): 519–26.

41 See for example McDonald et al., *Crisis in Health Care for Black and Poor Americans*, 18–20.

42 See American Hospital Association, *Health Care*, 20–22.

43 Quoted in ibid., 22.

44 Proceedings of the AHA House of Delegates, 1 September 1981 (Philadelphia), 27.

45 Bovbjerg and Holahan, *Medicaid in the Reagan Era*, 51, 52.

46 See ibid, 53.

47 Kenneth Noble, "Are Program Cuts Linked to Increased Infant Deaths?," *New York Times*, 13 February 1983, § E, 6; "On the Death of Poor Babies," *New York Times*, editorial, 19 March 1983.

48 John Iglehart, "Medicaid in Transition," *NEJM* 309 (1983): 868–72; "Rx for Medicaid: Major Surgery."

49 Higgins, "Time for a Second Opinion"; McDonald et al., *Crisis in Health Care for Black and Poor Americans*, 18.

50 McDonald et al., *Crisis in Health Care for Black and Poor Americans*, 18–19.

51 Data from the National Medical Care Expenditure Survey of 1977 support this claim. See the letter by John Iglehart under "Prepaid Care in Medicaid," NEJM 309 (1983): 1129.

52 Edward Yelin et al., "Is Health Care Use Equivalent across Social Groups? A Diagnosis-Based Study," AJPH 73 (1983): 563–70.

53 See "Response to the Children's Defense Fund Criticism," 5 June 1985, WR, box OA 12725, folder: "Infant Mortality (2)."

54 "Talking Points, Infant Mortality," WR, box OA 12725, folder: "Infant Mortality (2)."

55 AHA, "Medicaid Payment for Hospital Services: Plain Talk about What Has Happened and What Should Be Done," November 1983, 7–10.

56 Judith Feder, Jack Hadley, and Ross Mullner, "Poor People and Poor Hospitals: Implications for Public Policy," unpublished manuscript (Washington: Urban Institute, 1983), 4.

57 Daniel Seligman, "Twisting the Truth," *Fortune*, 11 June 1984, 208.

58 Ibid.

59 Interview with Ken Auletta, "Saving the Underclass," *Washington Monthly*, September 1985, 14.

60 Charles Murray, "Helping the Poor: A Few Modest Proposals," *Commentary*, May 1985, 28. In a later article Murray suggested that anti-poverty programs functioned so poorly at least partly because so few of the designers had ever been poor themselves and thus had little insight into the psychology of social mobility. See Charles Murray, "What's So Bad about Being Poor?," *National Review*, 28 October 1988, 36–59.

61 See Lemann, "The Future of Poverty," 29, 37.

62 Robert Morris, "Will the Growth of Health and Welfare Services Be Resumed?," AJPH 73 (1983): 733.

63 Minutes from the Cabinet Council on Human Resources, 17 November 1983, Paul Simmons Papers, Reagan Library, box OA 12174, folder: "Cabinet Council on Human Resources."

64 White House Office of Policy Information, "Ten Myths That Miss the Mark," 2 March 1983, WR, box OA 12725, folder: "Infant Mortality (2)."

65 Novak, "The Rich, the Poor, and the Reagan Administration," 30.

66 See for example Wayne Schramm, "WIC Participation and Its Relationship to Newborn Medicaid Costs in Missouri: A Cost/Benefit Analysis," AJPH 75, no. 8 (1985).

67 Copeland and Meier, "Gaining Ground," 268.

Chapter 10: Recovering the Cuts

1 Nicole Lurie et al., "Termination of Medi-Cal Benefits: A Follow-up Study One Year Later," NEJM 314 (1986): 1267. An alternative figure for the drop, from 63 to 46 percent, is cited in Robert Blendon et al., "Uncompensated Care by Hospitals or Public Insurance for the Poor: Does It Make a Difference?," NEJM 314 (1986): 1160.

2   Mary O'Neil Mundinger, "Health Service Funding Cuts and the Declining Health of the Poor," *NEJM* 313 (1985): 45, 47.

3   Editorial, "The Poor Get Poorer," *Los Angeles Times*, 29 May 1985.

4   Garland and DeGeorge, "A Welfare Mother's Battle to Clean Up the Medicaid Mess," 42.

5   Cited in Mundinger, "Health Service Funding Cuts and the Declining Health of the Poor," 46.

6   A useful summary of the provisions of these bills can be found in Charles Ogberg, "Medically Uninsured Children in the United States: A Challenge to Public Policy," *Journal of School Health* 60 (1990): 497. See also Deborah Chang and John Holahan, *Medicaid Spending in the 1980s* (Washington: Urban Institute Press. 1990), especially chapter 3.

7   See for example David Rogers, Robert Blendon, and Thomas Maloney, "Who Needs Medicaid?," *NEJM* 307 (1982): 15.

8   American Hospital Association, *Medicaid Options: State Opportunities and Strategies for Expanding Eligibility*, ed. Irene Fraser (Chicago: AHA, 1987), 6.

9   Ibid., 6, 7.

10 Projections from the Office of Management and Budget, cited in "Overview of Long Term Care," 26 February 1981, 2, RC, box OA 9586, folder: "Health: Long Term Care."

11 Quinn, "Family Obligations."

12 "Overview of Long Term Care," 9.

13 American Hospital Association, *Medicaid Options*, 7.

14 Quoted in Sandra Tanenbaum, "Medicaid Eligibility Policy in the 1980s: Medical Utilitarianism and the 'Deserving' Poor," *Journal of Health Politics, Policy, and Law* 20 (1995): 944. See also Agranoff and Pattakos, "Intergovernmental Management," 76–77.

15 From AHA annual survey data, reprinted in "Unsponsored Hospital Care and Medicaid Shortfalls, 1980–91: A Fact Sheet Update" (Chicago: AHA, 1991), 4.

16 Ibid., 8. The number of uninsured persons in the county had risen from 25 million in 1977 to 35 million by 1986.

17 David Ansell and Robert Schiff, "Patient Dumping: Status, Implications, and Policy Recommendations," *JAMA* 257 (1987): 1500. Also Rice, "The Urban Public Hospital," 67.

18 Arnold Relman, "Texas Eliminates Dumping: A Start toward Equity in Hospital Care," *NEJM* 314 (1986): 579.

19 Emily Friedman, "Public Hospitals Often Face Unmet Capital Needs, Underfunding, Uncompensated Patient-Care Costs," *JAMA* 257 (1987): 1701.

20 As quoted in Emily Friedman, "Problems Plaguing Public Hospitals: Uninsured Patient Transfers, Tight Funds, Mismanagement, and Misperception," *JAMA* 257 (1987): 1850.

21 Quoted in ibid.

22 S. Mohsin Shah, "Texas Eliminates Dumping," *NEJM* 315 (1986): 1422.

23 H. A. Tillman Hein, "The Effect of a Public Hospital's Transfer Policy on Patient Care," *NEJM* 316 (1987): 1551.

24 Ellison Weaver, "Caring for the Poor," *JAMA* 259 (1988): 2236.

25 E. E. Gilbertson, "The Dumping Problem: No Insurance, No Admission," *NEJM* 312 (1985): 1522; and David Coulter in ibid., 1523.

26 James Davis, "National Initiatives for Care of the Medically Needy," *JAMA* 259 (1988): 3172–73.

27 A good single-volume history of black northern migration is Nicholas Lemann, *The Promised Land: The Great Black Migration and How it Changed America* (New York: Alfred A. Knopf, 1991), especially 341–53.

28 For an account of black participation in industrialization see Thomas J. Sugrue, *The Origins of the Urban Crisis: Race and Inequality in Postwar Detroit* (Princeton: Princeton University Press, 1996).

29 National Center for Health Statistics, *Advance Report of Final Mortality Statistics, 1984* (Hyattsville, Md., 1986).

30 "Infant Mortality among Black Americans," *Morbidity and Mortality Weekly Report* 35 (1987): 598–99.

31 Gilbert Lewthwaite, "Infant Death Rate Study Cites Growing Racial Gap," *Baltimore Sun*, 6 January 1984.

32 Harry Schwartz, "Infant Death Rate Fell Again—Did You Hear?," *Wall Street Journal*, 24 April 1985.

33 For a case study of the effects of Medicaid cuts on the cities during the 1980s see James Fossett, Janet Perloff, John Peterson, and Phillip Kletke, "Medicaid in the Inner City: The Case of Maternity Care in Chicago," *Milbank Quarterly* 68 (1990): 111–38.

34 William Check, "Several Efforts Focus on Closing Black/White Health Gap," *JAMA* 255 (1986): 3342.

35 Harry Schwartz, "Narrowing the Black-White Health Gap," *Wall Street Journal*, 17 February 1984.

36 Eleanor Holmes Norton, "Restoring the Traditional Black Family," *New York Times*, 2 June 1985.

37 As quoted in William Raspberry, "Will the Underclass Be Abandoned?," *Washington Post*, 24 May 1985.

38 Ibid.

39 Victor Sidel, "Medical Technology and the Poor," *Technology Review*, May–June 1987, 24.

40 Robert Blendon, Linda Aiken, Howard Freeman, and Christopher Corey, "Access to Medical Care for Black and White Americans," *JAMA* 261 (1989): 280.

41 See Kenneth Ludmerer, *Time to Heal: American Medical Education from the Turn of the Century to the Era of Managed Care* (New York: Oxford University Press, 1999), 249–56.

42 Peter Wilson, John Griffith, and Philip Tedeschi, "Does Race Affect Hospital Use?," *AJPH* 75 (1985): 263–69.

43 Eric Munoz, "Care for the Hispanic Poor: A Growing Segment of American Society," *JAMA* 260 (1988): 2711–12.

44 See Blendon, Aiken, Freeman, and Corey, "Access to Medical Care for Black and White Americans," for a discussion of ethnic differences in the use of medical

resources. Significantly, blacks were far more comfortable than whites about seeing different medical care providers on subsequent visits for the same illness or condition.

45 Congressional Research Service and Congressional Budget Office, *Children in Poverty* (Washington: Government Printing Office, 1985).

46 As quoted in Robert Pear, "Study Finds Poverty among Children Is Increasing," *New York Times*, 23 May 1985.

47 The best study of deinstitutionalization and mental health policy in the United States during the postwar decades is Gerald Grob, *From Asylum to Community* (Princeton: Princeton University Press, 1991). See also Franklin Chu and Sharland Trotter, *The Madness Establishment: Report of the Nader Study on the Mentally Ill* (New York: Grossman, 1974).

48 See Richard Mollica, "From Asylum to Community: The Threatened Disintegration of Public Psychiatry," NEJM 308 (1983): 367–73.

49 Charles Marwick, "The 'Sizable' Homeless Population: A Growing Challenge for Medicine," JAMA 253 (1985): 3217.

50 While the litany of abuses sounds horrific, it is not an exaggeration. See Albert Deutsch, *The Shame of the States* (New York: Harcourt, Brace, 1948).

51 Andrew Nichols and Gail Silverstein, "Financing Medical Care for the Underserved in an Era of Federal Retrenchment: the Health Service District," PHR 102 (1987): 686–91. See also Mark Dettelbach, "Rural Areas Still Need Physicians," JAMA 260 (1988): 3214–15.

52 See C. Arden Miller, "Infant Mortality in the U.S.," *Scientific American*, July 1985, 31–37.

53 M. Grossman and S. Jacobowitz, "Variations in Infant Mortality Rates among Counties of the United States: The Roles of Public Policies and Programs," *Demography* 18 (1981): 695–713.

54 Wayne Schramm, "Prenatal Participation in WIC Related to Medicaid Costs for Missouri Newborns: 1982 Update," PHR 101 (1986): 607–15.

55 See for example the internal White House document responding to a report by the Institute of Medicine which called for increased federal funding for pre-natal care: "IOM Report on Preventing Low Birthweight," WR, box OA 12725, folder: "Infant Mortality (2)." White House staffers wrote, "This is not just a Federal responsibility. States and the private sector have major responsibilities in this area."

56 Ben Wattenberg, "No Crisis for Infants," *Washington Times*, 4 April 1985.

57 See Joseph Shapiro, "A Conservative War on Poverty," *U.S. News and World Report*, 27 February 1989, 20–23.

58 By 1985 Medicaid accounted for 55 percent of all public health expenditures for children (versus only 25 percent for the elderly). See P. Budetti, J. Butler, and P. McManus, "Federal Health Program Reforms: Implications for Child Health Care," MMFQ 60 (1982): 155–81.

59 In 1989 Representative Thomas Bliley (R., Va.) attempted to rectify EPSDT by introducing H.R. 2881, the "Consolidated Maternal and Child Health Services

Act of 1989," which would have broadened eligibility for all maternal and pediatric care programs, including Medicaid.

60 See John Iglehart, "Cutting Costs of Health Care for the Poor in California," *NEJM* 311 (1984): 745–48; Janet Reis and Lynn Olson, "The Medicaid Program and Consumer Needs: A Survey of a Poor Chicago Neighborhood," *PHR* 102 (1987): 530–38; Ashcraft and Berki, "HMOs as Medicaid Providers."

61 See Eli Ginzberg, "The Destabilization of Health Care," *NEJM* 315 (1986): 757–60, for one health scholar's early predictions on managed-care penetration in both private and government contracting. Ginzberg thought that managed-care penetration would top off at 25–33 percent nationally for all insured individuals. By 2001 the figure was closer to 95 percent.

62 For more on Medicare managed care, and to a lesser extent Medicaid managed care, see Roger Feldman, "Health Care: The Tyranny of the Budget," *Assessing the Reagan Years*, ed. David Boaz (Washington: Cato Institute, 1988), 223–41.

63 K. Melville and J. Doble, *The Public's Perspective on Social Welfare Reform* (New York: Public Agenda Foundation, 1988), 46–48.

64 American Hospital Association, *Medicaid Options*, 46–54.

65 Michael Whitcomb, "Health Care for the Poor: A Public Policy Imperative," *NEJM* 315 (1986): 1221.

66 K. E. Thorpe, J. E. Siegel, and T. E. Dailey, *Cost of Expanding Medicaid to the Uninsured Poor* (Chicago: Health Policy Agenda for the American People, 1989). See also Thorpe and Siegel, "Covering the Uninsured: Interactions among Public and Private Sector Strategies," *JAMA* 262 (1989): 2114–18.

67 M. LeClair, "The Canadian Health Care System," *National Health Insurance: Can We Learn From Canada?*, ed. S. Andreopoulos (New York: John Wiley and Sons, 1975), 11–92; Arnold Relman, "American Medicine at the Crossroads: Signs from Canada," *NEJM* 320 (1989): 590–91; Robert Dickman et al., "An End to Patchwork Reform of Healthcare," *NEJM* 317 (1987): 1086–88; Davis, "National Initiatives for Care of the Medically Needy."

68 See for example Harold Luft, "Regionalization of Medical Care," *AJPH* 75 (1985): 125–26.

69 See Daniel Hirshfield, *The Lost Reform* (Cambridge: Harvard University Press, 1970); also Ronald Numbers, *Almost Persuaded* (Baltimore: Johns Hopkins University Press, 1978), for accounts of battles over efforts to establish compulsory health insurance in the 1930s (Hirshfield) and 1910–14 (Numbers).

70 See Monte Poen, *Harry S. Truman versus the Medical Lobby* (Columbia: University of Missouri Press, 1979), 174–209.

71 Garland, "Health Care for All or an Excuse for Cutbacks?"

72 Ibid.

73 In his own analysis of the initial defeat of his proposal, Kitzhaber suggested that the ADA's concern was a contrived basis for the ACLU's challenge. Rather, the ACLU was simply uncomfortable with a system which explicitly mandated rationing. Author's interview, 29 September 2003.

74 Some of the original discussion of the Enthoven plan is outlined in Enthoven,

"Health Care for the Poor," 11 January 1985, WR, box OA 12725, folder: "Health Policy Folder: Three (5)." See also Enthoven to Charles Baker, 4 February 1985, same folder.

Chapter 11: Managed Medicaid

1   Erica Frank, "An Interview with Senator Edward Kennedy," *JAMA* 263 (1990): 2388.
2   Congressional Budget Office, "Selected Options for Expanding Health Insurance Coverage," July 1991, 10, 11. Data from CBO analysis of the 1990 Current Population Survey. See also U.S. General Accounting Office, "A Profile of the Uninsured," 8 February 1991, B-241836, 3–6.
3   Charles Oberg et al., "Prenatal Care Comparisons among Privately Insured, Uninsured, and Medicaid-Enrolled Women," *PHR* 105 (1990): 533–35.
4   M. Susan Marquis and Stephen Long, "Uninsured Children and National Health Reform," *JAMA* 268 (1992): 3473–77. Also Paul Newacheck, Jeffrey Stoddard, Dana Hughes, and Michelle Pearl, "Health Insurance and Access to Primary Care for Children," *NEJM* 338 (1998): 513–19.
5   Laura Montgomery, John Kiely, and Gregory Pappas, "The Effects of Poverty, Race, and Family Structure on U.S. Children's Health: Data from the NHIS, 1978 through 1980 and 1989 through 1991," *AJPH* 86 (1996): 1401–5. See also American Hospital Association, "Report and Position on Financing Care for Medically Indigent Children," 28 July 1990, 2–4.
6   American Hospital Association, "Report and Position on Financing Care for Medically Indigent Children," 4.
7   R. Burciaga Valdez et al., "Insuring Latinos against the Costs of Illness," *JAMA* 269 (1993): 889–94; Marsha Goldsmith, "Hispanic/Latino Health Issues Explored," *JAMA* 269 (1993): 1603.
8   Peter Margolis et al., "Factors Associated with Pediatricians' Participation in Medicaid in North Carolina," *JAMA* 267 (1992); Kevin Seitz, "Working to Build a Healthier Medicaid System," *Michigan Medicine*, September 1990, 35.
9   J. E. Pipas, "Access of Medicaid Recipients to Outpatient Care," *NEJM* 331 (1994): 878.
10   Jane Zanca, Letter to the Editor, *JAMA* 266 (1991): 2560.
11   Robert St. Peter, Paul Newacheck, and Neal Halfon, "Access to Care for Poor Children," *JAMA* 267 (1992): 2763.
12   Stephen Soumerai et al., "Effects of Medicaid Drug-Payment Limits on Admission to Hospitals and Nursing Homes," *NEJM* 325 (1991): 1072–77.
13   See Sparer, *Medicaid and the Limits of State Health Reform*, 47–49.
14   See Coughlin, Ku, and Holahan, *Medicaid since 1980*, 57–61.
15   See Gruber, "Medicaid and Uninsured Women and Children," 202–3.
16   U.S. General Accounting Office, "Potential Difficulties in Determining Eligibility for Low-Income People," 11 July 1994, GAO/HEHS-B-251424, 11.
17   John Holahan and David Liska, *Reassessing the Outlook for Medicaid Spending Growth* (Washington: Urban Institute Press, 1997).

18   John Iglehart, "The American Health Care System: Medicaid," NEJM 328 (1993): 898.

19   Gail Wilensky, "Financing Care for Patients with AIDS," JAMA 266 (1991): 3404.

20   Sparer, "Great Expectations," 193.

21   Sparer, *Medicaid and the Limits of State Health Reform*, 55.

22   Part of the funds spent on hospital care was going to waste and redundant services. See for example Regina Herzlinger, "The Quiet Health Care Revolution," *Public Interest*, spring 1994, 72–91.

23   Sparer, *Medicaid and the Limits of State Health Reform*, 56–57.

24   U.S. General Accounting Office, *Medicaid Financing*, 1 September 1994, GAO/HEHS-94-133, B-253837.

25   Shapiro, "How States Cook the Books," 25. See also Tucker, "A Leak in Medicaid," 46–47.

26   U.S. General Accounting Office, HCFA *Needs Authority to Enforce Third-Party Requirements on States*, 11 April 1991, GAO/HRD-91-60, B-241141.

27   See Robert Politzer, Dona Harris, Marilyn Gaston, and Fitzhugh Mullan, "Primary Care Physician Supply and the Medically Underserved," JAMA 226 (1991): 104–9.

28   See Dewitt, "Oregon's Bitter Medicine"; Robert Steinbrook and Bernard Lo, "The Oregon Medicaid Demonstration Project: Will It Provide Adequate Medical Care?," NEJM 326 (1992): 340–44; Morell, "Oregon Puts Bold Health Plan on Ice"; David Hadorn, "Setting Health Care Priorities in Oregon," JAMA 265 (1991): 2218–25.

29   Arnold Relman, "Is Rationing Inevitable?," NEJM 322 (1990): 1809–10.

30   John Lewin and Peter Sybinsky, "Hawaii's Employer Mandate and Its Contribution to Universal Access," JAMA 269 (1993): 2538–43; U.S. General Accounting Office, *Access to Health Care: States Respond*, GAO-HRD-92-70, 2–5.

31   Notably, several states which attempted to impose employer mandates at this time, such as Massachusetts and Washington, were thwarted by existing federal ERISA rules. Hawaii was largely exempted from these rules, and thus was uniquely successful in its mandate.

32   Barbara Yawn, William Jacott, and Roy Yawn, "MinnesotaCare," JAMA 269 (1993): 511–14; Steven Miles, Nicole Lurie, Lois Quam, and Arthur Caplan, "Health Care Reform in Minnesota," NEJM 327 (1992): 1092–95.

33   For detailed discussion of health care reform in New York, Massachusetts, Rhode Island, and New Hampshire see Robert Hackey, *Rethinking Health Care Policy*, particularly chapters 3–6.

34   Marilyn Moon and John Holahan, "Can States Take the Lead in Health Care Reform?," JAMA 268 (1992): 1588–94; L. Demkovich, *The States and the Uninsured: Slowly but Surely Filling the Gaps* (Washington: National Health Policy Forum, 1990); John Iglehart, "Health Care Reform: The States," NEJM 330 (1994): 76.

35   A Gray, "Directory to Free Medical Clinics in Virginia," *Virginia Medical Quarterly* 119 (1992): 238–50.

36 Bruce Harris, Letter to the Editor, *JAMA* 265 (1991): 2482.

37 For details on the history of the use of 1115 waivers see Schneider, "Medicaid Section 1115 Waivers"; also John Holahan, "Insuring the Poor through Section 11145 Medicaid Waivers," *Health Affairs* 14 (1995): 199–216.

38 Thomas Oliver and Karen Anderson Oliver, "Managed Care or Managed Politics? Medicaid Reforms in Maryland," *Medicaid Reform and the American States: Case Studies on the Politics of Managed Care*, ed. Mark Daniels (Westport: Auburn House, 1998), 136–40.

39 For more on the early forays into Medicaid managed care see Gregg Meyer and David Blumenthal, "TennCare and Academic Medical Centers," *JAMA* 276 (1996): 672–76; Jon Christianson et al., "Use of Community-Based Mental Health Programs by HMOs: Evidence from a Medicaid Demonstration," *AJPH* 82 (1992): 790–96; and James Fossett, "Managed Care and Devolution," *Medicaid and Devolution: A View From the States*, ed. Frank Thompson and John DiIulio Jr. (Washington: Brookings Institution, 1998), 106–53.

40 Penelope Lemov, "Nevada Finds a Way to Cut a Medicaid Bill," *Governing*, June 1993, 15–16.

41 A nice analysis of the health reform environment in 1990 can be found in Robert Hackey, "The Illogic of Health Care Reform: Policy Dilemmas for the 1990s," *Polity* 26, no. 2 (1993).

42 Congressional Budget Office, *Selected Options for Expanding Health Insurance Coverage* (Washington: Government Printing Office, 1991), 41–45.

43 A number of studies appearing in the early 1990s demonstrated the ill effects of receiving medical care through Medicaid, or indeed of being poor in the first place. See Maggi Machala and Margaret Miner, "Piecing Together the Crazy Quilt of Prenatal Care," *PHR* 106 (1991): 353–59; Ross, "Inequality"; Paul Buescher and Nancy Ward, "A Comparison of Low Birth Weight among Health Departments and Other Providers of Prenatal Care in North Carolina and Kentucky," *PHR* 107 (1992): 54–59.

44 *A Call for Action: Final Report of the Pepper Commission* (Washington: Government Printing Office, 1990).

45 "Proposal of the Conservative Democratic Forum Task Force on Health Care Reform," Conservative Democratic Task Force Files, Bush Library, box OA/ID, folder: 06983.

46 A very helpful listing of the many reform proposals floating around in 1991 can be found in Robert Blendon and Jennifer Edwards, "Caring for the Uninsured: Choices for Reform," *JAMA* 265 (1991): 2563–65. For evidence of Canadians' satisfaction with their health care see Robert Blendon et al., "Satisfaction with Health Systems in 10 Nations," *Health Affairs* 9 (1990): 185–92.

47 "Bush Health Plan, Please," *Atlanta Journal*, 20 March 1992.

48 Paul Cotton, "Less Is More and More Is Less in Health Care Proposals Offered in '92 Campaign," *JAMA* 268 (1992): 1635.

49 "The President's Comprehensive Health Reform Program," Conservative Democratic Task Force Files, Bush Library, box OA/ID, folder: 06983.

50 Louis Sullivan, "The Bush Administration's Health Care Plan," *NEJM* 327 (1992): 802.

51 See the GAO report on administrative costs, 1992.

52 For discussion of the conservative outlook toward social service legislation in the Bush administration see Matthew Moen and Kenneth Palmer, " 'Poppy' and His Conservative Passengers," *Leadership and the Bush Presidency*, ed. Ryan Barilleaux and Mary Stuckey (Westport: Praeger, 1992), 133–46; also "Bush and His Cabinet," *Policy Review*, winter 1990, 30–39.

53 Political correspondents familiar with the Clintons' love of bureaucracy, conversation, and expertise viewed the health reform debacle as a natural extension of the general chaos of the Clinton White House. For a good description of the culture of the first Clinton administration see Drew, *On the Edge*, especially chapters 1–3.

54 Floor debates on the Clinton plan led by George Mitchell (D., Me.) and Bob Dole (R., Kan.) can be found in "Should the Senate Approve the Mitchell Health Care Reform Plan," *Congressional Digest*, October 1994, 238–55.

55 Quoted in Paul Cotton, "Clinton Tinkers with Health System Status Quo: Critics Seek to Pick Apart Managed Competitions," *JAMA* 269 (1993): 1229.

56 It is important to realize that although Clinton's plan was maligned as radical and utopian, it was in many ways a highly pragmatic compromise between the single-payer and market-responsive proponents. It was daunting to Americans not so much in its essence as in its execution. See Skocpol, *Boomerang*, 17.

57 The best single-volume analysis of the failure of Clinton's plan is Joseph White, *Competing Solutions* (Washington: Brookings Institution, 1995). White faults the plan for not going far enough in embracing competition while employing universal rate-setting as a safety device, ultimately undermining its own potential efficacy in cost containment.

58 For analysis of the bureaucratic barriers facing the plan's implementation see Hacker, *The Road to Nowhere*, 157.

59 Galen, "Can the Poor Afford Health-Care Reform?"

60 Both Skocpol and Hacker attribute the Clinton plan's failure largely to the lack of *political* (as opposed to *policy*) planning within the White House during the bill's formative months. See Skocpol, *Boomerang*, 90, and Hacker, *The Road to Nowhere*, 179. Skocpol also sees the loss of elderly support (as articulated by the AARP) as another significant cause of the plan's downfall.

61 A great deal of post hoc analysis of the Clinton plan was conducted in the months and years following its demise. One of the most widely cited articles portrayed the debacle as a failure not of the plan itself but of political institutions incapable of rising above their immediate constituent pressures to achieve a far-reaching solution to America's health problems. See Sven Steinmo and Jon Watts, "It's the Institutions, Stupid: Why Comprehensive National Health Insurance Always Fails in America," *Journal of Health Politics, Policy, and Law* 20 (1995): 329–73.

62 S. G. Boodman, "The Dilemma of AZT: Who Can Afford It?," *Washington Post*, 8 August 1989, § H, 6.

63   Fred Hellinger, "Updated Forecasts of the Costs of Medical Care for Persons with AIDS, 1989–93," *PHR* 105 (1990): 1–12; for statistical modeling of the AIDS epidemic see Edward H. Kaplan and Margaret L. Brandeau, eds., *Modeling the AIDS Epidemic: Planning, Policy, and Prediction* (New York: Raven, 1994), 64, as quoted in Charles Marwick, "Congressional AIDS Commission in Limelight Likely to Remain There for Another Year," *JAMA* 266 (1991): 2050.

64   As quoted in Charles Marwick, "Congressional AIDS Commission in Limelight Likely to Remain There for Another Year," JAMA, 16 October 1991, 2050.

65   D. D. Chitwood et al., "HIV Seropositivity of Needles from Shooting Galleries in South Florida," *AJPH* 80 (1990): 150–52. See also S. R. Friedman and C. Casriel, "Drug Users' Organizations and AIDS Policy," *AIDS and Public Policy* 3 (1980): 30–36, for a detailed discussion of the response of intravenous drug users to anti-infection efforts.

66   See Jonathan Ellen et al., "Socioeconomic Differences in Sexually Transmitted Disease Rates among Black and White Adolescents, San Francisco, 1990–1992," *AJPH* 85 (1995): 1546–48; also J. S. Moran et al., "The Impact of Sexually Transmitted Disease on Minority Populations," *PHR* 104 (1989): 560–65.

67   John Aruffo, John Coverdale, and Carlos Vallbona, "AIDS Knowledge in Low-Income and Minority Populations," *PHR* 106 (1991): 115–19; D. J. Hum, R. Keller, and D. Fleming, "Communicating AIDS Information to Hispanics: The Importance of Language and Media Preference," *American Journal of Preventive Medicine* 5 (1989): 196–200.

68   Statistics are from the CDC report of March 1991, as cited in Priscilla Holman et al., "Increasing the Involvement of National and Regional Racial and Ethnic Minority Organizations in HIV Information and Education," *PHR* 106 (1991): 687–94. On New York City see "Overview of HIV/AIDS in New York City," White House policy memo, White House Office of Records Management, Bush Library, HE 001-01, box 23, folder: 314331–330898.

69   Jesse Green and Peter Arno, "The 'Medicalization' of AIDS," *JAMA* 264 (1990): 1261–66; F. J. Hellinger, "Forecasting the Medical Care Costs of the HIV Epidemic," *Inquiry* 28 (1991): 213–25; David Solomon and Andrew Hogan, "HIV Infection Treatment Costs under Medicaid in Michigan," *PHR* 107 (1992): 461–68.

70   The author worked as a consultant for the Newark Eligible Metropolitan Area planning council, 1995–98, and witnessed these biases in the funding delivery. See Newark Eligible Metropolitan Area Planning Council, *Local Area Needs Assessment* (1995, 1997) (Newark, N.J.).

71   See Robert Steinbrook, "Battling HIV on Many Fronts," *NEJM* 337 (1997): 779–80; Lawrence Altman, "AIDS Deaths Drop 19 Percent in U.S., Continuing a Heartening Trend," *New York Times*, 15 July 1997, § A, 1.

72   Michael Sparer and Lawrence Brown, "Nothing Exceeds Like Success: Managed Care Comes to Medicaid in New York City," *Milbank Quarterly* 77 (1999): 210. See also Sparer, "Medicaid Managed Care and the Health Reform Debate," 452–54.

73   Chartered Health Plan in Washington, D.C., was known for this practice, which it justified internally by noting that the cost of the transportation was more than offset by the savings brought by lower rates of no-show patients. For a good

overview of the early evolution of Medicaid managed care see Paul Offner, *Medicaid and the States* (New York: Century Foundation Press, 1999), 8–10.

74 As quoted in Ervin, "Door-to-Door HMO Scam."

75 John Iglehart, "The American Health Care System: Medicaid," *NEJM* 340 (1999): 407.

76 See Jane Mauldon et al., "Rationing or Rationalizing Children's Medical Care: Comparison of a Medicaid HMO with Fee-for-Service Care," *AJPH* 84 (1994): 899–904.

77 See John Holahan, Alison Evans, and Stephen Zuckerman, "Impact of the New Federalism on Medicaid," *Remaking Medicaid: Managed Care for the Public Good*, ed. Stephen Davidson and Stephen Somers (San Francisco: Jossey-Bass, 1998), 62–63.

78 Quoted in Iglehart, "The American Health Care System," 407.

79 For further discussion of Medicaid contracting in the late 1990s see James Fossett et al., "Managing Medicaid Managed Care: Are States Becoming Prudent Purchasers?," *Health Affairs* 19 (2000): 35–49; also Michael Sparer and Lawrence Brown, "Uneasy Alliances: Managed Care Plans Formed by Safety-Net Providers," *Health Affairs* 19 (2000): 23–35.

80 See Robert Morgan, Beth Virnig, Carolee DeVito, and Nancy Persily, "The Medicare-HMO Revolving Door: The Healthy Go In and the Sick Go Out," *NEJM* 337 (1997): 169–75.

81 Arlene Bierman, "Ensuring Health Care for the Uninsured," *JAMA* 276 (1996): 1804; Jerome Kassirer, "Is Managed Care Here to Stay?," *NEJM* 336 (1997): 1014. For retrospective analysis of the efficacy (and fairness) of Medicaid managed care in the 1990s see Landon and Epstein, "For-Profit and Not-For-Profit Health Plans Participating in Medicaid"; Hurley and Somers, "Medicaid and Managed Care"; and Bonnyman, "Stealth Reform."

82 Jerome Kassirer, "Our Ailing Public Hospitals," *NEJM* 333 (1995): 1349. See also Rebecca Voelker, "Are Medicaid Reforms on the Horizon?," *JAMA* 277 (1997): 697, for a discussion of DSH payments.

83 Finkelstein, "Bellevue's Emergency," 45.

84 Ibid., 46.

85 Quoted in Emily Friedman, "California Public Hospitals: The Buck Has Stopped," *JAMA* 277 (1997): 580.

86 For an interesting discussion of why private hospitals should continue to provide charity care, even in a Medicaid managed-care world, see Howard Tuckman and Cyril Chang, "A Proposal to Redistribute the Cost of Hospital Charity Care," *Milbank Quarterly* 69 (1991): 113–42.

87 J. W. Mason, "Triage: Who Gets In and Who's Left Out of the University of Chicago Hospitals," *Grey City Journal*, excerpted in "Double Standard," *Nation*, 9 January 1995, 52.

88 Congressional Budget Office, *Proposals to Subsidize Health Insurance for the Unemployed* (Washington: Government Printing Office, 1998), 5–11.

89 Jonathan Walters, "Kids and the Federal Trough," *Governing*, May 1998, 15. See also Susan Dentzer, "For Mercy's Sake, Let's Cover Kids," *U.S. News and World Report*, 21 October 1996, 69.

90 Figures are from Robert Pear, "A Million Parents Lost Medicaid, Study Says," *New York Times*, 20 June 2000.

91 Neal Halfon et al., "Medicaid Enrollment and Health Services Access by Latino Children in Inner-City Los Angeles," *JAMA* 277 (1997): 636–41.

92 See Showalter, "Physicians' Cost Shifting Behavior," 78–84.

93 See Magnusson, "Medicaid Is Getting Tough with Granny"; "Who Pays for Nursing Homes?"; and Pamela Farley Short, Peter Kemper, Llewellyn Cornelius, and Daniel Walden, "Public and Private Responsibility for Financing Nursing-Home Care: The Effect of Medicaid Asset Spend-Down," *Milbank Quarterly* 70 (1992): 277–98.

94 As of this writing, the SCHIP programs were overcoming their early lack of popularity, and were generally succeeding at enrolling greater numbers of eligible children.

Bibliography

Manuscript Collections

AMERICAN HOSPITAL ASSOCIATION LIBRARY
American Hospital Association Archives

LYNDON JOHNSON PRESIDENTIAL LIBRARY (AUSTIN, TEXAS)
Douglas Cater Papers
Fred Bohen Papers
James Gaither Papers
Task Force Reports
White House Central Files

JIMMY CARTER PRESIDENTIAL LIBRARY (ATLANTA)
Bunny Mitchell Papers
Chief of Staff Files
Domestic Policy Staff Files
President's Commission on Mental Health Files
White House Central Files

RONALD REAGAN PRESIDENTIAL LIBRARY (SIMI VALLEY, CALIF.)
Council of Economic Advisors Papers
Kenneth Crib Papers
Paul Simmons Papers
Robert Carleson Papers
White House Office of Records Management Files
William Roper Papers

GEORGE BUSH PRESIDENTIAL LIBRARY (COLLEGE STATION, TEXAS)
Conservative Democratic Task Force Papers

Gail Wilensky Papers
Johannes Kuttner Papers
White House Office of Records Management Files

RICHARD NIXON PRESIDENTIAL PAPERS PROJECT (COLLEGE PARK, MD.)
Domestic Policy Council Files
Emil Krogh Papers
John Ehrlichman Papers
White House Central Files

NATIONAL ARCHIVES AND RECORDS ADMINISTRATION
(COLLEGE PARK, MD.)
Healthcare Financing Administration Archives
Office of the Surgeon General Archives

Interviews

John Kitzhaber
Bruce Vladeck
Henry Waxman

Dissertations and Unpublished Manuscripts

Barrilleaux, Charles, "The Political Economy of Medicaid," State University of New York, 1984.

Berendt, Emil, "The Demand for Medicaid and AFDC," City University of New York, 1985.

Boyer, C. A., "Government Health Spending in the American Welfare State," Yale University, 1986.

Gilman, Jean Marie, "Medicaid and the Costs of Federalism 1984–1992," University of Virginia, 1996.

Jack, John, "Quality of Care under Medicaid: An Exploratory Analysis," State University of New York, 1980.

Satterthwaite, Shad, "Medicaid and the Politics of State Health Care Reform," University of Oklahoma, 1998.

Schmitz, Homer, "A Study of the Impact of Medicare and Medicaid on Financial Performance of St. Louis Area Hospitals," St. Louis University, 1983.

Twining, D. C., "The Politics of Health Care Reform: Health Planning for the Poor in Cleveland 1960–1982," Case Western Reserve University, 1988.

Books and Monographs

Abernathy, Glenn, ed., *The Carter Years: The President and Policy Making* (New York: St. Martin's, 1984).

American Hospital Association, *Health Care: What Happens to People When Government Cuts Back* (Chicago: AHA, 1982).

Barrileaux, Ryan, and Mary Stuckey, eds., *Leadership and the Bush Presidency: Prudence or Drift in an Era of Change?* (Westport: Praeger, 1992).

Bernstein, Irving, *Guns or Butter: The Presidency of Lyndon Johnson* (New York: Oxford University Press, 1996).

Blendon, Robert J., and Thomas W. Moloney, *New Approaches to the Medicaid Crisis: Proceedings of the 1981 Commonwealth Fund Forum* (New York: F&S, 1982).

Boaz, David, *Assessing the Reagan Years* (Washington: Cato Institute, 1988).

Bourne, Peter, *Jimmy Carter: A Comprehensive Biography from Plains to Post-presidency* (New York: Scribner, 1997).

Bovbjerg, Randall, and John Holahan, *Medicaid in the Reagan Era: Federal Policy and State Choices* (Washington: Urban Institute, 1982).

Brissenden, Robert, *Portrait of a Community Health Service* (Stockton, Calif.: San Joaquin County Medical Foundation, 1968).

Brown, Dorothy, and Elizabeth McKeown, *The Poor Belong to Us: Catholic Charities and American Welfare* (Cambridge: Harvard University Press, 1997).

Buchberger, Thomas, *Medicaid: Choices for 1982 and Beyond* (Washington: Congressional Budget Office, 1981).

Bush, George, and Brent Scowcroft, *A World Transformed* (New York: Alfred A. Knopf, 1998).

Campbell, Colin, and Bert Rockman, *The Bush Presidency: First Appraisals* (Chatham, N.J.: Chatham, 1991).

Catholic Health Association, *No Room in the Marketplace: Health Care for the Poor* (St. Louis: CHA, 1986).

Champagne, Anthony, *The Attack on the Welfare State* (Prospect Heights, Ill.: Waveland, 1984).

Cohen, Richard, *Changing Courses in Washington: Clinton and the New Congress* (New York: Macmillan, 1994).

Congressional Budget Office, *Health Differences between White and Nonwhite Americans* (Washington: Government Printing Office, 1977).

——. *Factors Contributing to the Growth of the Medicaid Program* (Washington: Government Printing Office, 1992).

Coughlin, Theresa, Leighton Ku, and John Holahan, *Medicaid since 1980: Costs, Coverage, and the Shifting Alliance between the Federal Government and the States* (Washington: Urban Institute Press, 1994).

Crenson, Matthew, *Building the Invisible Orphanage: A Prehistory of the American Welfare System* (Cambridge: Harvard University Press, 1998).

Dallek, Robert, *Flawed Giant: Lyndon Johnson and His Times, 1961–1973* (New York: Oxford University Press, 1997).

Daniels, Mark, *Medicaid Reform and the American States* (New York: Auburn, 1998).

David, S. I., *With Dignity: The Search for Medicaid and Medicare* (Westport: Greenwood, 1985).

Davidson, Stephen, *Remaking Medicaid: Managed Care for the Public Good* (San Francisco: Jossey-Bass, 1998).

Davis, Karen, and Cathy Schoen, *Health and the War on Poverty* (Washington: Brookings Institution, 1978).

Dodd, Lawrence, and Richard Schott, *Congress and the Administrative State* (New York: John Wiley and Sons, 1979).

Dowling, Harry, *City Hospitals: The Undercare of the Underprivileged* (Cambridge: Harvard University Press, 1992).

Drew, Elizabeth, *On the Edge: The Clinton Presidency* (New York: Simon and Schuster, 1994).

Feder, Judith, *Poor People and Poor Hospitals* (Washington: Urban Institute, 1983).

Fee, Elizabeth, and Daniel Fox, eds., *AIDS: The Making of a Chronic Disease* (Berkeley: University of California Press, 1992).

Fein, Rashi, *Medical Care, Medical Costs: The Search for a Health Insurance Policy* (Cambridge: Harvard University Press, 1986).

Foltz, Anne-Marie, *An Ounce of Prevention: Child Health Politics under Medicaid* (Cambridge: MIT Press, 1982).

Gardener, John, and Theodore Lyman, *The Fraud Game: State Responses to Fraud and Abuse in AFDC and Medicaid Programs* (Bloomington: Indiana University Press, 1985).

Gartner, Alan, ed., *What Reagan Is Doing to Us* (New York: Harper and Row, 1982).

Gilman, Jean Donovan, *Medicaid and the Costs of Federalism, 1984–1992* (New York: Garland, 1998).

Ginzburg, Benjamin, *Democrats Return to Power: Politics and Policy in the Clinton Era* (New York: W. W. Norton, 1994).

Goodwin, Doris Kearns, *Lyndon Johnson and the American Dream* (New York: Harper and Row, 1976).

Grannemann, Thomas, *Controlling Medicaid Costs: Federalism, Competition, and Choice* (Washington: American Enterprise Institute, 1993).

Greenberg, Stanley, *Middle Class Dreams: The Politics and Power of the New American Majority* (New York: Times Books, 1995).

Greenfield, Margaret, *MEDI-CAL: The California Medicaid Program (Title XIX), 1966–1967* (Berkeley: University of California, Institute of Governmental Studies, 1970).

Grimaldi, Paul, *Medicaid Reimbursement of Nursing Home Care* (Washington: American Enterprise Institute, 1982).

Grover, William, *The President as Prisoner: A Structural Critique of the Carter and Reagan Years* (Albany: State University of New York Press, 1989).

Hacker, Jacob, *The Road to Nowhere: The Genesis of President Clinton's Plan for Health Security* (Princeton: Princeton University Press, 1997).

——, *The Divided Welfare State* (New York: Cambridge University Press, 2002).

Hackey, Robert, *Rethinking Healthcare Policy: The New Politics of State Regulation* (Washington: Georgetown University Press, 1998).

Health Care Financing Administration, *Medicaid: An Overview* (Washington: HCFA, 1995).

———, *National Summary of State Medicaid Managed Care Programs* (Washington: HCFA, 1996).

Hoff, Joan, *Nixon Reconsidered* (New York: Basic Books, 1994).

Hoffman, Beatrix, *The Wages of Sickness: The Politics of Health Insurance in Progressive America* (Chapel Hill: University of North Carolina Press, 2001).

Holahan, John, *Financing Health Care for the Poor: The Medicaid Experience* (Lexington, Mass.: Lexington, 1975).

Howell, E., L. Corder, and A. Dobson, *Out-of-Pocket Health Expenses for Medicaid Recipients and Other Low-Income Persons* (Washington: U.S. Department of Health and Human Services, 1985).

Hynes, Margaret, *Who Cares for Poor People? Physicians, Medicaid, and Marginality* (New York: Garland, 1998).

Jacobs, Lawrence R., *The Health of Nations: Public Opinion and the Making of American and British Health Policy* (Ithaca: Cornell University Press, 1993).

Jahn, Dawn, and Thomas Ortiz, *The Texas Medicaid Program* (Austin: Policy Research Project on Health Care Cost and Access, 1992).

Johnson, Lyndon, *The Vantage Point: Perspectives of the Presidency, 1963–1969* (New York: Holt, Rinehart and Winston, 1971).

Katz, Michael, *Poverty and Policy in American History* (New York: Academic Press, 1983).

———, *In the Shadow of the Poorhouse* (New York: Basic Books, 1986).

Kaufman, Burton, *The Presidency of James Earl Carter* (Lawrence: University Press of Kansas, 1993).

Kentucky Commission on Indigent Care, *Medical Care for Indigent Persons in Kentucky* (Frankfort, 1957).

King, Anthony Stephen, *Both Ends of the Avenue: The Presidency, the Executive Branch, and Congress in the 1980s* (Washington: American Enterprise Institute, 1983).

Kissinger, Henry, *The White House Years* (Boston: Little, Brown, 1979).

Laham, Nicholas, *The Reagan Presidency and the Politics of Race* (Westport: Praeger, 1998).

Mansfield, Harvey, *Congress against the President* (New York: Academy of Political Science, 1975).

Marmor, Theodore, *The Politics of Medicare* (Chicago: Aldine, 1973).

———, *Understanding Healthcare Reform* (New Haven: Yale University Press, 1994).

Maryland State Planning Commission Committee on Medical Care, *Report of the Committee to Rescue the Medical Care Program* (Annapolis, 1953).

Matusow, Allen, *Nixon's Economy: Booms, Busts, Dollars, and Votes* (Lawrence: University Press of Kansas, 1998).

McDonald, Timothy, et al., *Crisis in Health Care for Black and Poor Americans: Report of the Southern Christian Leadership Conference* (Atlanta, 1984).

Moreno, Jonathan, *Paying the Doctor: Health Policy and Physician Reimbursement* (New York: Auburn, 1991).

Morone, James, *The Democratic Wish* (New York: Basic Books, 1990).

Nathan, Richard, *The Administrative Presidency* (New York: John Wiley and Sons, 1983).

New Jersey Commission to Study the Administration of Public Medical Care, *The Report and Recommendations of the NJCSMC* (Trenton, 1959).

Noble, Charles, *Welfare as We Knew It: A Political History of the Welfare State* (New York: Oxford University Press, 1997).

Norman, John C., ed., *Medicine in the Ghetto* (New York: Appleton-Century-Crofts, 1969).

Norsworthy, L. Alexander, *The Clinton Revolution: An Inside Look at the New Administration* (Lanham, Md.: University Press of America, 1993).

Oberlander, Jonathan, *The Political Life of Medicare* (Chapel Hill: University of North Carolina Press, 2003).

Opdyke, Sandra, *No One Was Turned Away: The Role of Public Hospitals in New York City since 1900* (New York: Oxford University Press, 1999).

Patterson, James, *America's Struggle against Poverty in the Twentieth Century* (Cambridge: Harvard University Press, 2000).

Peterson, Mark, *Legislating Together: the White House and Capitol Hill from Eisenhower to Reagan* (Cambridge: Harvard University Press, 1990).

Poen, Monte, *Harry S. Truman versus the Medical Lobby* (Columbia: University of Missouri Press, 1979).

Renshon, Stanley, *The Clinton Presidency: Campaigning, Governing, and the Psychology of Leadership* (Boulder: Westview, 1995).

Ripley, Randall, *Congress, the Bureaucracy, and Public Policy* (Homewood, Ill.: Dorsey, 1980).

Risse, Guenter, *Mending Bodies, Saving Souls* (New York: Oxford University Press, 1999).

Rosenbaum, Sara, Karen Silver, and Elizabeth Wehr, *An Evaluation of Contracts between State Medicaid Agencies and Managed Care Organizations for the Prevention and Treatment of Mental Illness and Substance Abuse Disorders* (Washington: U.S. Department of Health and Human Services, 1997).

Rosner, David, *A Once Charitable Enterprise: Hospitals and Health Care in Brooklyn and New York, 1885–1915* (New York: Cambridge University Press, 1982).

Rothman, David, *The Discovery of the Asylum: Social Order and Disorder in the New Republic* (Boston: Little, Brown, 1971).

Sardell, Alice, *The U.S. Experiment in Social Medicine: The Community Health Center Program 1965–1986* (Pittsburgh: University of Pittsburgh Press, 1988).

Schaller, Michael, *Reckoning with Reagan: America and Its President in the 1980s* (New York: Oxford University Press, 1992).

Shogan, Robert, *The Fate of the Union: America's Rocky Road to Political Stalemate* (Boulder: Westview, 1998).

Skocpol, Theda, *Protecting Soldiers and Mothers: The Political Origins of Social Policy in the United States* (Cambridge: Harvard University Press, 1992).

——, *Boomerang: Clinton's Health Security Effort and the Turn against Government in U.S. Politics* (New York: W. W. Norton, 1996).

Skocpol, Theda, and Dietrich Rueschemeyer, eds., *States, Social Knowledge, and the Origins of Modern Social Policy* (Princeton: Princeton University Press, 1996).

Solomon, Norman, *False Hope: The Politics of Illusion in the Clinton Era* (Monroe, Maine: Common Courage, 1994).

Sorkin, Alan, *Health Care and the Changing Economic Environment* (Lexington, Mass.: Lexington, 1986).

Sparer, Michael, *Medicaid and the Limits of State Health Reform* (Philadelphia: Temple University Press, 1996).

Spiegel, Allen D., ed., *The Medicaid Experience* (Germantown, Md.: Aspen Systems, 1979).

Starr, Paul, *The Social Transformation of American Medicine* (New York: Basic Books, 1982).

Stevens, Rosemary, *In Sickness and in Wealth: American Hospitals in the Twentieth Century* (New York: Basic Books, 1989).

Stevens, Rosemary, and Robert Stevens, *Welfare Medicine in America* (New York: Free Press, 1974).

Thornton, Richard, *The Carter Years: Toward a New Global Order* (New York: Paragon, 1991).

U.S. Department of Housing and Urban Development, *Affordable Health Insurance Is Now Here for Kids Who Need It* (Washington: U.S. Department of Housing and Urban Development, 1998).

U.S. General Accounting Office, *Medicaid: Early Implications of Welfare Reform for Beneficiaries* (Washington: GAO, 1998).

Vogel, Morris, *The Invention of the Modern Hospital* (Chicago: University of Chicago Press, 1980).

Weir, Margaret, Theda Skocpol, and Anna Shola Orloff, eds., *The Politics of Social Policy in the United States* (Princeton: Princeton University Press, 1988).

Journal Articles

Aday, Lu Ann, and Ronald Andersen, "Fostering Access to Medical Care," *Proceedings of the Academy of Political Science* 32 (1977): 29–41.

Agranoff, Robert, and Alex Pattakos, "Intergovernmental Management: Federal Changes, State Responses, and New State Initiatives," *Publius* 14 (1984): 49–84.

Altman, D., "Healthcare for the Poor," *Annals of the American Academy of Political and Social Science* 468 (1983): 103–21.

Ashcraft, Marie L., and S. E. Berki, "HMOs as Medicaid Providers," *Annals of the American Academy of Political and Social Science* 468 (1983): 122–31.

Bellush, Jewel, "Indispensable Facilities: In Defense of Municipal Hospitals," *New York Affairs* 5 (1979): 111–19.

Berkelhamer, J. E., E. J. Noyes, and R. T. Chen, "Child Health Policy: An Overview of Federal Involvement," *Advances in Pediatrics* 29 (1982): 211–18.

Blaisdell, F. W., "The Pre-Medicare Role of City/County Hospitals in Education and Health Care," *Journal of Trauma* 32 (1992): 217–28.

——, "Development of the City/County (Public) Hospital," *Archives of Surgery* 129 (1994): 760–64.

Blendon, Robert, "The Problems of Cost, Access, and Distribution of Medical Care," *Daedalus* 115 (1986): 119–35.

Bonnyman, G. Gordon, Jr., "Stealth Reform: Market-Based Medicaid in Tennessee," *Health Affairs* 15 (1996): 306–15.

Bradbury, Katharine, Sheldon Danziger, Eugene Smolensky, and Paul Smolensky, "Public Assistance, Female Headship, and Economic Well-Being," *Journal of Marriage and the Family* 41 (1979): 519–35.

Brieger, Gert, "The Use and Abuse of Medical Charities in Late 19th Century America," *American Journal of Public Health* 67 (1977): 264–67.

Buck, Peter, "Why Not the Best? Some Reasons and Examples of Child Health and Rural Hospitals," *Journal of Social History* 18 (1985): 413–31.

Cohen, Toby, "Medicaid Fraud Reconsidered: How the Hospitals Got on Welfare," *Dissent* 24 (1977): 390–98.

Cohen, Wilbur, "Reflections on the Enactment of Medicare and Medicaid," *Health Care Financing Review* 1985, supp., 3–11.

——, "The Twentieth Anniversary of Medicare and Medicaid: The Long, Difficult Road to Enactment," *Health Progress* 66 (1995): 22–23.

Conner, S. L., "The Sixties Medicare Debate Revisited," *Alabama Medicine* 61 (1991): 4–10.

Conover, C. J., W. G. Stumbo, and D. T. Allen, "Medicaid in Kentucky," *Journal of the Kentucky Medical Association* 79 (1981): 156–67.

Copeland, Gary, and Kenneth Meier, "Gaining Ground: The Impact of Medicaid and WIC on Infant Mortality," *American Politics Quarterly* 15 (1987): 254–73.

Coyne, J. S., and M. I. Roemer, "Paying For Hospital Care: Evolution and Implications," *Journal of Public Health Policy* 8 (1987): 65–85.

Davis, James E., "National Initiatives for Care of the Medically Needy," *Journal of the American Medical Association* 259 (1988): 3171–73.

Davis, R. G., "Congress and the Emergence of Public Health Policy," *Health Care Management Review* 10 (1985): 61–73.

Endquist-Seidenberg, Gretchen, "The States' Role in Health Care Cost Containment," *Policy Studies Review* 1 (1981): 275–87.

Ettner, Susan, "The Effect of the Medicaid Home Care Benefit on Long-Term Care Choices of the Elderly," *Economic Inquiry* 32 (1994): 103–27.

——, "Medicaid Participation among the Eligible Elderly," *Journal of Policy Analysis and Management* 16 (1997): 237–55.

Falk, Isidore, "Medical Care in the USA, 1932–1972: Problems, Proposals and Programs from the Committee on the Costs of Medical Care of the Committee for National Insurance," *Milbank Memorial Fund Quarterly* 51 (1973): 1–32.

Fine, Sidney, "The Kerr-Mills Act: Medical Care for the Indigent," *Journal of the History of Medicine* 53 (1998): 285–316.

Fox, Daniel, "Policy and Epidemiology: Financing Health Services for the Chronically Ill and Disabled," *Milbank Memorial Fund Quarterly* 67 (1989), suppl. 2, part 2:257–87.

Friedman, Emily, "Fifty Years of U.S. Health Policy," *Hospitals* 60 (1986): 95–104.

———, "The Compromise and the Afterthought: Medicare and Medicaid after 30 Years," *Journal of the American Medical Association* 274 (1995): 278–82.

Godfield, N., "Medicare and Medicaid: The First Successful Effort to Increase Access to Health Care," *Physician Executive* 19 (1993): 6–11.

Greenberg, D. S., "Bush Plays Safe on Healthcare Reform," *Lancet* 338 (1991): 561–62.

Gruber, Jonathan, "Medicaid and Uninsured Women and Children," *Journal of Economic Perspectives* 11 (1997): 199–208.

Hackey, Robert, "The Illogic of Health Care Reform: Policy Dilemmas for the 1990s," *Polity* 26 (1993): 233–57.

Hanson, Russell, "Medicaid and the Politics of Redistribution," *American Journal of Political Science* 28 (1984): 313–39.

Herman, Mary W., "The Poor: Their Medical Needs and the Health Services Available to Them," *Annals of the American Academy of Political and Social Science* 399 (1972): 12–21.

Hessler, R. K., "Citizen Participation in Neighborhood Health Centers for the Poor," *Human Organizations* 41 (1982): 245–55.

"History of the Provisions of the Old-Age, Survivors, Disability, and Health Insurance Program," *Social Security Bulletin*, 1980, Annual Statistical Supplement, 19–40.

Hurley, Robert, and Stephen Somers, "Medicaid and Managed Care: A Lasting Relationship," *Health Affairs* 22 (2003): 77–89.

"Iowa Physicians Want Medicaid to Operate Efficiently and Economically," *Journal of the Iowa Medical Society* 59 (1969): 859–64.

Jahn, David, and Thomas Ortiz, "The Texas Medicaid Program," LBJ School of Public Affairs Working Paper no. 65 (Austin: University of Texas, 1992).

Kim, H., "Oregon's Medicaid Architect," *Modern Healthcare* 19 (1989): 58.

Korcok, M., "Can Two-Tiered Healthcare Work?," *Canadian Medical Association Journal* 129 (1983): 629–35.

Landon, Bruce, and Arnold Epstein, "For-Profit and Not-for-Profit Health Plans Participating in Medicaid," *Health Affairs* 20 (2001): 162–72.

Leveson, Irving, "The Challenge of Health Services for the Poor," *Annals of the American Academy of Political and Social Science* 399 (1972): 22–29.

Lichter, Daniel, Diane McLaughlin, and David Ribar, "Welfare and the Rise in Female-Headed Families," *American Journal of Sociology* 103 (1997): 112–43.

Lusterman, E. A., "Medicaid: A History of Governmental Blunders and Misjudgments," *New York State Dental Journal* 34 (1968): 559–61.

Maioni, Antonia, "Parting at the Crossroads: The Development of Health Insurance in Canada and the United States, 1940–1965," *Comparative Politics* 29 (1997): 411–31.

"Medicaid in Michigan: Its Modest Beginnings, 1966–73," *Michigan Hospital* 14 (1978): 4–5.

Meier, Kenneth, and Thomas Holbrook, "No Longer Gaining Ground: An Update," *American Politics Quarterly* 19 (1991): 377–85.

Meyers, Beverlee, "Health Care for the Poor," *Proceedings of the Academy of Political Science* 32 (1977): 68–78.

Moreno, Lorenzo, and Sheila Hoag, "Covering the Uninsured through TennCare: Does It Make a Difference?," *Health Affairs* 20 (2001): 231–40.

Mowll, C. A., "Medicaid: Reviewing the Program," *Healthcare Financial Management* 42 (1988): 124–26.

Myers, B. A., "The Formulation of Federal Health Policy: Lessons from the Task Force on Medicaid and Related Programs," *Bulletin of the New York Academy of Medicine* 47 (1971): 1509–23.

Newman, Howard, "Medicaid and National Health Insurance," *Public Welfare* 32 (1974): 21–26.

Oberg, Charles N., "Medically Uninsured Children in the United States: A Challenge to Public Policy," *Journal of School Health* 60 (1990): 493–500.

Oliver, Thomas, "Health Care Market Reform in Congress: The Uncertain Path from Proposal to Policy," *Political Science Quarterly* 106 (1991): 453–78.

"Perspectives: Medicaid at 25: Rising Expectations," *Faulkner and Gray's Medicine and Health* 44 (1990), supplement 8.

"Perspectives: Twenty Years of Medicaid," *Washington Report on Medicine and Health* 39 (1985), supplement 4.

Politser, P., "American's Uninsured: Part I: A Long History, An Uncertain Future," *Bulletin of the American College of Surgeons* 75 (1990): 11–15.

Pontell, Henry, Paul Jesilow, and Gilbert Geis, "Practitioner Fraud and Abuse in Medical Benefit Programs," *Law and Policy* 6 (1984): 405–24.

Rice, Mitchell, "The Urban Public Hospital: Its Importance to the Black Community," *Urban League Review* 9 (1985–86): 64–70.

Rosner, David, "Social Control and Social Service: The Changing Use of Space in Charity Hospitals," *Radical History Review* 21 (1979): 183–97.

Rothman, David, "The Hospital as Caretaker: The Almshouse Past and Intensive Care Future," *Transactions and Studies of the College of Physicians of Philadelphia* 12 (1990): 151–74.

Russell, L. B., and C. S. Burke, "The Political Economy of Federal Health Programs in the United States: An Historical Review," *International Journal of Health Services* 8 (1978): 55–77.

Sager, A., "Why Urban Hospitals Close," *Health Services Research* 18 (1983): 451–75.

Schlesinger, M., T. Marmor, and R. Smithey, "Nonprofit and For-Profit Medical Care: Shifting Roles and Implications for Health Policy," *Journal of Health Politics, Policy, and Law* 12 (1987): 427–57.

Schneider, Saundra, "Medicaid Section 1115 Waivers: Shifting Health Care Reform to the States," *Publius* 27 (1997): 89–109.

Showalter, Mark, "Physicians' Cost Shifting Behavior: Medicaid versus Other Patients," *Contemporary Economic Policy* 15 (1997): 78–84.

Siefert, K., "An Example of . . . : The Sheppard-Towner Act of 1921," *Social Work in Health Care* 9 (1983): 87–103.

Silver, George, "The Route to a National Health Policy Lies through the States," *Yale Journal of Biology and Medicine* 64 (1991): 443–53.

Sloan, Frank, et al., "The Demise of Hospital Philanthropy," *Economic Inquiry* 28 (1990): 725–43.

Sparer, Michael S., "Great Expectations: The Limits of State Healthcare Reform," *Health Affairs* 14 (1995): 191–202.

——, "Medicaid Managed Care and the Health Reform Debate: Lessons from New York and California," *Journal of Health Politics, Policy, and Law* 21 (1996): 433–60.

Sparer, M. S., et al., "Promising Practices: How Leading Safety-Net Plans Are Managing the Care of Medicaid Clients," *Health Affairs* 21 (2002): 284–92.

Stevens, Rosemary, "Health Care in the Early 1960s," *Health Care Financing Review* 18 (1996): 11–22.

Stuart, Bruce C., "Who Gains From Public Health Programs?," *Annals of the American Academy of Political and Social Science* 399 (1972): 145–50.

Tannenbaum, S. J., "Medicaid Eligibility Policy in the 1980s: Medical Utilitarianism and the 'Deserving' Poor," *Journal of Health Politics, Policy, and Law* 20 (1995): 933–54.

Wagner, L., "Running the Medicaid Bureau," *Modern Healthcare* 20 (1990): 52.

Wetstein, Matthew, "The Abortion Rate Paradox: The Impact of National Policy Change on Abortion Rates," *Social Science Quarterly* 76 (1995): 607–18.

Wolski, P. R., "Kevin Seitz: Working to Build a Healthier Medicaid System," *Michigan Medicine* 89 (1990): 35.

Selected Newspaper and Magazine Articles

Albanese, G. J., "Medicaid," *Vital Speeches*, 1 February 1985, 236–39.

Arnold, M. R., "Prescription for Health Care," *Commonweal*, 9 September 1974, 423–26.

Auletta, K., "Saving the Underclass," *Washington Monthly*, September 1985, 12–16.

Barnes, F., "Prince of Poverty," *New Republic*, 8 October 1990, 10.

Bates, A., "Golden Girls," *New Republic*, 3 February 1992, 17–18.

Bethell, Tom, "Inciting Poverty," *Harper's*, February 1980, 161.

"Billions in Medicaid Ripoffs: Can Anyone Stop It?," *U.S. News and World Report*, 22 March 1976, 18–20.

Boffey, Phillip, "Federal Health Programs: A Major Reorganization Is under Way," *Science* 160 (1968): 1429–31.

Braham, Robert, and Thomas Lee, "The Worst Care Money Can Buy," *Washington Monthly*, June 1981, 28–30.

"Bringing Down-to-Earth Medical Care to Areas without Doctors," *U.S. News and World Report*, 31 December 1979, 76–77.

Budish, A. D., "Medicaid: Middle Class Need Not Apply," *Modern Maturity*, June 1994, 48–51.

Castelli, Jim, "Will Health Beat Nixon in '72?," *Commonweal*, 9 April 1971, 108–12.

Clark, Wayne, and Joseph Huttie Jr., "New Federalism in the Delta," *Progressive*, April 1974, 24–25.

Cohen, T., "Medical Class Struggle," *Nation*, 21 February 1981, 203–4.

Coles, Robert, "What Poverty Does to the Mind," *Nation*, 20 June 1966, 746–48.

Dentzer, S., "For Mercy's Sake: Let's Cover Kids," *U.S. News and World Report*, 21 October 1996, 69.

Derks, Scott, "Sort of Dampens Your Spirits: Suit against Dr. C. H. Pierce for Sterilizing Welfare Patients," *Nation*, 16 December 1978, 675–76.

Dewitt, P. E., "Oregon's Bitter Medicine," *Time*, 17 August 1992, 45.

"Don't Give Up: Poverty Programs That Work," *Washington Monthly*, June 1988, 28–40.

Dreifus, C., "Sterilizing the Poor," *Progressive*, February 1976, 46–47.

Edwards, M. D., "Medical Care for the Young," *Nation*, 28 September 1974, 275–76.

Ervin, M., "Door to Door HMO Scam," *Progressive*, September 1997, 18.

Finkelstein, Katherine Eban, "Bellevue's Emergency," *New York Times Magazine*, 11 February 1996, 44–50.

Fleming, R., "Eugenic Sterilization: Great for What Ails the Poor," *Encore*, June 1980, 17–19.

Frankel, M., "What the Poor Deserve," *New York Times Magazine*, 22 October 1995, 46.

Galbraith, J. K., "Let Us Begin: An Invitation to Action on Poverty," *Harper's*, March 1964, 16.

——, "The Heartless Society," *New York Times Magazine*, 2 September 1984, 20–21.

Galen, Michele, "Can the Poor Afford Health Care Reform?," *Business Week*, 4 October 1993, 31–32.

Gardner, W. D., "Running Out of Money, Not Patients: New York State's Medicaid Program," *New Republic*, 17 February 1968, 19.

Garland, Susan B., "Health Care for All or an Excuse for Cutbacks?," *Business Week*, 26 June 1989, 68.

Garland, Susan B., and Gail DeGeorge, "A Welfare Mother's Battle to Clean Up the Medicaid Mess," *Business Week*, 21 December 1987, 42.

Graber, S., "Clinics, Toilets, and Black Management," *Nation*, 26 June 1976, 785–88.

Higgins, Thomas, "Time for a Second Opinion," *Commonweal*, 17 June 1983, 365–67.

Hodgson, Geoffrey, "The Politics of American Health Care" and "Discussion," *Atlantic*, October 1973, 45–61.

"Income, Illness, and the Health Gap," *Science News*, 24 January 1981, 59.

Keyserling, L. H., "Reply to Tobin," *New Republic*, 10 June 1967, 33–34.

Klass, P., "Tackling Problems We Thought We Solved," *New York Times Magazine*, 13 December 1992, 54–58.

Koretz, G., "Medicaid's Baby Boon," *Business Week*, 19 January 1998, 24.

Lemann, Nicholas, "The Future of Poverty," *Atlantic*, September 1984, 26–27.

——, "The Unfinished War," *Atlantic*, January 1989, 52–56.

Lemov, P., "Nevada Finds a Way to Cut a Medicaid Bill," *Governing*, June 1993, 15–16.

Lenkowsky, Leslie, "Welfare Reform and the Liberals," *Commentary*, March 1979, 56–61.

Lewis, Irving J., "Government Investment in Health Care," *Scientific American*, April 1971, 17–25.

Magnusson, Paul, "Medicaid Is Getting Tough with Granny," *Business Week*, 30 September 1996, 145.

Mason, J. W., "Double Standard," *Nation*, 9 January 1995, 32.

Mayer, J. L., "Time Out: Pediatrician's Experience with the Poor in Vermont," *New York Times Magazine*, 19 October 1986, 96.

McCullough, B. L., "Demise of Rural Medicine," *Vital Speeches*, 15 June 1971, 517–18.

"Medical Pains," *Time*, 2 March 1981, 27–28.

Morell, Virginia, "Oregon Puts Bold Health Plan on Ice," *Science* 249 (1990): 468–71.

"Mt. Bayou's Crisis," *Time*, 25 November 1974, 107.

Murray, C. A., "Helping the Poor: A Few Modest Proposals," *Commentary*, May 1985, 27–34.

——, "What's So Bad about Being Poor?," *National Review*, 28 October 1988, 36–39.

Myrdal, G., "War on Poverty," *New Republic*, 8 February 1964, 14–16.

Nixon, R., "Food, Nutrition and Health," *Vital Speeches*, 1 January 1970, 162–65.

Novak, Michael, "The Rich, the Poor, and the Reagan Administration," *Commentary*, August 1983, 27–31.

Oransky, I., "Losing Patients," *New Republic*, 17 November 1997, 16–17.

Peterson, O. L., "How Good Is Government Medical Care?," *Atlantic*, September 1960, 29–33.

Pooley, E., "Everybody Hurts," *New York*, 13 March 1995, 24.

Quinn, Jane Bryant, "Family Obligations," *Newsweek*, 29 August 1983, 56.

"Reading the Ghetto: Clinic Referral Plan of St. Francis X. Cabrini Hospital," *Time*, 12 November 1973, 121.

Reisman, F., "Mental Health of the Poor," *New Republic*, 6 February 1965, 21–23.

Rorty, R., "What's Wrong with Rights?," *Harper's*, June 1996, 15–18.

Ross, Philip E., "Inequality," *Forbes*, 31 January 1994, 81.

"Rural Health Care in Dire Straits, *Science Digest*, September 1976, 20–21.

"Rx for Medicaid: Major Surgery," *U.S. News and World Report*, 13 February 1984, 9.

Samuelson, R., "RIP: The War on Poverty," *Newsweek*, 9 October 1995, 59.

——, "The Culture of Poverty," *Newsweek*, 5 May 1997, 49.

Saunders, M. K., "Doctor Meets the People: Neighborhood Health Center of Montefiore Hospital," *Harper's*, January 1968, 56–62.

Schwartz, W. B., "Policy Analysis and the Health Care System," *Science*, 15 September 1972, 967–69.

Seligman, D., "Twisting the Truth," *Fortune*, 11 June 1984, 205.

Shapiro, Joseph P., "A War on Poverty," *U.S. News and World Report*, 27 February 1989, 20–23.

——, "How States Cook the Books," *U.S. News and World Report*, 29 July 1991, 24–25.

——, "To Ration or Not to Ration," *U.S. News and World Report*, 10 August 1992, 24.

Shepherd, "Birth Control for the Poor," *Look*, 7 April 1964, 63–67.

Sidel, V., "Medicaid, Technology, and the Poor," *Technology Review*, May–June 1987, 24–25.

Titmus, R. M., "What British Doctors Really Think about Socialized Medicine," *Harper's*, February 1963, 16.

Tobin, J., "It Can Be Done: Conquering Poverty in the U.S. by 1976," *New Republic*, 3 June 1967, 14–18.

TRB, "The War on Poverty," *New Republic*, 14 March 1964, 2.

——, "Heavy Warm Inflation," *New Republic*, 8 March 1969, 6.

——, "Health Care Crisis in the U.S.," *New Republic*, 18 October 1969, 4.

Tucker, William, "A Leak in Medicaid," *Forbes*, 8 July 1991, 46.

Tunley, R., "America's Unhealthy Children: An Emerging Scandal," *Harper's*, May 1966, 41–46.

Walters, J., "Kids and the Federal Trough," *Governing*, May 1998, 15.

Watson, Thomas J., Jr., "Health Service: Is the Next Step to Socialism?," *Vital Speeches*, 1 February 1971, 249–51.

Webb, G. S., "Poor Health," *Progressive*, May 1988, 17–19.

"What's Fair," *Time*, 16 April 1984, 23.

"Who Pays for Nursing Homes?," *Consumer Reports*, September 1995, 591–97.

Index

Alabama, 141–42, 201–2

Alcoholism, 95

Alienation, medical, 76

All Workers Act (1987), 205

Almshouses, 11

AMA. *See* American Medical Association

American Civil Liberties Union, 207

American Hospital Association (AHA): cost control and, 148; Kerr-Mills Act and, 35–36; on Medicaid, 66–67, 204–5; on nursing home care, 186, 188; on Reagan's policies, 176, 179

American Medical Association (AMA): All Workers Act and, 205; community health centers movement and, 101; cost control and, 148; federal programs and, 64; King-Anderson Bill and, 39; Medicaid and, 59, 64–65; Medicare and, 47–48, 59, 64–65; on OBRA cuts, 171; rural physicians and, 77–78

American Psychiatric Association, 104

American Public Health Association, 229

Americans with Disabilities Act (ADA), 207

An American Dilemma (Myrdal), 26

Anderson, Albert, 135

Anderson, Clinton, 38–39, 46–47

Annis, Edward, 39

Antibiotics, 94

Appalachia, 41–42

Appalachian Regional Hospital system, 77

Appel, James, 64

Appointment scheduling, 239–40

Arizona, 202

Arkansas, 229

Aronovits, Leslie, 215

Asset transfers, 187

Associated Health Care Insurance Plan (AHIP), 120

Attitudes toward health, 24–25, 75–76

Autonomy, professional, 93

Avalanche phenomenon, 24

Balanced Budget Act (1997), 242

Ball, Robert, 31–32

Baltimore, 70, 71

Bamberger, Lisbeth, 54

Basic health care, 17

Bellevue Hospital, 238–39

Bellin, Lowell, 161

Bellush, Jewel, 166

Berry, Theodore, 54

Biemiller, Andrew, 31–32

Bierman, Jessie, 159

Birth rates, 42

Bismark, Leonard, 35

Blacks. *See* African Americans

Blind persons, 186–87

Block grants, 149, 166–68, 173, 175–76

Blue Cross, 4, 32, 55, 110–11

Blue Shield, 55

Blum, Henrik, 190

Boland, James, 65

Bourne, Peter, 152–53

Boyd, Don, 241

Breathitt, Edward, 42

Breslow, Lester, 87

Brownfeld, Allan, 180

Burns, Arthur, 110

Burns, Eveline, 53

Bush, George H. W., 229–30

Bush, George W., 242–43

Cain, James, 121–22

Cal-Med, 62–63, 108, 109

Califano, Joseph, 151, 152, 153, 158

California: capitation programs in, 202; HMOs in, 137–38, 236; hospital debt in, 190; hospital payments in (1990s), 216; Medi-Cal, 62–63, 108, 109; Medicaid in, 128, 163; per capita spending in (1980s–1990s), 215–16; physician ratio in, 70; San Francisco Health Department plan, 222; welfare reform in (1996), 241

Canadian health care, 120–21, 205–6

Capitation, 145, 149–50, 202, 224, 237

Caplan, Arthur, 207

Cardwell, Horace, 66
Caregivers, family, 187–88
Caretaking services, 188
Carleson, Robert, 170
Carter, Jimmy: attitude toward health care of, 144–46; Child Health Assessment Program and, 159–62; comprehensive reform and, 151–55; hospital cost control and, 146–48; Medicaid and, 148–51, 161–62; urban areas and, 193; welfare reform and, 155–59
Castro, Raul, 147
Catastrophic care, 3, 117–18, 154
Cater, Douglass, 51, 64
Catholic Hospital Association, 204
Caudill, Harry, 56
Cavanaugh, James, 96
CCMC (Committee on the Costs of Medical Care), 4–5, 131
Celebrezze, Anthony, 19
Certificate of need (CON) process, 133–35, 147
Chafee, John, 205
CHAP (Child Health Assessment Program), 159–62
Charity care: in 1950s, 30; in 1960s, 17–18, 107–8; in 1980s, 208; ambivalence toward, ix–xi; early history of, xi–xii, 7–10; government-provided, 245–47; historical attempts to provide, 244–45; interest groups and, xvii; mass immigration and, 8; modern provision of, 245–47; national health care and, 120; perceptions of poverty and, 27; by physicians, 13–15, 191–92; physicians' attitudes toward, 111–12, 223, 246–47; racial breakdown of, 17–18; in rural areas, 139; scientific, 11, 13; state programs for, 17–19; very poor and, 5. *See also specific programs*
Charlottesville Free Clinic, 222
Chicago: appointment scheduling in, 239–40; community health centers in, 102; Cook County Hospital, 190; physician ratio in, 70; three-echelon system of care in, 71
Child Health Assessment Program (CHAP), 159–62
Child Health Insurance Program (CHIP), 88–89
Children: access to care for, 5, 18–19, 213; African American, 80–81, 173–74, 197; chronic illness in, 86; crippled children's programs, 18, 21, 86; dental care for, 86; Early and Periodic Screening, Diagnosis and Treatment Program and, 128–29, 165; early federal programs for, 15–16; health status of (1960s), 18–19, 49, 85–88; health status of (1980s), 165–66, 173–74, 199–202; Hispanic, 197; immunization of, 108; malnutrition in, 87; Medicaid eligibility and, 85–88, 163; mortality rates for (1981), 165–66; orphaned, 21; physician visits by, 123; in poverty, 86, 211; primary care for, 214; Reagan's policies and, 184; Ribicoff children, 204–5; in rural areas, 74–75; SCHIP for, 241; spending on (1967), 87; uninsured, 211–12; of unwed mothers, 194–95, 211
Children's Defense Fund, 160, 173–74, 178, 179
CHIP (Child Health Insurance Program), 88–89
CHIP (Comprehensive Health Insurance Plan), 120–21
Choice: denial of, 145; free, 180–81
CHPS (Community Health Partnerships), 227
Chronic illness, 7, 18–19, 30–31, 86
Cigarette taxes, 222
Clinical care, 11–12, 29
Clinics: establishment of, 17; free, 222, 223; neighborhood, 54, 90, 130. *See also* Community health centers
Clinton, Bill, 229, 230–32
Cobbs, Price, 82
COBRA (Consolidated Omnibus Reconciliation Act), 185, 208, 240, 243

Coffey, Gladys, 54

Cohen, Wilbur: on community health programs, 58; on expanding federal programs, 40; Forand Bill and, 31–32, 33; Medicaid and, 48, 60, 64; Medicare and, 47, 48; on poverty, 6, 21

Colorado, 102, 222

Committee for National Health Insurance, 229

Committee on Health Care for the Disadvantaged, 67

Committee on the Costs of Medical Care (CCMC), 4–5, 131

Community action programs, 55, 58, 60–61, 100–101

Community health centers: funding for, 103; hospitalization and, 136; Medicaid and, 249; movement for, 98–103, 106; outcomes of, 135–36; physicians and, 136–37; Reagan's cuts in, 184; success of, 103

Community Health Partnerships (CHPS), 227

Community health programs: early history of, 7; environmental health and, 130–31; establishment of, 53–55; lack of, 12; in New York City, 72; in rural areas, 8, 77; section 2176 waivers and, 188–89; War on Poverty and, 58

Community Health Service, 101

Community medicine, 131, 138–39

Community mental health centers, 103–6, 142

Community Mental Health Centers Act (1963), 38, 103–4

Comprehensive Health Insurance Plan (CHIP), 120–21

Comprehensive Health Planning and Public Health Service Act (1966), 96–97

Compulsory health insurance, 118–19

Congenital disorders, 18–19

Congressional Budget Office, 225–26

CON (certificate of need) process, 133–35, 147

Conservative Democratic Forum, 227–28

Consolidated Omnibus Reconciliation Act (COBRA), 185, 208, 240, 243

Consumer choice, 207–8

Cook County Hospital, 190

Cooper, Edward, 84

Cooper, Samuel, xii

Co-payments, 169, 175

Corbett, Robert, 134

Cornely, Paul, 82, 85

Cost-benefit ratio, 206–7

Cost control: George H. W. Bush and, 230; Carter and, 146–48, 149; Clinton's health plan and, 232; for hospitals, 146–48; for Medicaid, 149–51; physicians and, 148; specialist access and, 145; state reform plans for, 223–25

Costs: Canadian health care and, 121; catastrophic, 3; increase in (1965–76), 130; Kerr-Mills Act and, 39–40; Medicaid overruns, 62–63, 108–10, 224; in 1960s, 2–3, 62–63, 98; in 1970s, 115–17, 146–47; reasonable cost principle and, 169; of small, rural hospitals, 140–41. *See also* Inflation

County reform plans, 222–23

Crippled children's programs, 18, 21, 86

Cruikshank, Nelson, 31–32

Cubans, 212

Cultural identity, 82

Cultural lag, 75, 78

Culture: access to care and, 91; African American, 82; health, 77, 78; of poverty, 19–22, 52–53, 67–68, 112

Davis, James, 192

Davis, Karen, 123, 131

Dean, Howard, 241

Deficit Reduction Act (DEFRA), 185

Deinstitutionalization, 38, 104–5, 142

Delivery of care. *See* Health care delivery

Dental care, 6, 74, 86, 173–74

Dentists, 85

Denver, 102

Department of Health, Education and Welfare (HEW): on child health, 18; community health centers movement and, 98; Community Health Service, 101; Early and Periodic Screening, Diagnosis and Treatment Program and, 128–29

Depression, 17

Deregulation, 171

Deschin, Celia, 95

DeVise, Pierre, 195

Diabetes, 174

Diagnostic related groups (DRGS), 171–72, 177

Disabled persons, 164, 186–87

Disease model of health, 92–93

Disproportionate share hospitals, 238–40

Dole, Bob, 231

Domke, Herbert, 54

Draft-age men, 18–19, 45

DRGS (diagnostic related groups), 171–72, 177

Dublin, Louis, 16

Duhl, Leonard J., 44, 92

Dumping, 189–92, 213

Early and Periodic Screening, Diagnosis and Treatment Program (EPSDT), 128–29, 165, 201–2

Economic factors. See Income; Socio-economic factors

Economic Opportunity Act (1964), 56, 57, 60, 98–103, 100–101

Edelman, Marian Wright, 160

Education: for African Americans, 79, 81, 83–85; health manpower program for, 88–89; pediatric and obstetric, 90. See also Medical schools

EHIP (Employee Health Care Insurance Plan), 120

Eizenstat, Stuart, 150

Eldercare, 59

Elderly: asset transfers by, 187; chronic illness and, 30–31; family respon-sibility for, 187–88; federal programs for, 30–39; health insurance for, 31–32; high-risk status of, 32; hospital insur-ance for (1960s), 4; income of, 35; indigent, 50; Kerr-Mills Act and, 34–40; King-Anderson Bill and, 38–39; nursing home expenditures for, 125, 128, 164, 186–87, 186–87; quality of life of, 6; spending on (1967), 87; under-writing care for, 32; well-to-do, 242. See also Medicare

Eliastam, Michael, 134

Ellwood, Paul, 230

Emergency Medical Service Systems Act (1973), 134

Emergency medical systems planning, 134

Emergency rooms: Medicaid patients diverted from, 238–39; primary care in, 70–71, 177, 196

Emotional maladjustment, 18–19

Employee Health Care Insurance Plan (EHIP), 120

Employer-based health insurance, 3–4, 30, 207–8, 220–21, 226–27

Employment: Aid to Families with Dependent Children (AFDC) and, 156–57; full-time, 228; guaranteed income and, 180; part-time, 210; uninsured Americans and, 210–11, 212

England, 75–76, 97, 153

Enthoven, Alain, 207–8, 230

Environmental health, 95, 130–31

EPSDT (Early and Periodic Screening, Diagnosis and Treatment Program), 128–29, 165, 201–2

Ethnic groups, 24–25

European health care systems, xii–xiii, 75–76, 97, 153

Falk, I. S., 31–32, 60

Families: as caregivers, 187–88; poverty and, 53, 129; private health insurance and, 210; two-parent, 140; unwed mothers and, 194–95

22; in 1990s, 226–32, 240–42; public
health and, 95; state legislation for
(1990s), 218–25
Health care utilization, 6, 174
Health education, 53
Health-enhancing behavior, 144
Health insurance: access to care and, 15;
for catastrophic coverage, 154; Comprehensive Health Insurance Plan
and, 120–21; compulsory, 118–19;
development of, 3–4; for elderly, 31–
32; government-provided, 29; middle
class and, 30; postwar growth in, 15;
for prenatal and postnatal care, 87–88;
sliding scale for, 221. *See also* National
health care; Private health insurance
Health Insurance Association of America, 231
Health Insurance Portability and
Accountability Act (HIPAA), 240–41
Health Insurance Purchasing Cooperatives (HIPCS), 227, 230, 231
"Health Is a Community Affair," 45
Health maintenance organizations
(HMOS): in California, 137–38, 236;
consumer choice health plan and,
207–8; declining use of, 172–73; Med-
icaid and, 137–38, 202–3
Health manpower: health planning and,
97–98; Johnson's program for, 88–89;
lack of, 117. *See also* Physicians
Health Manpower Shortage Areas, 198
Health of Regionville, The (Koos), 75
Health planning: centralized, 96–98; cer-
tificate of need process for, 133–35; for
emergency medical systems, 134; by
Johnson, 44–45; national model for,
132; opposition to, 134–35
Health planning agencies, 96
Health Services Corporation (New
York), 72
Health status: of African Americans,
173–75, 193–97; of children (1960s),
18–19, 49, 85–88; of children (1980s),
165–66, 173–74, 199–202; of draft-age

men, 18–19, 45; of mentally ill, 197–98;
in 1960s, 1–5; in 1974, 138; poverty and,
24–25; rich vs. poor, 165–66; in rural
areas (1960s), 40–43, 74–75; in rural
areas (1980s), 198–99; socioeconomic
factors and, 193; of United States, 182;
in urban areas, 193–97
Health Systems Agency (HSA), 133
Hein, Tillman, 191
Henderon, C. R., 11
Heroic medicine, 14
HEW. *See* Department of Health, Educa-
tion and Welfare
High blood pressure, 174, 195
Hill-Burton hospital construction pro-
gram, 41, 43, 140
HIPAA (Health Insurance Portability and
Accountability Act), 240–41
HIPCS (Health Insurance Purchasing
Cooperatives), 227, 230, 231
Hippocratic Oath, 111–12, 131
Hispanics: AIDS and, 233–34; health sta-
tus of, 196, 197; uninsured, 210, 211–12;
welfare reform (1996) and, 241
HMOS. *See* Health maintenance
organizations
Hodgson, Godfrey, 73, 115
Home care, 188–89
Homeless persons, 197–98
Hospital construction programs, 41, 43,
140
Hospitalization: community health centers and, 136; cost of, 2–3; in Hawaii,
220; Medicaid and, 108; poverty and,
24–25; of uninsured Americans, 4
Hospitals: AIDS and, 234; community
medicine departments in, 138–39; cost
control for, 146–48; disproportionate
share, 238–40; early history of, 8–13;
in early 1960s, 1–2; inflation and, 146–
48; Kerr-Mills Act and, 37–38; physicians' control of, 66; prestige of, 13;
Reagan and, 176–77, 179; research, 11–
12; in rural areas, 41, 140–41; sectarian,
8–13; tax on, 217; Veterans Admin-

Hospitals (*continued*)
    istration, 21. *See also* Private hospitals;
    Public hospitals
Howard University Dental School, 85
HSA (Health Systems Agency), 133
Hughes, James, 86
Humphrey, Hubert, 95
Hunt, James, Jr., 170
Hunter, R., 11
Hypertension, 174, 195

Identity, cultural, 82
Illness: chronic, 7, 18–19, 30–31, 86; pov-
    erty and, 6–7, 24–25
Immigration, mass, 7–8
Immunization, 108
Income: access to care and, 4–5; of Afri-
    can Americans, 79–80; elderly, 35;
    guaranteed, 180; inadequate, 5; Medic-
    aid eligibility and, 48–49, 51; mini-
    mum, 159; nurses', 116; physicians', 116;
    two-tiered system of care and, 119–20;
    of uninsured Americans, 114; utiliza-
    tion of care and, 6; of whites, 80
Indigent care. *See* Charity care
Infant health, 80, 87, 88
Infant mortality: of African American
    babies, 83, 179, 193–94; Child Health
    Insurance Program and, 89–90; com-
    munity health centers and, 136; early
    federal programs for, 15–16; interna-
    tional rates of, 199; in 1969, 107; in
    1980s, 199–201; racial disparity in, 179;
    Reagan and, 182–83, 193–94, 200–201;
    in rural areas, 139; socioeconomic fac-
    tors and, 200; of white babies, 179,
    193–94
Infectious disease, 94–95
Inflation: health care and, 73, 98, 115–17,
    218, 250–51; health care reform and,
    122; hospital cost control and, 146;
    managed care and, 202–3, 237–38;
    Medicaid and, 109, 148; prospective
    payment systems and, 176–77
Influenza, 174

Infrastructure, 133–35
Inner city. *See* Urban areas
Insurance industry, 33, 35
Interest groups, xvii
Intermediate care facilities, 187
Intravenous drug users, 233–34
IQ (Intelligence quotient), 81
Isolation, 20, 79

Jackson, Jesse, 195
Jacobowitz, Steven, 200
James, George, 20, 24, 92
Japan, 153
Jobs-oriented welfare, 157–58
Joe, Tom, 169–70
Johns Hopkins Medical School, 14
Johnson, Lyndon: Child Health Insur-
    ance Program and, 88–91; Great
    Society programs of, 112–13, 179–82,
    201; policy planning by, 44–45; on
    right to health care, 93; War on Pov-
    erty of, 25–27, 55–59
Johnson, Pearlie, 136
Johnson, William O., 181
Jones, Edith, 194

Kassirer, Jerome, 238
Kelly, Florence, 16
Kemp, Jack, 201
Kennedy, Edward, 60, 101, 205, 209
Kennedy, John, 46, 48
Kentucky, 62, 77, 142
Kentucky Medical Assistance Pro-
    gram, 62
Kentucky Medical Care Program, 62
Kerr, Robert, 34
Kerr-Mills Act, 4, 34–40, 39–40, 46
Kiddycare, 88–89
King, Cecil, 38–39, 46–47
King, Edward, 170
King-Anderson Bill, 38–39, 46
Kitzhaber, John, 206–7, 219
Klark, Sidney, 139
Koos, Earl, 75
Kristol, Irving, 180

Medicaid (*continued*)
224; Nixon on, 113, 114; nursing home
expenditures and, 125, 128, 164, 186–
87; Omnibus Budget Reconciliation
Act and, 168–72, 175–76; opposition
to, 58–59, 64–68; prescription drug
program of, 242–43; primary care
and, 107–8; private charity care and,
249; prospective payment systems for,
149–50, 176–77; quality of care and,
107–8, 118; racial disparity and, 60–61;
Reagan and, 168–72, 175–79, 181, 184–
85, 208; reform plans for (1980s), 203–
8; in rural areas, 76–78, 139; spending
on (1988–92), 215–17; success of, xviii,
142–43, 249–50; War on Poverty and,
59–61
Medi-Cal, 62–63, 108, 109
Medical alienation, 76
Medical Assistance to the Aged (MAA),
34–35, 36–37
Medically Underserved Areas, 198
Medical schools: African Americans in,
25, 83–85, 196; foreign, 126–28;
research focus of, 121–22; scholarships
to, 217–18
Medicare: diagnostic related groups for,
171–72, 177; establishment of, 46–49;
fee schedules for, 177; opposition to,
47–48, 59, 64–68; provision of care
and, 97; reimbursement for, 110
Medicare Catastrophic Coverage Act
(1988), 185
Medicine: heroic, 14; mission of, 130;
research-driven, 14–15; rights-based,
132; scientific, 1, 13, 245; socialized, 47,
195
Mental health centers, community, 103–
6, 142
Mental health programs, 38, 142
Mental illness, 197–98
Metzler, Dwight, 95
Michigan, 213
Middle class, 30
Migrant care, 40

Milio, Nancy, 82
Mills, Wilbur, 34, 48
Miluszusky, Brian, 239
Minnesota, 221, 222
MinnesotaCare, 221
Minority groups, 18, 103, 210, 211–12. *See
also* African Americans; Hispanics
Mississippi, 74–75, 76, 141–42, 215
Mitchell, Maria, 239
Montefiore Center, 102, 103
Morris, Robert, 181
Mothers, unwed, 194–95, 211
Muller, Charlotte, 5, 37–38
Mundinger, Mary O'Neil, 184
Municipal hospitals. *See* Public hospitals
Murray, Charles, 180–81
Muskie, Edmund, 92
Myers, Beverly, 125
Myrdal, Gunnar, 26

Nathan, Richard, 170
National Advisory Commission on
Health Manpower, 97–98
National Commission on Community
Health Services, 45, 99, 130
National health care: attempts to pro-
vide, 247; in Canada, 120–21, 205–6;
charity care vs., 120; Child Health
Insurance Program and, 89; early
opposition to, 29–30; in Europe, xii–
xiii, 75–76, 97, 153; Kennedy's proposal
for, 46; Medicaid and, 60; reform
plans for (mid-1980s), 205–6; in
United Kingdom, 97
National Health Care Reform Act (1981),
164
National Health Plan (1979), 154
National Health Planning and Resources
Development Act (1974), 133
National Health Service (United King-
dom), 75–76, 97
National Health Service Corps, 198, 217
National Medical Association, 25, 84
National Study Group on State Medicaid
Strategies, 178

Nebraska, 141

Neighborhood health centers, 54, 90, 130. *See also* Community health centers

Neoconservatives, 180–81

Nevada, 177, 224–25

Newark, 102

New Deal, 113, 157, 179–82

New Federalism, 113

New Hampshire, 215, 216

New Jersey, 102, 222

Newman, Howard, 120

New York City: Bellevue Hospital crisis in, 238–39; Medicaid cost overruns in, 109–10; Medicaid eligibility in, 163; Medicaid programs in, 71–72; medical purchasing by, 125

New York State, 210, 213, 215, 216, 235–36

Night Comes to the Cumberlands (Caudill), 56

Nixon, Richard, 105, 112–15, 120–21

Noble, Charles, xiv, xv–xvi, 56

North Carolina, 45, 76, 124, 213

Norton, Eleanor Holmes, 194

Novak, Michael, 182

Nuclear families, 194–95

Nursing homes: asset transfers and, 187; eligibility for, 169; Medicaid expenditures for, 125, 128, 164, 186–87; reasonable cost principle and, 169; well-to-do elderly in, 242

Nutrition, 75. *See also* Malnutrition

OAA (Old Age Assistance), 34, 36

OASI (Old Age, Survivors and Disability Insurance), 46

OBRA. *See* Omnibus Budget Reconciliation Act

Obstetric care, 90

Office of Equal Opportunity (OEO), 89, 101

Office of Health Affairs, 101

Okun, Arthur, 131

Old Age Assistance (OAA), 34, 36

Old Age, Survivors and Disability Insurance (OASDI), 46

Omnibus Budget Reconciliation Act (OBRA), 168–72, 175–76; access to care and, 208; community health centers and, 184; dumping and, 189–90; Medicaid capitation and, 202; section 2176 waivers, 188–89

Open-door policy, 238–39

Oregon, 207, 219–20, 222

Organized medicine, 32–34, 35, 47–48, 101. *See also* American Medical Association

Orphans, 21

Other America, The (Harrington), 56

Paris, Martin, 161

Parkland Memorial Hospital, 189–90

Part-time employment, 210

Pauperism, 11, 20–21

Pay-or-play schemes, 120, 222, 228, 229

Payroll tax, 39

PBJI (Program for Better Jobs and Income), 157–58, 159

Pediatric care, 18–19, 90, 213. *See also* Children

Pennsylvania, 229, 232

Pensions, xiv, 80

Pepper, Claude, 227

Peterson, Osler, 34

Philanthropy, 3, 176

Physician hospital organizations (PHOs), 138

Physician organizations, 32–34, 35, 47–48, 101. *See also* American Medical Association

Physicians: African American, 25, 61, 82–85, 174–75, 195–96; autonomy of, 93; on Canadian health care, 205; on charity care, 111–12, 223, 246–47; charity care by, 13–15, 191–92; community health centers and, 136–37; cost control and, 148; cost of, 2; early fees of, 14; in early hospitals, 8, 10; fee schedules for, 177; health care inflation and, 116; hospital control by, 66; income increases for, 116; on managed

Physicians (*continued*)
care, 237–38; Medicaid and, 65–66,
67–68, 107–8; medical education for,
83–85; on OBRA cuts, 171; primary-
care, 121, 196, 217–18; Reagan and,
184–85; reimbursements to, 216–17;
in rural areas, 41–42, 76, 77–78;
Sheppart-Towner Act and, 16; in
urban areas, 70; visits to, 123. *See also*
Specialists
Physicians' assistants, 141
Physicians for a National Health Pro-
gram, 228–29
Pickett, George, 132
Pipas, J. E., 213
Planning. *See* Health planning
Planning commissions, 74
Pneumonia, 174
Policy planning. *See* Health planning
Poor care. *See* Charity care
Porter, Sylvia, 170
Poulos, Peter, 93
Poverty: access to care and, 4–5; African
American rates of, 78–79, 197; attitudes and behavior of poor, 54; causes
of, 21; children in, 86, 211; culture of,
19–22, 52–53, 67–68, 112; defined, 5–6;
deserving poor, 9–10, 21; dumping of
poor, 189–92; family dysfunction and,
53; feminization of, xiv–xv; geographic difference in, 23–24; health
status and, 24–25, 165–66; hospitalization and, 24–25; illness and, 6–7, 24–
25; isolation and, 20; length of stay
and, 24–25; in 1960s, 5–7; Nixon on,
112–13; pauperization and, 20–21;
pauperism vs., 11; poor as blameless
victims, 21; poor as caretakers, 164–65;
preventive care and, 52–53; public attitudes toward, 56–57; public health
and, 93, 95; racial breakdown of, 17–
18, 22–24, 60–61; rates of, 5–6, 22–24,
129, 163; in rural areas, 17–18, 22, 40–
42, 74–78; social order and, 54–55;
structural origins of, 21–22, 26–27; in

urban areas, 17–18, 22, 69–74; war on,
25–27, 55–59, 129; working poor, 161
Poverty trap, 180
Pregnancy: private health insurance and,
87–88; teenage, 194–95, 211
Prenatal care, 107, 123; for African Americans, 80, 83, 195; Child Health Insurance Program and, 88; infant mortality and, 16; private health insurance
and, 87–88; in rural areas, 140; voluntary sterilization and, 124
Prepaid Health Care Act (Hawaii), 221
Prescription drug program, 242–43
Preventive care, 52–53, 203, 220
Primary care: for children, 214; in emergency rooms, 70–71, 177, 196; in
Hawaii, 220; for Medicaid patients,
107–8; in New York City, 72; scholarships for, 217–18
Primary care physicians, 121, 196, 217–18
Private health insurance: compulsory
insurance and, 118–19; dominance of,
118–19; employer-based, 3–4, 30, 207–
8, 220–21, 226–27, 228; families and,
210; health care inflation and, 117; hospital, 3–4; national health care plans
and, 206; prenatal care and, 87–88;
quality of care and, 118; single-payer
plans and, 229
Private hospitals: charity care by, 246–
47; dumping by, 189–90, 191, 213;
establishment of, 8–9, 11; health care
inflation and, 116; Medicaid and, 66–
68, 72–73, 126, 213; revenue increases
for, 116; state cost-control plans and,
225
"Problem of Poverty in America, The"
(Lampman), 56
Pro bono care. *See* Charity care
Pro-family welfare programs, 181–82, 183
Professional autonomy, 93
Professional Standards Review Organizations, 116
Program for Better Jobs and Income
(PBJI), 157–58, 159

Prospective payment systems, 149–50, 176–77
Provider-driven health care delivery, 138
Provision of care. *See* Health care delivery
Psychiatric patients, 197–98
Psychiatrists, 104, 105–6
Public Agenda Foundation, 203
Public good, 134
Public health: accomplishments of, 94; community health centers movement and, 99–100; environmental health and, 95, 130–31; expanding vision of, 94–96; poverty and, 93
Public Health Service (PHS), 28–29, 42, 43, 198, 199
Public hospitals: bad debt held by, 190; changes in (1975), 125–26; charity care by (1982), 166; city, 126; closings of (1990s), 239; declining patient populations in, 72–73; dumping to, 189–92; early history of, 10–13; managed care and, 238–40; Medicaid and, 67, 125–26, 249; open-door policy of, 238–39; primary care in, 70–71; state closure of, 225; uninsured Americans and, 240; in urban areas, 69–74, 126; working poor in, 161
Puerto Ricans, 70

Quality of care: graduates of foreign medical schools and, 127–28; Medicaid and, 66, 107–8; private vs. Medicaid, 118; uninsured Americans and, 119
Quality of life, 6
Quie, Albert, 170
Quinn, Jane Bryant, 187

Rabin, David, 139
Race: life expectancy and, 179; Medicaid benefits and, 125; physician selection and, 85; poverty and, 17–18, 22–24; wealth and, 60–61
Raspberry, William, 195
Rationing, 207, 219

Reagan, Ronald: block grants and, 166–68; on catastrophic care, 117–18; on deregulation, 171; diagnostic related groups and, 171–72; health care delivery changes and, 179–83; HMOs and, 172; infant mortality and, 193–94, 200–201; Medicaid changes by, 168–72, 175–79; Medi-Cal and, 63, 109–10; National Health Service Corps and, 198; tax policies of, 176; welfare programs and, 179–83
Referrals, 67
Reform. *See* Health care reform
Reimbursement. *See* Third-party reimbursement
Reitz, H. Lewis, 35
Relman, Arnold, 190, 219
Research, 14–15, 119, 121
Research hospitals, 11–12
Retirement, 80, 135
Reuther, Walter, 33
Ribicoff, Abraham, 39
Ribicoff children, 204–5
Right to health, 131–32
Right to health care, 203
Robert Wood Johnson Foundation, 138, 202
Rockefeller, John D., 227
Rockefeller, Nelson, 7, 63–64
Roosevelt, Franklin, 29
Rosenbaum, Sara, 178
Rosenberg, Charles, 190
Rothman, David, xii
Rubenstein, Daniel, 133
Rural areas: African Americans in, 76, 175; birth rates in, 42; charity care in (1965–78), 139; children in, 74–75; community health programs in, 8, 77; dental care in, 74; health services in (1975), 132–33; health status in (1960s), 40–43, 74–75; health status in (1980s), 198–99; hospitals in, 41, 140; infant mortality in, 139; Medicaid in, 76–78, 139; mental health services in, 142; physicians in, 41–42, 77–78; poverty

Jonathan Engel is an associate professor in the Department of
Public and Healthcare Administration at Seton Hall University.

Library of Congress Cataloging-in-Publication Data
Engel, Jonathan.
Poor people's medicine : Medicaid and American
charity care since 1965 / Jonathan Engel.
p. cm.
Includes bibliographical references and index.
ISBN 0-8223-3683-9 (cloth : alk. paper) —
ISBN 0-8223-3695-2 (pbk. : alk. paper)
1. Medicaid—History. 2. Medicare—History. 3. Poor—Medical care.
4. Health services accessibility. I. Title. [DNLM: 1. Medicaid—history.
2. Health Policy—United States. 3. Health Services Accessibility—
United States. 4. Poverty—United States.
W 250 AA1 E57p 2006]
RA412.4.E54 2006
368.4'2'00973—dc22   2005021133